'Dr Josephs' book illustrates a novel approach to help psychotherapy patients manage their weight by using the power of the therapeutic relationship as a fulcrum of change. In psychotherapy, patients have the opportunity to figure out how to manage their weight when one-size-fits-all approaches may not apply and work through their indecision when they are of two minds about how to go about it. Josephs not only recounts the many challenges patients and their therapists are likely to encounter on patients' weight-management journeys but also offers unique pathways to navigate those challenges. Vivid case illustrations bring this approach to life'.

Geoff Goodman, *PhD, ABPP, FIPA, CST, CSAT-S, CPTT-S, RPT-S,*
professor, Emory University Psychoanalytic Institute, Department of
Psychiatry and Behavioral Sciences, Emory University School of Medicine

'Dr Josephs tackles a common clinical concern and does so with a unique and rich consideration. He addresses the relational/cultural dimensions of weight management and examines the ways the patient-therapist relationship can be strained or ruptured when approaching it in psychotherapy. Clinicians across levels and traditions will greatly appreciate this significant contribution with its many insights and illustrations'.

J. Christopher Muran, *PhD, dean and professor, The Gordon F. Derner*
School of Psychology, Adelphi University, principal investigator,
Mount Sinai Beth Israel Psychotherapy Research Program

The Relational Dimensions of Weight Management

The Relational Dimensions of Weight Management is a book for nonspecialist psychotherapists of any theoretical orientation to help patients concerned with weight management. Psychotherapy patients use their therapists as sounding boards to help them answer two questions: Do I need to lose weight? And, if I do need to lose weight, how should I go about it? Chapters provide therapists with the tools they need to help patients find personalized solutions to their weight loss concerns, to boost their self-image, and to deal with the judgment that is sometimes imposed by others, regardless of which weight management approach patients eventually embrace.

Lawrence Josephs, PhD, is a professor at the Derner School of Psychology at Adelphi University. He also offers individual and couples therapy in private practice in New York City.

The Relational Dimensions of Weight Management

A Therapist's Guide to Helping Patients Resolve Weight Concerns

Lawrence Josephs

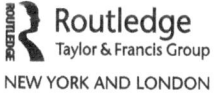

Routledge
Taylor & Francis Group

NEW YORK AND LONDON

Designed cover image: wragg © Getty Images

First published 2025
by Routledge
605 Third Avenue, New York, NY 10158

and by Routledge
4 Park Square, Milton Park, Abingdon, Oxon, OX14 4RN

Routledge is an imprint of the Taylor & Francis Group, an informa business

© 2025 Lawrence Josephs

The right of Lawrence Josephs to be identified as author of this work has been asserted in accordance with sections 77 and 78 of the Copyright, Designs and Patents Act 1988.

ISBN: 978-1-032-50379-0 (hbk)
ISBN: 978-1-032-50378-3 (pbk)
ISBN: 978-1-003-40233-6 (ebk)

DOI: 10.4324/9781003402336

Typeset in Janson MT Std
by Apex CoVantage, LLC

In memory of Jonathan Josephs

Contents

Acknowledgments   xi

Introduction   1

Overview   5

Part I: Relational Dimensions of Eating Behavior   **21**

1   Internalized Weight Stigma and the Desire to Diet   23

2   Behavioral Weight Loss Intervention and the
    Consumer Culture   37

3   When Food is Love and Food Choice is Autonomy:
    The Relational Dynamics of Emotional Eating   51

4   Food Addiction and Divergent Weight Management Stigma   66

5   The Evolution of Human Food Sharing and Feasting   82

6   Who to Believe? The Confusing Nature of Dietary Reality
    and Epistemic Trust   97

**Part II: Patients' Weight Management Journeys and
         the Therapeutic Relationship**   **113**

7   Kill the Messenger: Helping Patients Deal with 'Bad Numbers'
    (i.e., weight, BMI, calories, blood glucose, cholesterol, blood pressure)   115

8   Recommending or Demanding? Helping Patients Choose
    an Approach to Weight Management   131

9   Coaching or Policing? Helping Patients Self-Monitor   143

10 Accepting or Judging? Weight Cycling and Relapse Recovery   154

11 Empowering or Pressuring? Helping Patients Deal with Prejudice   163

Conclusion   178

Index   184

Acknowledgments

Many thanks go to my wife, Dr. Laura Josephs, who has provided unfailing support for my own weight management efforts as well as support for writing this book. I thank my adult children, Aaron, Matthew, and Sam (all excellent cooks), for also supporting my weight management efforts and for not making too much fun of me for being on an old person's diet although I am a senior citizen. I owe a debt of gratitude to all my patients who allowed me to accompany them on their weight management journeys and help them with their weight management struggles. All the case studies in this book are based on composite portraits based on multiple patients in which names, ages, occupations, marital status, parental status, sometimes gender and sexual orientation have been changed to protect patients' confidentiality. The research and clinical experiences presented in this book are up to date but do not reflect the impact of the newest generation of weight loss drugs like Ozempic, Wegovy, or Mounjaro. It remains to be seen if such drugs will eventually lessen or entirely obviate the kind of clinical challenges that confront psychotherapists in addressing patients' weight management concerns.

Introduction

The Relational Dimensions of Weight Management: A Therapist's Guide to Helping Patients Resolve Weight Concerns is a book intended for psychotherapists of all theoretical orientations. Most psychotherapists are not trained weight loss experts but nevertheless do end up working with patients that are concerned about their weight but who may have originally sought psychotherapy for other reasons like relationship problems, anxiety, or depression. Patients concerned about their weight will invariably utilize their psychotherapists as sounding boards for their weight concerns and solicit their therapists' feedback on that issue looking for emotional support and practical guidance.

Many patients who are concerned about their weight do not necessarily possess a diagnosable eating disorder like anorexia, bulimia, or binge eating and their weight is not sufficient that they would be considered candidates for bariatric surgery. They are typically individuals who have gained weight over the years and worry that they weigh too much because they believe that they overeat without necessarily binging. They wonder if they need to lose weight to improve their appearance or decrease their health risks. The health risks of high body weight may be more salient for older patients who discover that they have elevated blood sugar, high cholesterol, and/or high blood pressure. Their physicians have recommended losing weight to treat those conditions.

Patients concerned about their weight often deliberate on two challenging questions for which they seek their therapists' input: 1) Do I need to lose weight? And 2) If I do indeed need to lose weight, what is the best way to go about it? Those two questions are emotionally fraught and may be difficult to discuss openly. Perceiving oneself as overweight is a highly shame sensitive issue due to 'internalized weight stigma' (Ratcliffe & Ellison, 2015). The desire to lose weight may be driven by 'fat phobia' and a dread of 'fat shaming' due to the cultural idealization of thinness. There is a perspective that one can be 'healthy at any size' if one eats healthful foods and exercises regularly (O'Hara, Ahmed, & Elashie, 2021). Yet research also suggests that a high body mass index (BMI) is associated with a variety of 'metabolic syndromes' such as Type 2 diabetes and heart disease for which weight loss is recommended (Lee, 2020). Losing weight is emotionally challenging. Individuals often 'yo-yo' between losing weight and regaining it due to stress induced relapse (Hutchinson, 2011).

Psychotherapists, as sounding boards who are not weight management specialists, will find themselves playing a central role in patients' efforts to find a sustainable approach to weight management that they can feel good about. Weight management may mean learning how to lose weight and keep it off by learning to accept and adhere to reasonable dietary restrictions. Weight management can mean learning to accept one's weight for what it is without self-flagellation. Weight management can mean learning an approach to eating that

DOI: 10.4324/9781003402336-1

is less obsessed with faulting oneself for failing to adhere to dietary restrictions and is more intuitive or mindful.

Being a constructive sounding board who provides useful feedback to patients struggling with weight management concerns is not easy. Therapists can readily be perceived as taking sides in an inner conflict of which the patient is of two minds. Patients may receive contradictory weight management advice. Some weight management specialists are anti-diet, support 'body positivity', and the belief that one can be healthy at any size (O'Hara, Ahmed, & Elashie, 2021). Such specialists could be perceived as unsupportive of patients' weight loss goals that seem legitimate to them. In contrast weight management specialists who endorse cognitive behavioral approaches to weight loss goals could be perceived as implicitly reinforcing internalized weight stigma (Ratcliffe & Ellison, 2015), that patients are not acceptable as they are. Therapists who recommend weight loss strategies like counting calories could be perceived as policing patients' eating behavior and making patients feel badly about themselves when they fail to follow those strategies.

How people feel about their weight and how people manage their weight is influenced by the relational/cultural context in which they are embedded. In the culture-at-large 'fat shaming' and 'fat phobia' resulting in internalized weight stigma make it difficult to feel good about oneself unless one possesses a thin body (Ratcliffe & Ellison, 2015). Yet the culture also makes it difficult for many people to maintain a thin body if they so desired because consumption is encouraged of highly processed calorie-dense comfort foods like pizza and ice cream that may possess addictive qualities (Moss, 2014). Compliance with dietary restrictions is not easy when subject to 'divergent weight management stigma' (Romo, 2018), being shamed for being too rigid and too self-depriving when trying to count calories or abstain from certain calorie-dense foods. Thus, individuals concerned about their weight can feel judged for their weight and how much they eat yet also judged for their restrictive approach to dieting if it strikes others as excessively rigid to the point of obsession.

These sociocultural dynamics can play out in the therapeutic relationship in ways that strain the therapeutic alliance. Therapists can easily be experienced as rationalizing and enabling 'bad' eating habits to help patients feel better about themselves as they are without having to make any serious changes in their eating habits or as the exact opposite, as judging patients for failing to change their 'bad' eating habits when they should. It behooves therapists to repair any ruptures to the therapeutic alliance (Eubanks, Sergi, & Muran, 2021) to ensure a positive outcome as a positive working alliance is one of the best predictors of psychotherapy outcome (Flückiger, Del Re, Wampold, & Horvath, 2019). Relational/cultural factors such as 'internalized weight stigma' and 'divergent weight management stigma' make patients highly sensitive to their therapists' explicit, implicit, and/or imagined judgments in ways that may result in ruptures to the therapeutic relationship.

Help with weight management means helping patients come to a place where they feel good about their current weight, feel good about their appearance and health, feel good about their current eating habits, and have acquired the relational skills to deal effectively with judgmental individuals who appear to be making them feel badly about their weight and eating habits. There may be no one-size-fits-all approach to achieving such goals given the plethora of contradictory weight management advice. Part of psychotherapy is helping patients find their own individual solutions that work at least for them if not for others. Finding individual solutions is challenging when patients are confused by conflicting advice and are consequently of two minds about what to do. When it comes to weight loss it's not clear that there are any evidence-based solutions that work for everyone. Many approaches appear to yield short-term results that don't hold up in the long-term (Langeveld & de Vries, 2013).

There may be a division of labor between psychotherapists and other healthcare professionals such as personal trainers who help patients with exercise, nutritionists who help patients with diet, physicians who may offer medication or even bariatric surgery, and/or other psychotherapists who might specialize in approaches like mindfulness meditation or behavior modification that could be a helpful adjunct to more exploratory approaches to psychotherapy. Psychotherapists may be called upon to help patients with the emotional and relational challenges of compliance with a recommended approach to eating, dieting, or exercising.

Though generalist psychotherapists are not necessarily weight management specialists, it behooves them to be aware of the range of options as well as the pros and cons of various treatment options. There is considerable controversy in the field as to the best approach to weight management. Is it best to learn to eat intuitively or to count calories, is it best to learn to eat calorie-dense foods in moderation or to abstain from such foods, is the best diet low-fat or low-carbohydrate, is the goal to achieve a normal body mass index (BMI) or to accept being healthy at any size, when is a dietary approach too restrictive or too permissive? Patients turn to their therapists as sounding boards when they are of two minds about such pressing dieting dilemmas.

This book will review the range of weight management options and the pros and cons of such options so psychotherapists can be better informed sounding boards when patients deliberate such dieting dilemmas and are looking for guidance in resolving such weight management concerns. Psychotherapists can help patients with the emotional and relational dimensions of implementing such options though other professionals might be the ones helping patients with other important aspects of weight management such as working out a daily menu, monitoring their weight, monitoring their daily caloric intake, facilitating a regular exercise routine, prescribing medication, performing bariatric surgery, or learning to meditate.

Psychotherapists also have a central role to play in patients' weight management when patients fail to lose weight when the goal is weight loss, when patients regain lost weight, or when patients are trying to maintain their current weight but keep gaining further weight. Patients become demoralized when they fail to achieve their weight management goals despite having made a considerable sacrifice of time and effort to achieve such goals. Patients may find it difficult to have self-compassion when failing to achieve their weight management goals despite having given it their best effort.

The serenity prayer suggests that serenity is achieved when patients change what they can, accept what they can't, and possess the wisdom to know the difference. Yet sometimes when it comes to weight management patients get stuck in a frustrating place where they can't seem to change what it seems they should be able to change, cannot seem to learn to accept what they can't change, and can't figure out exactly why that is. Were the goals unrealistic, was the approach not right for them, was their implementation faulty, is successful and enduring weight management beyond their ability no matter what approach they try, and is self-acceptance impossible to achieve without possession of a thin and healthy body?

When psychotherapy is long-term, psychotherapists embark on a long journey with patients of failed weight management experiments in search of a sustainable approach.

Patients turn to their therapists when deliberating whether to give up the search for a sustainable approach to weight management or to continue to stubbornly persevere in a seemingly endless test of endurance until a sustainable approach is finally discovered. The therapeutic relationship will have its ups and downs as patients learn through trial and error what works for them given their unique individuality and life circumstances.

References

Eubanks, C. F., Sergi, J., & Muran, J. C. (2021). Responsiveness to ruptures and repairs in psychotherapy. In J. C. Watson & H. Wiseman (Eds.), *The responsive psychotherapist: Attuning to clients in the moment* (pp. 83–103). American Psychological Association.

Flückiger, C., Del Re, A. C., Wampold, B. E., & Horvath, A. O. (2019). Alliance in adult psychotherapy. In J. C. Norcross & M. J. Lambert (Eds.), *Psychotherapy relationships that work: Evidence-based therapist contributions* (pp. 24–78). Oxford University Press.

Hutchinson, E. (2011). Systems neuroscience: The stress of dieting. *Nature Reviews Neuroscience, 12*(2), 65. https://doi.org/10.1038/nrn2985

Langeveld, M., & de Vries, J. H. (2013). Het magere resultaat van diëten [The mediocre results of dieting]. *Nederlands tijdschrift voor geneeskunde, 157*(29), A6017.

Lee, J. (2020). Influences of cardiovascular fitness and body fatness on the risk of metabolic syndrome: A systematic review and meta-analysis. *American Journal of Health Promotion, 34*(7), 796–805. https://doi.org/10.1177/0890117120925347

Moss, M. (2014). *Salt sugar fat: How the food giants hooked us.* New York: Random House.

O'Hara, L., Ahmed, H., & Elashie, S. (2021). Evaluating the impact of a brief Health at Every Size®-informed health promotion activity on body positivity and internalized weight-based oppression. *Body Image, 37,* 225–237. https://doi.org/10.1016/j.bodyim.2021.02.006

Ratcliffe, D., & Ellison, N. (2015). Obesity and internalized weight stigma: A formulation model for an emerging psychological problem. *Behavioural and Cognitive Psychotherapy, 43*(2), 239–252. https://doi.org/10.1017/S1352465813000763

Romo L. K. (2018). An examination of how people who have lost weight communicatively negotiate interpersonal challenges to weight management. *Health Communication, 33*(4), 469–477. https://doi.org/10.1080/10410236.2016.1278497

Overview

Psychological problems can be associated with worries about being overweight and per-ceiving oneself as overweight may exacerbate such psychological problems if such self-perception contributes to poor body image and insecure attachment (Gravina, Palla, Piccione, & Nebbiai, 2015). Culturally prevalent 'fat shaming' and 'fat phobia' contribute to 'internalized weight stigma', so that regardless of whether a patient needs to lose weight, weight is a shame-sensitive topic that is difficult to discuss openly. It can be challenging to have such discussions in ways that don't further reinforce patients' internalized weight stigma. Though some individuals may be able to remain 'healthy at any size', weight contributes with advancing age to weight-related metabolic syndromes like heart disease and Type 2 diabetes (Lee, 2020). Thus, weight presents itself in psychotherapy as a shame-sensitive issue with some ambiguity as to whether there is a legitimate need to lose weight to be attractive and healthy.

Looking at weight management from an evidence-based perspective reveals equivocal conclusions. Weight loss research suggests that most approaches to dieting appear to work in the short-term, but patients tend to regain weight in the long-term (Langeveld & de Vries, 2013). Contributing to regaining lost weight are factors like stress-induced relapse (Hutchinson, 2011) and that the rewards of weight loss maintenance do not appear to be as reinforcing as the rewards of the initial weight loss (Perri & Ariel-Donges, 2018). Motivation to stick with a diet that has worked appears to diminish over time.

Behavioral approaches to weight loss obtain the best results. Behavioral approaches may limit patients' daily caloric intake (i.e., often 1,800 calories/day for men and 1,500 calories/day for women) concurrent with a regular exercise routine. Such behavioral approaches result in significant weight loss, about 8–10%, and that 4–5% weight loss is maintained in the long-term up to eight years (Gomez-Rubalcava, Stabbert, & Phelan, 2018).

Research on weight loss maintenance suggest a need for extended continuous care for prevention of relapse (Perri & Ariel-Donges, 2018). Some individual difference variables have emerged as to which individuals are best able keep the weight off after losing it. Individuals who are high on conscientiousness, high on self-monitoring their weight and caloric intake, and who exercise regularly seem to do best with weight loss maintenance (Gold, Carr, Thomas, Burrus, O'Leary, Wing, & Bond 2020; Gomez-Rubalcava, Stabbert, & Phelan, 2018; Jakicic, Rogers, Sherman, & Kovacs, 2018). Research has suggested that significant weight loss that falls short of achieving a normal body mass index can result in significant health benefits (Gomez-Rubalcava, Stabbert, & Phelan, 2018).

DOI: 10.4324/9781003402336-2

Behavioral approaches have been integrated with approaches such as motivational interviewing and acceptance and commitment therapy to see if such integrative approaches might make weight loss treatment more effective. Motivational interviewing assumes that patients can be of two minds about losing weight and tries to reinforce patients' motivation to change. (Burrows, Collins, Rollo, Leary, Hides, & Davis, 2021). Patients often know quite well what they 'should' do to lose weight and keep it off (i.e., eat more fruits and vegetables, control portion size, exercise more regularly) and often criticize themselves quite harshly for not doing what they know they 'should' be doing. Yet there is a concurrent mindset that questions whether the privations of weight control are worth the benefits, that questions if it's worth it to fight a losing battle, that wonders if the motivation for losing weight derives from a lack of self-acceptance, that likes having a big, hefty body, that believes that a healthy diet is a boring diet, etc.

Motivational interviewing, given its derivation from Roger's client-centered therapy (Miller & Moyers, 2017), requires that therapists have equal empathy and respect for both points of view when patients are of two minds about something. The patient may need help articulating all the 'valid' reasons the patient has for not losing weight and not keeping it off when the reasons for losing weight and keeping it off are obvious and do not need to be belabored. The patient's autonomy must be respected as they struggle to make up their mind.

Power struggles could ensue when therapists are perceived as campaigning too vociferously for the point of view that the therapist favors. Patients might rebel against behavioral approaches if such approaches seem too structured, too strict, too demanding, and too rigid. Motivational interviewing recognizes and addresses that ambivalence.

Acceptance and commitment therapy tries to help patients accept and learn to tolerate their negative internal reactions to behavioral weight loss treatment. It accepts the fact that adhering to onerous dietary restrictions can be distressing but distress tolerance can be increased. Reinforcement of patients' acceptance of and commitment to their long-term weight loss goals and valuation of a healthful lifestyle increases patients' self-determination to stick with the program despite their internal discomfort (Butryn, Schumacher, & Forman, 2018).

Due to the great difficulty patients have in adhering to dietary restrictions in the long-term and the problem of weight cycling, other approaches to weight management such as intuitive eating have been developed that reject adherence to dietary restrictions. The key principle of intuitive eating is to only eat when one is physiologically hungry, to discern genuine physiological hunger and satiety through greater attention to bodily sensations, and to remove concern with externally imposed dietary rules and a weight-normative mindset (Tylka, 2006). The term mindful eating has often been used interchangeably with intuitive eating as they both teach nonjudgmental awareness of the experience of eating (Zhang, Hugh-Jones, & O'Connor, 2022). Mindful eating entails attention to external eating cues, to the inner states such cues trigger, and the degree to which one eats in a distracted frame of mind.

Approaches such as intuitive and mindful eating that reject dietary restriction and a weight-normative mindset are often associated with the philosophy of health at any size. Such approaches encourage 'body positivity' (O'Hara, Ahmed, & Elashie, 2021), concurrent with facilitating what is considered a more healthful attitude towards eating. Such approaches construe excessive concern with dietary restriction as a kind of psychopathology called 'orthorexia nervosa' which is basically the opposite of intuitive eating (Novara, Pardini, Maggio, Mattioli, & Piasentin, 2022). Orthorexia nervosa is reflected in excessive self-flagellation any time one goes over one's calorie count or consumes a 'bad' food that is considered fattening from which one should abstain. Such diets could lead to rebound effects if excessively self-depriving (Coelho, 2003).

Meta-analyses of studies of intuitive eating (Linardon, Tylka, & Fuller-Tyszkiewicz, 2021) and mindful eating (Yu, Song, Zhang, & Wei, 2020) do not show significant weight loss. These results should not be surprising as the goals of intuitive and mindful eating, when associated with promoting the notion of being healthy at any size, are not necessarily to lose weight but primarily to decrease obsessive self-critical concern with weight and dietary restrictions.

These meta-analyses suggest that these approaches do succeed with their stated goals. A meta-analysis of mindful-based interventions (MBI) for problematic eating behavior suggested that MBI groups showed significant reduction in emotional eating, external eating, binge eating, and weight and shape concern (Yu, Song, Zhang, & Wei, 2020). Meta-analyses of intuitive eating suggest improvement in body image, self-esteem, well-being, and intuitive eating (Braun, Unick, Abrantes, Dalrymple, Conboy, Schifano, Park, C. & Lazar, 2022; Linardon, Tylka, & Fuller-Tyszkiewicz, 2021). As such these approaches offer an alternative approach to weight management than behavioral weight loss treatment.

The concept of health at any size has been questioned. Weight does seem to be an independent determinant of metabolic syndromes such as heart disease, regardless of how much one exercises (Valenzuela, Santos-Lozano, et al., 2022). In addition, for some individuals, permission to relinquish dietary restrictions might be interpreted as a license to eat more than they already do thus resulting in further weight gain (Sainsbury & Hay, 2014). The evidence that weight cycling is hazardous to one's health as sometimes claimed is questionable (Elfhag & Rössner, 2010).

Another challenge to the concept of intuitive eating derives from the possibility that higher BMIs might be a product of food addiction as well as genetic predisposition. Food addiction is not an official DSM eating disorder and there is controversy as to whether it should be. The argument against food addiction as an eating disorder is that some find it hard to imagine how something that is necessary for survival, eating when hungry, could be pathogenic. Others might concede that eating might constitute a behavioral addiction like a sex or gambling addiction, a kind of compulsive behavior disorder.

Others have argued that food addiction should be made an official eating disorder and the Yale Food Addiction Scale has been developed to assess that eating disorder (Vasiliu, 2022). There is some research that suggests that foods such as sugar do function like addictive substances and that having a small taste of an addictive food has a priming effect that increases the craving for that food (Ahmed, 2012). Approaches, like Overeaters Anonymous, that view frequent consumption of calorie-dense food as a symptom of food addiction believe that losing weight may require abstaining from trigger foods such as sugar and white flour (Blumenthal, DuPont, & Gold, 2012). A 12-step type approach requires overcoming one's withdrawal from addictive trigger foods and learning to live without. The assumption is that over time cravings would incrementally subside for foods one no longer eats.

From this perspective, one's intuitive food preferences are not to be trusted because the cravings for one's trigger foods have become excessive. Eating such foods until one is sated or even trying to learn to eat such foods in moderation may simply prime and reinforce the craving for calorie-dense foods whose frequent consumption results in weight gain. Controversy remains in the treatment of addiction in general whether abstinence or moderation constitutes the most viable approach to recovery (Eddie, Bergman, Hoffman, & Kelly, 2022).

The evidence-based weight management outcome literature does not reveal any universally effective one-size-fits-all approach. Outcome studies look at group averages. That means that on average individuals do well with a given strategy, but some do poorly or drop out prior to study completion. Participation in a weight management study implies some motivation to seek help with weight management. Therefore, those studies do not examine the many individuals with elevated BMIs who do not seek help with weight management but who might benefit from such help. Some weight management specialists acknowledge that no evidence-based one-size-fits-all approach has yet to be discovered. Such specialists see a need for a science and practice of 'personalized obesity treatment' that unfortunately is only in the earliest stages of development (Bakizada, Wadden, Wadden, & Alamuddin, 2018).

Patients may draw their psychotherapists into their dieting dilemmas when patients with weight management concerns have difficulty making up their minds about which approaches to try, and which approaches to stick with when the currently embraced approach isn't yielding the anticipated results. When it comes to patients' dieting dilemmas there is uncertainty and ambiguity as to what are the healthiest or most effective options (i.e., achieve a normal BMI or embrace being healthy at any size). Traditional psychodynamic approaches have recommended a stance of neutrality when patients grapple with such inner conflicts. Yet contemporary psychodynamic approaches question to what degree therapists can transcend their implicit biases (Mitchell, 1997). Thus, patients may be reactive to therapists' implicit weight management biases.

Patients look to their psychotherapists for help making up their minds. They want to know what their psychotherapists think and what their therapists would recommend if they were in their patients' shoes. Patients may resent therapists who decline to disclose their point of view or give advice when they wish guidance and coaching with their dieting dilemmas. Patients may resent therapists who try to help patients accept their body sizes as they are when they want a therapist who will support their weight loss goals. Patients may resent therapists who offer a structured approach to weight loss that strikes patients as excessively rigid (like abstaining from trigger foods), overly demanding (regular exercise and counting calories), and too depriving to be tolerable (like sticking to a daily calorie budget). Thus, addressing patients' dieting dilemmas is likely to strain the therapeutic relationship regardless of the psychotherapists' approach to weight management because patients can be of two minds regarding whatever treatment approach their therapists offer.

Perusal of the clinical literature shows that therapists of most theoretical orientations have made promising attempts to address patients' weight management issues; be it psychodynamic (Schwartz, Nickow, Arseneau, & Gisslow, 2015), cognitive-behavior therapy (Comşa, David, & David, 2020), dialectical behavior therapy (Braden & O'Brien, 2021), acceptance and commitment therapy (Lillis, Dunsiger, Thomas, Ross, & Wing, 2021), or teaching mindfulness, self-compassion, and intuitive eating (Schnepper, Richard, Wilhelm, & Blechert, 2019).

A consistent finding of psychotherapy outcome research is that all approaches appear to be equally successful for the clinical conditions that have been studied. That consistent finding has been called 'the dodo bird hypothesis' (Marcus, O'Connell, Norris, & Sawaqdeh, 2014). Even though psychotherapy might be generally effective it is not effective with all patients and patients who initially improve may relapse (Shedler, 2020). This situation has led to the search for common relationship factors that may best predict psychotherapy outcome (Finsrud, Nissen-Lie, Vrabel, Høstmælingen, Wampold, & Ulvenes, 2022).

The quality of the therapeutic alliance is the common relationship factor that best predicts psychotherapy outcome (Flückiger, Del Re, Wampold, & Horvath, 2019). The alliance can be defined as a purposeful collaboration on the tasks and goals of therapy and the presence of a positive affective bond between patient and therapist (Safran & Muran, 2000). Psychotherapists whatever their theoretical orientation achieve better results with the establishment of a positive therapeutic alliance. The therapeutic alliance may be an evidence-based therapeutic relationship that is a common factor present in any successful psychotherapy regardless of therapists' theoretical orientation or patients' clinical problem (Norcross & Lambert, 2019). There is some evidence that the therapeutic alliance can be therapeutic in and of itself (Zilcha-Mano & Ben David-Sela, 2022).

For this reason, some therapeutic approaches focus on addressing ruptures to the therapeutic alliance to ensure that the factor most predictive of a successful outcome is effectively cultivated (Eubanks, Sergi, & Muran, 2021). Ruptures in the working alliance between the patient and therapist can be defined as a disagreement on the goals of therapy, a lack of collaboration on therapy tasks, or a strain in the therapeutic dyad's affective bond (Eubanks, Muran, & Safran, 2019). Two types of ruptures have been described: Confrontation ruptures, in which there is movement against the other or the work of therapy, and withdrawal ruptures, in which there is movement away from the other or the work of therapy (Eubanks, Muran, & Safran, 2019). Repairing ruptures to the therapeutic relationship is an evidence-based therapeutic process that may be a common therapeutic factor that can be operative in any approach to psychotherapy (Eubanks, Muran, & Safran, 2019).

Confrontation ruptures are likely to occur when therapists recommend a weight management goal for treatment that patients reject or to which they respond ambivalently, when therapists address patients' noncompliance with a weight management strategy to which they consented, and when patients relapse, and fear being blamed. Confrontation ruptures generally tend to occur when therapists offer weight management advice that patients are not ready to implement.

Withdrawal ruptures occur when patients deliberate about whether they need to lose weight, which approach to try, implementation difficulties, or why a particular approach isn't working and their therapists, despite being sympathetic, are not perceived as providing any actionable feedback or practical guidance that will help them resolve the dieting dilemmas by which patients feel stymied. Withdrawal ruptures generally occur when patients seek guidance in trying to make up their minds about some pressing dieting dilemma and therapists are perceived as withholding the advice and guidance that they believe they need to make up their minds and move forward. Patients may seek alternative sounding boards if their therapists fail to meaningfully connect to them on this shame-sensitive issue.

Some general guidelines have been developed for repairing ruptures to the therapeutic relationship (Eubanks, Muran, & Safran, 2019). Ruptures can be repaired explicitly by exploring patients' thoughts and feelings about the rupture. It is recommended that therapists nondefensively acknowledge their role in precipitating a rupture. Ruptures can also be repaired implicitly when therapists intuitively adjust their therapeutic approach (backing off if therapists are perceived as too challenging or providing more feedback if therapists are perceived as too passive).

Outcome research has hardly begun to explore whether the quality of the therapeutic relationship is also the best predictor of outcome when it comes to weight management (Krukowski, West, Priest, Ashikaga, Naud, & Harvey, 2019). One intriguing finding is that the therapeutic relationship does not predict outcome until the patient is ready to lose weight (Larocque, Lecomte, Savard, Stotland, & Sadikaj, 2015). Part of the therapeutic alliance is goal consensus (Tryon, Birch, & Verkuilen, 2018) and it might take some time with patients concerned about their weight before goal consensus is achieved as to the optimum weight management strategy given their unique personality, individual circumstances, and time of life.

Psychotherapy research is beginning to move away from an emphasis on developing specific treatments for specific clinical conditions (i.e., the medical model). Instead, psychotherapy research is moving towards an 'idionomic approach to processes of change' to establish a 'unified personalized science of human improvement' (Hayes, Ciarrochi, Hofmann, Chin, & Sahdra, 2022). In other words, clinicians will be called upon to individually tailor evidence-based processes of change, including evidence-based therapeutic relationships, to unique patients in unique circumstances who might not be amenable to any one-size-fits-all approach to treatment. This personalized approach to change is especially pertinent to weight management given the equivocal results of the various approaches to weight management.

Goal consensus when it comes to weight management may have to be continually reevaluated and reestablished as patients go through different phases of their weight management journeys with its successes and failures. Ruptures are likely any time patients' and therapists' goals begin to diverge, sometimes without awareness by either party that the two have begun to work at cross-purposes. Patients may remain ambivalent about sticking with a weight management approach as well as choosing a particular approach with which to begin. Ruptures can arise as therapists are working towards goals to which patients are ambivalently committed.

An important aspect of the therapeutic alliance is the extent to which patients feel validated and affirmed by their psychotherapists (Bate, Prout, Rousmaniere, & Vaz, 2022). Validation is an important therapeutic technique in psychodynamic psychotherapy (Kohut, 1971), humanistic psychotherapy (Rogers, 1961), and dialectical behavior therapy (Linehan, 2015). Patients need to feel understood, supported, and affirmed in their relationships with their therapists as that is an essential element of the therapeutic alliance (Bedi & Hayes, 2020). Nevertheless, practitioners of Dialectical Behavior Therapy have noted that as important as it is to validate patients, it is also important to avoid inadvertently validating the invalid (Fruzzetti & Ruork, 2019). In the psychodynamic tradition it is important to analyze defense mechanisms like denial and rationalization that preserve a maladaptive status quo rather than to unwittingly collude with and support such defenses (Gray, 1987).

It is a complex clinical judgment to ascertain to what extent the patient's approach to weight management is misguided and what to do when the patient looks to the therapist to validate an approach the therapist believes has been or will prove to be ineffective. Such situations are fertile soil for confrontation ruptures. How do patient and therapist negotiate a serious difference of opinion regarding the most sustainable approach to weight management when the patient seeks validation of an approach to which the therapist does not subscribe?

Such confrontation ruptures may be unavoidable unless the therapist's approach is to always validate the patient's viewpoint regardless of the therapist's personal belief. Yet therapist authenticity is also an important element of the therapeutic alliance (van Vreeswijk, 2020). Therapist inauthenticity if detected may result in a withdrawal rupture. The therapist is not perceived as being genuine and seems to be concealing what they truly believe. It can be tempting to validate the invalid to avoid a confrontation rupture though avoiding confrontation might result in an implicit withdrawal rupture because of the therapist's inauthenticity.

Assisting patients with their dieting dilemmas means helping patients look at their weight management strategies honestly with self-compassion rather than self-flagellation as they deliberate about whether they need to lose weight. When there is goal consensus for weight loss it means helping patients choose a diet and exercise program that has the best chance of being sustainable given their unique personality and individual circumstances. And finally, it requires helping patients respond with self-compassion when their weight management strategies fail. These are all shame-sensitive issues and helping patients with any shame-sensitive issue over which there is considerable ambivalence and defensiveness is fertile ground for ruptures to the therapeutic relationship.

Patients tend to assume that therapists are as critical of them as they are of themselves. Patients concerned about their weight tend to be harshly self-blaming for their failures to lose weight or continuing to gain weight due to internalized weight stigma (Himmelstein, Puhl, Pearl, Pinto, & Foster, 2020). Therapists can be perceived as reinforcing patients' internalized weight stigma whenever trying to help patients lose weight or prevent further weight gain regardless of the approach to weight management as weight is being treated as a problem to be solved rather than as a self-attribute to be accepted. Patients may assume there is implicit moralistic judgment any time a therapist is an advocate of any type of behavior change that patients resist. Patients whose therapists promote self-acceptance might assume that their therapists are frustrated with them if they continue to give voice to their self-flagellating self-talk despite considerable efforts to reduce self-critical self-talk. The patient may assume that any behavior that the therapist is helping the patient change is 'bad' behavior. Therefore, the patient is 'bad' if they fail to make the desired change.

Many aspects of dietary reality are known but much remains unknown. What is known is that people gain weight when the number of calories consumed is greater than the number of calories utilized (Marlatt & Ravussin, 2018). What is known is the calorie count, macro-nutrient composition (i.e., percentage of carbohydrates, protein, fat, and fiber), and glycemic index (i.e., how much a food spikes one's blood sugar) of various foods (Astrup, 2018). What is known is that there tends to be incremental weight gain with age as metabolism slows down and individuals become more sedentary (Rejeski & Williamson, 2018). What is known from research on identical versus fraternal twins is that there is a strong hereditable pre-disposition to developing a high BMI (Farooqi, 2018). What is known is that the risk of acquiring a metabolic syndrome like heart disease or Type 2 diabetes increases with weight gain (Colditz & Dart, 2018). What is known is that cultural factors like the availability of cheap highly palatable refined foods is correlated with weight gain (Moss, 2014). And what is known is that when the number of calories consumed is less than the number of calories utilized people lose weight (Marlatt & Ravussin, 2018).

What remains unknown is the extent to which one can remain healthy at any size and how that is moderated by BMI, exercise, food choices, age, and genetic predisposition. When weight loss is the goal the outcome literature is equivocal as to the most sustainable approach to enduring weight loss for different individuals in different circumstances given the high rates of regaining lost weight (Gomez-Rubalcava, Stabbert, & Phelan, 2018;

Hutchinson, 2011). Consequently, there are a dizzying array of commercial weight-loss diets (i.e., Paleo, Keto, Mediterranean, etc.) from which to choose and of psychological/behavioral approaches to weight management. Some diets advocate low-fat while others advocate low carbohydrates (Gardner, Trepanowski, Del Gobbo, Hauser, Rigdon, Ioannidis, Desai, & King, 2018). Some weight management strategies advocate complete abstinence from trigger foods such as sugar and flour (Blumenthal, DuPont, & Gold, 2012) while other approaches recommend doing away with all dietary restrictions whatsoever as one learns intuitive eating (Matz & Frankel, 2014). Some cognitive-behavioral approaches recommend vigilant self-monitoring of daily weight and caloric intake (Gomez-Rubalcava, Stabbert, & Phelan, 2018) while other approaches advocate letting go of obsessions with weight, calories, and food restrictions as one learns to eat intuitively or mindfully (Conason, 2015). Some approaches recommend analyzing the emotional traumas underlying emotional eating (Strodl & Wylie, 2020) while other approaches utilize behavior chain analysis to unlearn conditioned eating behavior (Gomez-Rubalcava, Stabbert, & Phelan, 2018).

Helping patients negotiate these dieting dilemmas when it comes to choosing a weight management strategy is challenging when there is a tendency to idealize various weight management strategies with considerable ideological zeal and respond dismissively to the competition. Weight management specialists tend to possess vested interests in the approaches of which they are proponents. Research has found associations between dietary adherence and ideological belief for practices like veganism (Krizanova, Rosenfeld, Tomiyama, & Guardiola, 2021). Whether a given diet is considered pathogenic or healthy can be influenced by ideological belief as diets based on food restrictions can be seen as reflecting a 'hegemonic anti-obesity ideology' (Rodney, 2018) while others view such restrictive diets as a medical necessity. Adopting a more ecumenical or neutral attitude towards these weight management controversies puts one in the minority and makes one vulnerable to being attacked by all sides for assuming a middle ground.

Therapists' cultural humility has been associated with client perceived working alliance (Dixon, Kivlighan, Hill, & Gelso, 2022). Patient and therapist may live in conflicting food cultures with conflicting food beliefs. Therapists may need to cultivate humility about their own approach to helping patients with their dieting dilemmas given the uncertain nature of many aspects of dietary reality. Patients possess dietary beliefs, some conducive to weight loss and some not (Storm, Reinwand, Wienert, Kuhlmann, De Vries, & Lippke, 2017). Motivated reasoning may sustain false dietary beliefs in the face of contradictory evidence (Gold, 2013). Yet patients may resent the implication that their dietary beliefs are not factually objective but tainted by wishful thinking (i.e., food myths) when therapists try to educate patients as to the dietary beliefs that appear to be better supported by the research literature or therapists' clinical/personal experiences (i.e., a confrontation rupture).

There can be significant cross-cultural differences about not only what is an attractive appearance but also about what constitutes a healthy weight and way of eating (Puhl, Lessard, Pearl, Himmelstein, & Foster, 2021). Patients could experience it as a lack of cultural humility if therapists assume that their evidence-based and/or clinical/personal experience–based dietary beliefs are more objective than patients' discrepant dietary beliefs (i.e., a withdrawal rupture that leads to a cultural disconnect). Patients may appreciate a therapist who provides an alternative perspective in a respectful way but may resent it if they feel implicit coercive pressure to adopt their therapists' way of thinking about weight management.

Some research suggests that patients may require long-term treatment to make signifi-cant changes in health compromising behavior (Jyrä, Knekt, & Lindfors, 2017). First, it may take time to make up one's mind about a particular dieting dilemma and then commit to an actionable weight management strategy. Once committing to a particular weight manage-ment strategy, it may take time to ascertain whether it will yield the desired results. It may be difficult to try something quite different when the current approach is not yielding the hoped-for results after a reasonable amount of time and effort. Loss aversion can keep indi-viduals committed to endeavors that are proving to be losing propositions and loss aversion appears to be higher in individuals with addictions (Thrailkill, DeSarno, & Higgins, 2022).

Psychotherapy could be seen as facilitating a process of dietary self-discovery as patients learn through trial and error which individualized approach is most sustainable for them in the long-term. Psychotherapy then must facilitate brutally honest reality-testing about what does and doesn't work despite what may be patients' tendencies to rationalize the status quo due to loss aversion. Psychotherapy must facilitate self-compassion in the face of weight management failure – a weight management approach that isn't working despite consider-able sacrifice of time and effort or after experiencing substantial success with a particular approach that no longer appears to be working. Psychotherapy must facilitate acceptance and commitment if it turns out that the most sustainable diet is one that requires ongoing and onerous dietary restrictions and high levels of self-monitoring and exercise when less restrictive approaches have proven ineffective.

Some of what may contribute to the uncertainty around the most sustainable approach to weight management is the scientific uncertainty about the determinants of body weight. There is research that suggests a strong heritable component to body weight (Farooqi, 2018). Possibly high weight individuals for genetic reasons just need more calories to feel sated than do slimmer individuals and it becomes near impossible to feel sated on the limited number of calories that could be ingested and still maintain a BMI within the normal range. Other research links weight gain to psychological trauma as eating 'comfort foods' becomes a maladaptive emotion regulation strategy (i.e., emotional eating) (Dawson, Strodl, & Kitamura, 2022). Treating overeating then requires treating the underlying psycho-logical trauma. Other research views weight gain as a result of conditioned eating habits to be unlearned through various cognitive behavioral techniques (Boutelle & Bouton, 2015, Gomez-Rubalcava, Stabbert, & Phelan, 2018). Yet other research suggests that weight gain may be a symptom of food addiction as refined foods like sugar and flour may constitute addictive substances for some individuals (Ahmed, 2012). Treatment then requires absti-nence from the addictive substances. There may also be cultural elements to weight gain as higher body weight seems to be more prevalent in some cultures than others as some cul-tural cuisines and cultural traditions may result in more weight gain than others. In the con-temporary American context, cheap freely available 'fast foods' made of highly processed ingredients may contribute to weight gain (Moss, 2014).

The role of exercise in weight management is also debatable. Exercise by itself does not seem to lead to considerable weight loss while diet plus exercise seems to do better than diet alone (Jakicic, Rogers, Sherman, & Kovacs, 2018). Advocates of health at any size view regular exercise as an important component of being able to remain healthy at any size (O'Hara, Ahmed, & Elashie, 2021). The question then becomes how much exercise and what kind of exercise best contributes to weight management. Must psychotherapy not only have to help patients concerned about their weight stick with a weight management strategy despite their ambivalence but also help sedentary patients exercise more regularly despite their reluctance to do so, regardless of whether they aspire to lose weight?

Part I of the book will address the theories behind the different approaches to weight management and the relational dimensions of the various approaches. Chapter 1 addresses the cultural dimension. Why is body weight such a shame-sensitive issue that is so difficult to discuss openly without fear of judgement? Chapter 2 examines behavioral theories of weight gain and reviews cognitive behavioral approaches to weight loss. Eating is in part a conditioned response that has been learned so it can be unlearned. Yet when eating behavior is a response to cultural conditioning it is not so easy to learn to go against the current of culturally conditioned eating habits. Chapter 3 explores psychodynamic theories of weight gain. Eating can be a form of emotion regulation to downregulate negative emotions (i.e., emotional eating). Alleviating emotional eating may require helping patients better deal with the negative emotions that eating serves to downregulate. Yet since emotion dysregulation is often a result of trauma, childhood adversity, and/or insecure attachment alleviating emotional eating may require facilitating secure attachment and healing trauma, a relational challenge.

Chapter 4 addresses the controversial topic of food addiction and the recommendation to abstain from trigger foods like sugar. It discusses the 'divergent weight management stigma' that individuals are subject to who subscribes to strict dietary restrictions. They may be judged for being too rigid and too self-denying thereby undermining their weight management strategy.

Chapter 5 addresses evolutionary theories of weight gain. Evolutionary psychology explains the innate preference for calorie-dense foods that were scarce in the environment-of-evolutionary adaptedness but abundant in contemporary environments. Since feasting on calorie-dense food to cement social bonds may be part of our evolutionary heritage, it may be a difficult relational challenge to learn to refrain from such feasting without feeling socially disconnected.

Chapter 6 addresses the confusing plethora of dietary approaches from which patients must choose, the rationales of the various approaches, and the pros and cons of those approaches. It is a relational challenge to know who to trust and believe when receiving contradictory advice by weight management specialists.

Part II examines the kinds of ruptures to the therapeutic relationship that can arise when therapists are trying to help patients with weight management and offer therapists guidance on how to address such ruptures. Chapter 7 examines the ways that the therapeutic relationship can be strained when patients are deliberating whether they need to lose weight and using their therapists as a sounding board. Patients may get upset with therapists who seem to be the bearers of bad news when it comes to 'bad' numbers related to body mass index, calorie count, blood glucose, cholesterol, and blood pressure. Chapter 8 examines the ways that the therapeutic relationship can be strained as patients are trying to decide on a weight management strategy to which they will commit. Patients may get upset with therapists who fail to give advice or provide advice patients aren't ready to implement.

Chapter 9 examines the ways the therapeutic relationship can be strained when patients look to the therapist to help them implement a particular weight management strategy. Therapists can be perceived as 'the food police' if therapists appear to be monitoring patients' implementation of a weight management strategy and judging them for its faulty implementation. Chapter 10 examines the ways that the therapeutic relationship is strained when patients are failing with their current weight management strategy. Patients worry that their therapists will be disappointed with them if they fail or relapse in their weight management strategy. Chapter 11 examines the ways that the therapeutic relationship can be strained when therapists are helping patients deal with judgmental individuals who are making patients feel badly about their weight and eating habits. Therapists can be perceived as 'pushy' when they are encouraging them to assert themselves with 'judgy' people who are undermining their weight management strategies. The conclusion summarizes the implications of the book for helping patients resolve their weight management concerns.

References

Ahmed, S. H. (2012). Is sugar as addictive as cocaine? In K. D. Brownell & M. S. Gold, *Food and addiction: A comprehensive handbook* (pp. 232–237). Oxford University Press. https://doi.org/10.1093/med:psych/9780199738168.003.0035

Astrup, A. (2018). Dietary treatment of overweight and obesity. In T. A. Wadden & G. A. Bray (Eds.), *Handbook of obesity treatment.* (pp. 309–321). The Guilford Press.

Bakizada, Z. M., Wadden, T. A., Wadden, S. Z., & Alamuddin, N. (2018). An overview of the treatment of obesity in adults. In T. A. Wadden & G. A. Bray (Eds.), *Handbook of obesity treatment* (pp. 283–308). The Guilford Press.

Bate, J., Prout, T. A., Rousmaniere, T., & Vaz, A. (2022). Exercise 5. Empathic validation. In J. Bate, T. A. Prout, T. Rousmaniere, & A. Vaz, *Deliberate practice in child and adolescent psychotherapy* (pp. 67–75). American Psychological Association. https://doi.org/10.1037/0000288-007

Bedi, R., & Hayes, S. (2020). Clients' perspectives on, experiences of, and contributions to the working alliance: Implications for clinicians. In J. N. Fuertes (Ed.), *Working alliance skills for mental health professionals* (pp. 111–136). Oxford University Press. https://doi.org/10.1093/med-psych/9780190868529.003.0006

Blumenthal, K., DuPont, R. L., & Gold, M. S. (2012). Treatment of alcohol and drug dependence in 2011 and relevance to food addiction. In K. D. Brownell & M. S. Gold, *Food and addiction: A comprehensive handbook* (pp. 318–328). Oxford University Press. https://doiorg/10.1093/med:psych/9780199738168.003.0048

Boutelle, K. N., & Bouton, M. E. (2015). Implications of learning theory for developing programs to decrease overeating. *Appetite, 93,* 62–74. https://doi.org/10.1016/j.appet.2015.05.013

Braden, A., & O'Brien, W. (2021). Pilot study of a treatment using dialectical behavioral therapy skills for adults with overweight/obesity and emotional eating. *Journal of Contemporary Psychotherapy: On the Cutting Edge of Modern Developments in Psychotherapy, 51*(1), 21–29. https://doi-org/10.1007/s10879-020-09477-1

Burrows, T., Collins, R., Rollo, M., Leary, M., Hides, L., & Davis, C. (2021). The feasibility of a personality targeted intervention for addictive overeating: FoodFix. *Appetite, 156,* 104974. https://doi.org/10.1016/j.appet.2020.104974

Butryn, M. L., Schumacher, L. M., & Forman, E. M. (2018). Alternative behavioral weight loss approaches: Acceptance and commitment therapy and motivational interviewing. In T. A. Wadden & G. A. Bray (Eds.), *Handbook of obesity treatment* (pp. 508–521). The Guilford Press.

Braun, T. D., Unick, J. L., Abrantes, A. M., Dalrymple, K., Conboy, L. A., Schifano, E., Park, C. L., & Lazar, S. W. (2022). Intuitive eating buffers the link between internalized weight stigma and body mass index in stressed adults. *Appetite*, 169, 105810. https://doi.org/10.1016/j.appet.2021.105810

Coelho, J. (2003). *Psychological and Behavioral Consequences of Selective Food Restriction* [Conference session abstract]. https://doi-org/10.1037/e350572004–001

Colditz, G. A., & Dart, H. (2018). Epidemiology and health and economic consequences of obesity. In T. A. Wadden & G. A. Bray (Eds.), *Handbook of obesity treatment* (pp. 3–23). The Guilford Press.

Comşa, L., David, O., & David, D. (2020). Outcomes and mechanisms of change in cognitive-behavioral interventions for weight loss: A meta-analysis of randomized clinical trials. *Behaviour Research and Therapy*, 132, 103654. Advance online publication. https://doi.org/10.1016/j.brat.2020.103654

Conason, A. (2015). The influence of dieting (hedonic deprivation) on food intake, how it can promote hedonic overeating, and mindful-eating interventions. In N. M. Avena, *Hedonic eating: How the pleasure of food affects our brains and behavior* (pp. 147–161). Oxford University Press.

Dawson, D., Strodl, E., & Kitamura, H. (2022). Childhood maltreatment and disordered eating: The mediating role of emotion regulation. *Appetite*, 172, 105952. https://doi.org/10.1016/j.appet.2022.105952

Dixon, K. M., Kivlighan, D. M., Hill, C. E., & Gelso, C. J. (2022). Cultural humility, working alliance, and Outcome Rating Scale in psychodynamic psychotherapy: Between-therapist, within-therapist, and within-client effects. *Journal of Counseling Psychology*, 69(3), 276–286. https://doi.org/10.1037/cou0000590

Eddie, D., Bergman, B. G., Hoffman, L. A., & Kelly, J. F. (2022). Abstinence versus moderation recovery pathways following resolution of a substance use problem: Prevalence, predictors, and relationship to psychosocial well-being in a U.S. national sample. *Alcoholism: Clinical and Experimental Research*, 46(2), 312–325. https://doi-org/10.1111/acer.14765

Elfhag, K., & Rössner, S. (2010). Weight loss maintenance and weight cycling. In P. G. Kopelman, I. D. Caterson, & W. H. Dietz (Eds.), *Clinical obesity in adults and children* (pp. 351–365). Wiley Blackwell.

Eubanks, C. F., Muran, J. C., & Safran, J. D. (2019). Repairing alliance ruptures. In J. C. Norcross & M. J. Lambert (Eds.), *Psychotherapy relationships that work: Evidence-based therapist contributions* (pp. 549–579). Oxford University Press.

Eubanks, C. F., Sergi, J., & Muran, J. C. (2021). Responsiveness to ruptures and repairs in psychotherapy. In J. C. Watson & H. Wiseman (Eds.), *The responsive psychotherapist: Attuning to clients in the moment* (pp. 83–103). American Psychological Association.

Farooqi, I. S. (2018). Genetics of obesity. In T. A. Wadden & G. A. Bray (Eds.), *Handbook of obesity treatment* (pp. 64–74). The Guilford Press.

Finsrud, I., Nissen-Lie, H. A., Vrabel, K., Høstmælingen, A., Wampold, B. E., & Ulvenes, P. G. (2022). It's the therapist and the treatment: The structure of common therapeutic relationship factors. *Psychotherapy Research: Journal of the Society for Psychotherapy Research*, 32(2), 139–150. https://doi.org/10.1080/10503307.2021.1916640

Flückiger, C., Del Re, A. C., Wampold, B. E., & Horvath, A. O. (2019). Alliance in adult psychotherapy. In J. C. Norcross & M. J. Lambert (Eds.), *Psychotherapy relationships that work: Evidence-based therapist contributions* (pp. 24–78). Oxford University Press.

Fruzzetti, A. E., & Ruork, A. K. (2019). Validation principles and practices in dialectical behaviour therapy. In M. A. Swales (Ed.), *The Oxford handbook of dialectical behaviour therapy* (pp. 325–344). Oxford University Press.

Gardner, C. D., Trepanowski, J. F., Del Gobbo, L. C., Hauser, M. E., Rigdon, J., Ioannidis, J. P. A., Desai, M., & King, A. C. (2018). Effect of low-fat vs low-carbohydrate diet on 12-month weight loss in overweight adults and the association with genotype pattern or insulin secretion: The DIETFITS Randomized Clinical Trial. JAMA, 319(7), 667–679. https://doi.org/10.1001/jama.2018.0245

Gold, J. M., Carr, L. J., Thomas, J. G., Burrus, J., O'Leary, K. C., Wing, R., & Bond, D. S. (2020). Conscientiousness in weight loss maintainers and regainers. *Health Psychology*, 39(5), 421–429. https://doi-org/10.1037/hea0000846

Gold, R. S. (2013). Perceived likelihood of experiencing a desirable versus undesirable outcome. *Psychological Reports*, 113(2), 525–527. https://doi.org/10.2466/04.07.PR0.113x18z5

Gomez-Rubalcava, S., Stabbert, K., & Phelan, S. (2018). Behavioral treatment of obesity. In T. Wadden & G. A. Bray (Eds.), *Handbook of obesity treatment* (pp. 336–348). The Guilford Press.

Gravina, G., Palla, M., Piccione, C., & Nebbiai, G. (2015). Therapeutic education and psychotherapy. In A. Lenzi, S. Migliaccio, & L. M. Donini (Eds.), *Multidisciplinary approach to obesity: From assessment to treatment* (pp. 219–232). Springer International Publishing.

Gray, P. (1987). On the technique of analysis of the superego: An introduction. *The Psychoanalytic Quarterly*, 56(1), 130–154.

Hayes, S. C., Ciarrochi, J., Hofmann, S. G., Chin, F., & Sahdra, B. (2022). Evolving an idionomic approach to processes of change: Towards a unified personalized science of human improvement. *Behaviour Research and Therapy*, 156, 104155. https://doi.org/10.1016/j.brat.2022.104155

Himmelstein, M. S., Puhl, R. M., Pearl, R. L., Pinto, A. M., & Foster, G. D. (2020). Coping with weight stigma among adults in a commercial weight management sample. *International Journal of Behavioral Medicine*, 27(5), 576–590. https://doi.org/10.1007/s12529-020-09895-4

Hutchinson E. (2011). Systems neuroscience: The stress of dieting. *Nature Reviews Neuroscience*, 12(2), 65. https://doi.org/10.1038/nrn2985

Jakicic, J. M., Rogers, R. J., Sherman, S. A., & Kovacs, S. J. (2018). Physical activity and weight management. In T. A. Wadden & G. A. Bray (Eds.), *Handbook of obesity treatment* (pp. 322–335). The Guilford Press.

Jyrä, K., Knekt, P., & Lindfors, O. (2017). The impact of psychotherapy treatments of different length and type on health behaviour during a five-year follow-up. *Psychotherapy Research: Journal of the Society for Psychotherapy Research*, 27(4), 397–409. https://doi.org/10.1080/10503307.2015.1112928

Kohut, H. (1971). *The analysis of the self: A systematic approach to the psychoanalytic treatment of narcissistic personality disorders.* University of Chicago Press.

Krizanova, J., Rosenfeld, D. L., Tomiyama, A. J., & Guardiola, J. (2021). Pro-environmental behavior predicts adherence to plant-based diets. *Appetite*, 163, 105243. https://doi.org/10.1016/j.appet.2021.105243

Krukowski, R. A., West, D. S., Priest, J., Ashikaga, T., Naud, S., & Harvey, J. R. (2019). The impact of the interventionist–participant relationship on treatment adherence and weight loss. *Translational Behavioral Medicine*, 9(2), 368–372. https://doi-org. /10.1093/ tbm/iby007

Langeveld, M., & de Vries, J. H. (2013). Het magere resultaat van diëten [The mediocre results of dieting]. *Nederlands tijdschrift voor geneeskunde*, 157(29), A6017.

Larocque, C., Lecomte, C., Savard, R., Stotland, S., & Sadikaj, G. (2015). Alliance thérapeutique, état de préparation psychologique et perte de poids [Therapeutic alliance, psychological readiness and weight loss]. *Annales Médico-Psychologiques*, 173(8), 665–674. https://doi-org/ 10.1016/j.amp.2015.01.007

Lee, J. (2020). Influences of cardiovascular fitness and body fatness on the risk of metabolic syndrome: A systematic review and meta-analysis. *American Journal of Health Promotion*, 34(7), 796–805. https://doi.org/10.1177/0890117120925347

Lillis, J., Dunsiger, S., Thomas, J. G., Ross, K. M., & Wing, R. R. (2021). Novel behavioral interventions to improve long-term weight loss A randomized trial of acceptance and commitment therapy or self-regulation for weight loss maintenance. *Journal of Behavioral Medicine*, 44(4), 527–540. https://doi-org.libproxy.adelphi.edu/10.1007/ s10865-021-00215-z

Linardon, J., Tylka, T. L., & Fuller-Tyszkiewicz, M. (2021). Intuitive eating and its psychological correlates: A meta-analysis. *The International Journal of Eating Disorders*, 54(7), 1073–1098. https://doi.org/10.1002/eat.23509

Linehan, M. M. (2015). *DBT skills training manual (2nd ed.)*. New York: Guilford Press.

Marcus, D. K., O'Connell, D., Norris, A. L., & Sawaqdeh, A. (2014). Is the Dodo bird endangered in the 21st century? A meta-analysis of treatment comparison studies. *Clinical Psychology Review*, 34(7), 519–530. https://doi.org/10.1016/j.cpr.2014.08.001

Marlatt, K. L., & Ravussin, E. (2018). Energy expenditure and obesity. In T. A. Wadden & G. A. Bray (Eds.), *Handbook of obesity treatment* (pp. 38–63). The Guilford Press.

Matz, J., & Frankel, E. (2014). *Beyond a shadow of a diet: The comprehensive guide to treating binge eating disorder, compulsive eating, and emotional overeating* (2nd ed.). Routledge/Taylor & Francis Group.

Miller, W. R., & Moyers, T. B. (2017). Motivational interviewing and the clinical science of Carl Rogers. *Journal of Consulting and Clinical Psychology*, 85(8), 757–766. https://doi. org/10.1037/ccp0000179

Mitchell, S. A. (1997). *Influence and autonomy in psychoanalysis*. Analytic Press.

Moss, M. (2014) *Salt sugar fat: How the food giants hooked us*. New York: Random House.

Norcross, J. C. & Lambert, M. J. (2019). *Psychotherapy relationships that work: Evidence-based therapist contributions*. Oxford University Press.

Novara, C., Pardini, S., Maggio, E., Mattioli, S., & Piasentin, S. (2022). Orthorexia nervosa: Over concern or obsession about healthy food? *Eating and Weight Disorders*, 26(8), 2577–2588. https://doi-org/10.1007/s40519-021-01110-x

O'Hara, L., Ahmed, H., & Elashie, S. (2021). Evaluating the impact of a brief Health at Every Size®-informed health promotion activity on body positivity and internalized weight-based oppression. *Body Image*, 37, 225–237. https://doi.org/10.1016/j.bodyim.2021.02.006

Perri, M. G., & Ariel-Donges, A. H. (2018). Maintenance of weight lost in behavioral treatment of obesity. In T. A. Wadden & G. A. Bray (Eds.), *Handbook of obesity treatment* (pp. 393–410). The Guilford Press.

Puhl, R. M., Lessard, L. M., Pearl, R. L., Himmelstein, M. S., & Foster, G. D. (2021). International comparisons of weight stigma: Addressing a void in the field. *International Journal of Obesity* (2005), 45(9), 1976–1985. https://doi.org/10.1038/s41366-021-00860-z

Rejeski, W. J., & Williamson, D. A. (2018). Effects of lifestyle interventions on health-related quality of life and physical functioning. In T. A. Wadden & G. A. Bray (Eds.), *Handbook of obesity treatment* (pp. 223–240). The Guilford Press.

Rodney A. (2018). Pathogenic or health-promoting? How food is framed in healthy living media for women. *Social Science & Medicine* (1982), 213, 37–44. https://doi.org/10.1016/j.socscimed.2018.07.034

Rogers, C. R. (1961). *On becoming a person.* Houghton Mifflin.

Safran, J. D., & Muran, J. C. (2000). *Negotiating the therapeutic alliance: A relational treatment guide.* Guilford Press.

Sainsbury, A., & Hay, P. (2014). Call for an urgent rethink of the 'health at every size' concept. *Journal of Eating Disorders*, 2, 8. https://doi.org/10.1186/2050-2974-2-8

Schnepper, R., Richard, A., Wilhelm, F. H., & Blechert, J. (2019). A combined mindfulness–prolonged chewing intervention reduces body weight, food craving, and emotional eating. *Journal of Consulting and Clinical Psychology*, 87(1), 106–111. https://doi-org/10.1037/ccp0000361

Schwartz, D. C., Nickow, M. S., Arseneau, R., & Gisslow, M. T. (2015). A substance called food: Long-term psychodynamic group treatment for compulsive overeating. *International Journal of Group Psychotherapy*, 65(3), 386–409. https://doi.org/10.1521/ijgp.2015.65.3.386

Shedler, J. (2020). Where is the evidence for "evidence-based" therapy? In M. Leuzinger-Bohleber, M. Solms, & S. E. Arnold (Eds.), *Outcome research and the future of psychoanalysis: Clinicians and researchers in dialogue* (pp. 44–56). Routledge/Taylor & Francis Group. https://doi-org.libproxy.adelphi.edu/10.4324/9780429281112-5

Storm, V., Reinwand, D., Wienert, J., Kuhlmann, T., De Vries, H., & Lippke, S. (2017). Brief report: Compensatory health beliefs are negatively associated with intentions for regular fruit and vegetable consumption when self-efficacy is low. *Journal of Health Psychology*, 22(8), 1094–1100. https://doi.org/10.1177/1359105315625358

Strodl, E., & Wylie, L. (2020). Childhood trauma and disordered eating: Exploring the role of alexithymia and beliefs about emotions. *Appetite*, 154, 104802. https://doi-org/10.1016/j.appet.2020.104802

Thrailkill, E. A., DeSarno, M., & Higgins, S. T. (2022). Loss aversion and risk for cigarette smoking and other substance use. *Drug and Alcohol Dependence*, 232, 1–8. https://doi-org/10.1016/j.drugalcdep.2022.109307

Tryon, G. S., Birch, S. E., & Verkuilen, J. (2018). Meta-analyses of the relation of goal consensus and collaboration to psychotherapy outcome. *Psychotherapy* (Chicago, Ill.), 55(4), 372–383. https://doi.org/10.1037/pst0000170

Tylka, T. L. (2006). Development and psychometric evaluation of a measure of intuitive eating. *Journal of Counseling Psychology*, 53(2), 226–240. https://doi.org/10.1037/0022-0167.53.2.226

Valenzuela, P. L., Santos-Lozano, A., Barrán, A. T., Fernández-Navarro, P., Castillo-García, A., Ruilope, L. M., Ríos Insua, D., Ordovas, J. M., Ley, V., & Lucia, A. (2022). Joint association of physical activity and body mass index with cardiovascular risk: A nationwide population-based cross-sectional study. *European Journal of Preventive Cardiology*, 29(2), e50–e52. https://doi.org/10.1093/eurjpc/zwaa151

van Vreeswijk, M. (2020). Authenticity and personal openness in the therapy relationship. In G. Heath & H. Startup (Eds.), *Creative methods in schema therapy: Advances and innovation in clinical practice* (pp. 237–252). Routledge/Taylor & Francis Group.

Vasiliu, O. (2022). Current status of evidence for a new diagnosis: Food addiction—A literature review. *Frontiers in Psychiatry*, 12, 824936. https://doi-org/10.3389/fpsyt.2021.824936

Yu, J., Song, P., Zhang, Y., & Wei, Z. (2020). Effects of mindfulness-based intervention on the treatment of problematic eating behaviors: A systematic review. *Journal of Alternative and Complementary Medicine*, 26(8), 666–679. https://doi.org/10.1089/acm.2019.0163

Zhang, Q., Hugh-Jones, S., & O'Connor, D. B. (2022). Investigation of psychometric properties of the mindful eating questionnaire in Chinese adolescents and young adults using mixed methods. *Appetite*, 176, 1–10. https://doi-org/10.1016/j.appet.2022.106097

Zilcha-Mano, S., & Ben David-Sela, T. (2022). Is alliance therapeutic in itself? It depends. *Journal of Counseling Psychology*, 69(6), 786–793. https://doi.org/10.1037/cou0000627

Relational Dimensions of Eating Behavior

part I

Internalized Weight Stigma and the Desire to Diet

1

The first question that patients concerned about their weight pose is whether they need to lose weight. The answer to that question is not without ambiguity. Patients may want to lose weight to be more physically attractive as they believe that 'thin' is more attractive than 'fat'. Patients may want to lose weight as preventative medicine as they believe it will lower the risk of acquiring a metabolic syndrome such as heart disease or Type 2 diabetes. Patients may want to lose weight because they have acquired a metabolic syndrome and their physician has prescribed weight loss as well as medication to treat their medical condition.

From a certain perspective these all seem like perfectly sensible reasons to lose weight. Given the positive bias towards physically attractive individuals [i.e., the beauty is good stereotype (Dion, Berscheid, & Walster, 1972)] why not make oneself as physically attractive as possible. It will improve one's self-esteem and contribute to greater success in one's work and love life. If remaining physically fit and trim is health promoting behavior that will contribute to greater longevity and lessened physical disability with advancing age one would be remiss to remain a sedentary high weight individual given the health risks. And if one is taking medication for a metabolic syndrome whose progression will result in early disability and demise, why not lose weight if losing weight might slow down or arrest the disease process beyond what is achievable by taking medication alone. From this perspective it's understandable that one might become frustrated with oneself and demoralized if unable to achieve one's weight loss goals.

All the 'good' reasons for losing weight are regularly reinforced by cultural messages that remaining fit and trim throughout the lifespan are key to looking attractive and remaining healthy. Such cultural messages come from everyday people, such as friends and colleagues, who tell us we look good when they notice that we lost weight, from parents and romantic partners who feel free to engage in explicit 'fat shaming' by noting critically or mockingly one's increasingly large body size, and by the media that presents physically fit and trim individuals as role models to emulate.

Despite the apparent cultural hegemony of what has been called an 'anti-obesity ideology' (Rodney, 2018) there is an emergent viewpoint that offers an alternative perspective buttressed by empirical support. The alternative viewpoint is that culture significantly influences attractiveness ratings of different body sizes (Puhl, Lessard, Pearl, Himmelstein, & Foster, 2021) and that one can be 'healthy at any size' as well as physically attractive at any size (Tylka & Wood-Barcalow, 2015). Therefore, the desire to lose weight may derive from 'internalized weight stigma' which reflects the mistaken belief that only thin people are attractive and healthy. The alternative to losing weight is then to develop 'body positivity', (O'Hara, Ahmed, & Elashie, 2021) acceptance of one's body no matter what the

DOI: 10.4324/9781003402336-4

size, and to appreciate that if one is physically fit from living a reasonably active lifestyle and if the biomarkers of a metabolic syndrome like blood glucose levels, blood cholesterol levels, and blood pressure look good one is healthy at one's current size (Tylka & Wood-Barcalow, 2015).

Weight Bias and Internalized Weight Stigma

In a systematic literature review Pearl and Puhl (2018) defined weight bias as negative attitudes directed toward individuals who are perceived to have excess body weight. These prejudicial attitudes are rooted in negative stereotypes suggesting that people perceived as obese are lazy, incompetent, and lack willpower (Puhl & Brownell, 2001) Weight bias can result in discriminatory treatment in employment, education, and health care, as well as stigma in interpersonal relationships and the mass media (Puhl & Brownell, 2006). Weight bias is associated with negative health consequences such as maladaptive eating, low physical activity, physiological stress, weight gain, and body dissatisfaction (Puhl, Himmelstein, & Pearl, 2020).

Individuals that have been subject to prejudicial treatment for their perceived weight may internalize that stigmatization. That process has been referred to as internalized weight stigma, weight bias internalization, self-directed weight stigma, or internalized weight-based oppression (Pearl & Puhl, 2018). When weight bias has been internalized there is awareness of the negative stereotypes to which one has been subjected, some degree of agreement with those stereotypes, the application of those negative stereotypes to oneself, and low self-esteem as a result (Pearl & Puhl, 2018). Pearl and Puhl (2018) noted that a high percentage of overweight and obese individuals internalize the weight stigma to which they have been subjected.

Internalized weight stigma appears to be associated with many of the same adverse consequences that result from weight bias. In a systematic review Pearl and Puhl (2018) found that internalized weight stigma was associated with depression, anxiety, low self-esteem, poor body image, disordered eating such as binge eating and food addiction, high body weight, and greater weight regain. Consequently, regardless of whether patients aspire to lose weight, alleviating internalized weight stigma appears to be an important goal for treatment. Patients who choose not to lose weight may need to learn to accept their bodies and appetites for what they are and patents who do choose to lose weight may need help overcoming their self-disparagement when failing to achieve what may be unrealistic weight loss goals like achieving a fat-free body. Self-disparagement because of internalized weight stigma may impede weight loss efforts because it increases the tendency towards emotional eating (Dawson, Strodl, & Kitamura, 2022).

Ruptures to the therapeutic relationship will arise whenever therapists interact with patients in ways that convey weight bias and when therapists engage patients in ways that trigger patients' internalized weight stigma. Since therapists' biases are often implicit (Meulman, 2019), the therapist might have thought their comment was neutral or supportive when they said it but upon reflection it may emerge that it did indeed express implicit bias. Freud (1911) noted long ago in a discussion of paranoid dynamics that when patients project their own thoughts and feelings on to others (i.e., negative mind reading), they do not project into a vacuum or on to a blank screen. They hang their projection on a piece of reality so there is at least a kernel of truth in the patient's projection. It behooves therapists to acknowledge not only that something they did precipitated an alliance rupture but that at least some implicit level of bias was expressed if the patient is feeling shamed by the therapist for their weight or eating habits.

Arthur was a single young adult who felt that he couldn't date until he lost weight. He hadn't dated in several years because he hadn't lost weight in several years and was feeling lonely for lack of a love life. I noted that his love life need not be held hostage to losing weight as women seemed to be attracted to both his body and his personality when he was out socializing with friends. Arthur retorted that he would have a better selection of women if he lost weight. He said the therapy sessions would be better spent helping him lose weight rather than trying to get him to resume dating at his current weight. To provide autonomy support, achieve goal consensus, and avoid working at cross-purposes I made it clear that I would support his weight loss goals. Arthur was happy about that.

Arthur came up with a weight loss plan that involved eating out less, drinking less alcohol, and eliminating junk food. I was supportive of that plan of action. Arthur would have 'good' weeks and 'bad' weeks following his dieting plan. I approached the bad weeks in a problem-solving way to see if we could collaboratively tweak his plan so he could better stick to it, a kind of relapse prevention. But I noticed that Arthur didn't want to dwell on what he didn't do correctly but simply wanted validation of what he still did right.

Initially I went along with that but after several months I realized that Arthur wasn't losing weight. He was simply losing a little weight during the good weeks and gaining it back during the bad weeks. I pointed out that pattern and Arthur responded angrily that I was just making him feel badly about himself. I tried to clarify that my rationale was relapse prevention, to keep the 'good' weeks going without falling back into his old eating habits. Arthur responded defensively saying: 'I know but I don't have to be perfect and sometimes I just need a break'.

Upon reflection I realized that consciously I didn't think I possessed weight bias because I was supportive of his dating without having to lose weight. But I realized that I did have the implicit weight-related bias that Arthur was being 'lazy', not taking responsibility for working on relapse prevention as much as he should have given his own stated goals for treatment. My relentlessly problem-solving approach, more often appreciated than not, was implicitly reinforcing his internalized weight stigma by making him feel like a lazy and irresponsible overweight person who just wanted to indulge his appetites rather than work on consistently implementing his own dieting plan. I came to appreciate that for Arthur simply maintaining his current weight was an achievement. His good weeks stemmed the tide of further weight gain and I needed to be appreciative of that.

Body Positivity

Tylka and Wood-Barcalow (2015) proposed that positive body image is a multifaceted construct.

> The facets include body appreciation, body acceptance and love, adaptive appearance investment, broadly conceptualizing beauty, inner positivity that radiates outward and manifests as adaptive behavior, and filtering information in a body-protective manner.
> (p. 127)

Positive body image will be constructed differently for different people given their particular social identities and unique individuality. Social support of that individual construction contributes to positive body image whereas social critique for failure to conform to some normative standard of appearance undermines that positive construct and contributes to negative body image.

'Body positivity' has been proposed as an antidote to internalized weight stigma. Body positivity means cultivating fat acceptance, appreciation for body diversity, and appreciating that one can be 'healthy at any size' (Watkins, Clifford, & Souza, 2018). Individuals with large bodies could perceive that difference as something that makes them special and unique in a good way. High weight individuals might perceive themselves as high status in cultures in which all the poor people are thin because they don't have enough to eat and only the rich people are well-fed. 'Dad bods' or 'mom bods' might convey that one is a loving and devoted nurturing caretaker who is not vain when it comes to appearance. What is or isn't physically attractive might be a matter of perspective rather than something essential about the individual's appearance.

Most clinical approaches have techniques that could help facilitate positive body image. Psychodynamic approaches might examine identification with negative parental attitudes towards body size and childhood experiences of being teased, criticized, and rejected for one's large body size. Cognitive approaches might utilize cognitive reappraisal to help high weight individuals see that from an alternative perspective their bodies can be perceived as attractive. Feminist approaches might help patients perceive that normative standards of beauty are a form of weight-based discrimination and oppression (Pearl & Puhl, 2018). Mindfulness can help high weight individuals learn to look at their bodies without judgment (Schnepper, Richard, Wilhelm, & Blechert, 2019).

Humanistic approaches (Adame, 2022) might help individuals honor and cultivate their individual uniqueness in terms of physical appearance (a look that expresses their true inner selves). A large body may be a statement to the world of one's values and a courageous assertion of one's core values in cultures where weight stigma is prevalent. Thus, the integrative psychotherapist has a wide armamentarium of approaches from which to choose to help patients acquire a positive body image despite internalized weight stigma.

Daphne Merkin (2010), a writer, discussed her consultation with a psychiatrist for her chronic treatment resistant depression. The therapist was known for his confrontational approach, but Merkin did not anticipate being confronted with his weight loss agenda:

> He wondered, for instance, whether I thought of losing weight. Dumbstruck, I momentarily lost my footing, and then I answered that I had. He nodded and then coldly observed, "But you lack the motivation." No, I said, I didn't lack the motivation forever, I just lacked it for right now. Dr. F. looked entirely unconvinced and went on to ask me if I didn't long to be part of a couple, to have someone to visit art galleries with . . . His tone was smug and self-congratulatory.

The implication was that Merkin was depressed because she didn't have a good love life and she didn't have a good love life because she was overweight. Fortunately, Merkin was sufficiently self-accepting and assertive that she did not return for further treatment after being subjected to weight stigma during the initial consultation. Years later Merkin (2014) wrote about seeking weight loss treatment after learning that she had diabetes.

Respect for patients' autonomy is a cardinal value in psychotherapy (Miller & Moyers, 2017). Patients set the goals of treatment. Therapists are free to suggest alternative goals for treatment but not to impose alternative goals. Patients and therapists are working at cross purposes when they possess divergent goals but lack awareness of that discrepancy and fail to discuss it. Working at cross purposes is fertile ground for ruptures to the therapeutic relationship that can only be resolved when goal consensus is achieved through a respectful dialogue about the difference of opinion about the goals for treatment, be it acceptance of patients' current weight or weight loss.

Gordon was a very large man married to a large woman with two sons who came for therapy because he was confused about his sexuality. He didn't know what to do. Gordon's weight never came up as an issue until he came out as gay and decided to divorce his wife so he could live as an openly gay man. At that point Gordon decided that he would be more successful with the thin physically fit men to whom he was attracted if he was thinner, and more muscle bound. Sometimes patients feel that life is easier if they conform to the normative standards of beauty within a certain subculture rather than combat such standards as oppressive as such standards can be. Since Gordon had failed with dieting in the past, he decided that he would seek bariatric surgery.

I inquired why Gordon wouldn't first try to lose weight through diet and exercise before resorting to bariatric surgery which initially struck me as a radical form of body modification. Gordon clarified that being in his mid-thirties he worried that he was starting to look old so that he couldn't waste precious time with dieting and exercise that had not worked in the past. Now that Gordon wanted to be with men, he didn't want to limit himself to men who were attracted to big bearish men like himself since that wasn't his type. Consequently, bariatric surgery was the pragmatic solution. We avoided a more serious rupture because I could support his weight loss strategy as he helped me see that conforming to my preferred weight management strategy would have been counter-productive in his circumstances. After the surgery Gordon would attend sessions beaming with pride showing off his slimmed down body and flexing his biceps.

Applying the principles of Dialectical Behavior Therapy (Braden & O'Brien, 2021) can help patients learn to live with the dialectical tensions between acceptance and change and of seemingly contradictory goals for treatment. Therapists require the cognitive flexibility to see the inner logic and kernel of truth in contrary points of view and work towards synthesis even when the synthetic solution is not readily apparent. On the one hand alleviation of internalized weight stigma and fat acceptance is crucial because achieving a fat-free body is unattainable for most individuals. Why feel badly about oneself for failure to conform to unrealistic and oppressive beliefs about ideal bodies? Lack of fat acceptance is associated with maladaptive eating (Puhl, Himmelstein, & Pearl, 2020).

Yet on the other hand, losing weight may be part of a medically recommended treatment plan for those who have acquired a metabolic syndrome to which weight is contributory. It may also seem like a practical necessity for large individuals who are attracted to only thin partners and believe that they must be thin to attract a thin partner. The challenge for clinicians is to not fall into dichotomous (i.e., either/or) thinking about this clinical issue and to recover a more dialectical way of thinking when starting to fall into potentially polarizing rupture-inducing debates with patients on this shame-sensitive topic.

Sometimes achieving body acceptance is supporting patients' efforts to achieve the body they want rather than the body they already have and to which they don't want to have to reconcile themselves. That may involve hormone supplements and/or plastic surgery as in gender affirming care. When it comes to weight not all high weight patients want to learn to love their high weight bodies. Samantha Irby (2023), a 300-pound African American lesbian comedy writer, 'says it's OK to hate your body' when you feel that your body does not work correctly, and then people unfairly judge you for your 'fat struggle' over which you have little control. Irby believes that 'the tyranny around loving yourself is bonkers' so she doesn't think that 'we all have to love our bodies'. Yet Irby is happy for those who do achieve fat acceptance and can publicly celebrate their high weight bodies.

Health at any Size

One part of fat acceptance is believing that one can be beautiful at any size. Another part of fat acceptance is believing that one can be 'healthy at any size' (Watkins, Clifford, & Souza, 2018). Considerable research suggests that various illnesses, most notably Type 2 diabetes, and heart disease, are associated with high weight (Colditz & Dart, 2018). This is correlational research and correlation does not equal causation. There are plausible theories of how high weight might 'cause' various metabolic syndromes such as adipose tissue secreting inflammatory hormones (Adams, Stears, Savage, & Deaton, 2018). Yet none are firmly established.

High weight may also be associated with behaviors such as lack of physical exercise, smoking, high alcohol consumption, and/or consuming highly processed foods that could also be contributory to various metabolic syndromes. Not all high weight individuals will suffer such metabolic syndromes since genetic predispositions towards such syndromes might also be contributory. Sometimes average weight individuals acquire such syndromes because of a strong genetic predisposition and/ or smoking and drinking too much. Consequently, high weight individuals could be healthy if they exercise regularly, don't smoke, don't drink, consume more whole foods than highly processed foods, and lack the genetic predisposition towards various metabolic syndromes. Losing weight as preventative medicine, especially if there is not a family history of heart disease or diabetes, may be unwarranted if the biomarkers of such metabolic syndromes (i.e., blood glucose, blood cholesterol, blood pressure) all look good in yearly checkups.

One could spend one's entire life enduring the privations of dieting to prevent a medical event that might never happen. Such preventative medicine could have unintended negative psychological consequences. Every time one consumes a high fat food it might trigger a worry about clogging one's arteries and every time one consumes a sweet it may trigger a worry about spiking one's blood sugar. Every time one looks in the mirror and sees one's body fat one sees a medical catastrophe in the making. There is also concern that dieting could have unintended negative physical consequences. Excessively restrictive and unsustainable diets may result in rebound effects in which one regains more weight than one had originally lost (Campos, 2004).

Weight does seem to be an independent determinant of metabolic syndromes such as heart disease regardless of how much one exercises (Valenzuela, Santos-Lozano et al., 2022). Perhaps not everyone can be healthy at every size forever. If high weight is indeed contributory to the development of such medical conditions, it is still unclear exactly how much weight loss is necessary to minimize the risk. Will being of average, if not below average weight, significantly contribute to longevity? Or is it good enough in terms of one's health prospects if one's BMI descends from morbid obesity to obesity or from obesity to overweight without ever making it into the normal BMI range? Sustained weight loss maintenance of as little as 3–5% can produce clinically meaningful health benefits (Jensen et al., 2014) and the greater the weight loss the greater the health benefits (Wing et. al., 2011).

Clinicians have noted that some high weight individuals acquire the same unhealthy attitudes towards food, eating, and bodily appearance that individuals with eating disorders such as anorexia and bulimia possess (Novara, Pardini, Maggio, Mattioli, & Piasentin, 2022). They may believe that only a fat-free body is attractive and healthy. To achieve a fat-free body they may obsessively weigh themselves, count calories to limit themselves to a very low-calorie diet, discriminate between good foods (i.e., low calorie) and bad foods (i.e., fattening). Self-flagellation is intense with any weight gain or any transgressions of the rules of dieting.

Such unhealthy attitudes may contribute to eating disorders. Starving oneself in the case of anorexia but increased emotional eating in the case of high weight may be compensatory reactions to fat phobia and the consequent self-disgust at the detection of body fat [i.e., fat phobia (Bacon, Scheltema, & Robinson, 2001)]. Such unhealthy attitudes towards eating and one's own body may need to be alleviated regardless of whether one is underweight, or overweight, hoping to lose weight or hoping to acquire greater acceptance of one's current weight.

To counter these unhealthy attitudes towards body size and eating Robison (1999) proposed an alternative paradigm that highlighted that individual variations in body shape and size are natural and that thin bodies are not inherently healthy or appealing, nor are fat bodies inherently unhealthy or unappealing. The goal is to empower individuals to lead healthy lives caring for and appreciating the bodies they presently have regardless of size. Burgard (2009) explained that the Health at Every Size model is about enhancing physical, emotional, and spiritual health without focusing on weight loss. It encourages eating based on internal hunger cues, satiety, appetite, nutrition, and enjoyment rather than externally imposed dietary rules. It encourages physical activity for pleasure and health benefits rather than for weight loss. Advocates of Health at Every Size cite research that suggests that their approach provides equal or better physiological and psychological outcomes compared to control conditions largely composed of weight loss interventions (Watkins, Clifford, & Souza, 2018). Patients in health at any size programs on average don't lose weight nor do they gain weight.

In terms of psychotherapy, advocates of Health at Any Size recommend that high weight individuals seeking treatment for depression, anxiety, or post-traumatic stress disorder should be treated in the same way as would average weight patients (Mizock, 2015). Weight loss should not be the recommended treatment for those emotional problems. In addition, such patients may need to be taught skills to contend with weight stigma and fat phobia outside of the treatment setting. Like members of any other minority group subject to discrimination there is a level of minority stress (Cardoso, Paim, Catelan, & Liebross, 2022) that high weight patients may need help managing.

Though some people may be able to remain healthy at any size throughout the lifespan it's not clear that all people can do so. For example, Kelly deVos (2018), a life-long advocate of body positivity discussed an adjustment in her thinking when she developed rapidly advancing Type 2 diabetes at age 41 and was told she had ten years left to live if she didn't lose weight. deVos had taught her average size teenage daughter body positivity so was stunned when her daughter blurted out one day that she wanted to lose weight. deVos felt that there must be a way to support her daughter's and now her own weight loss goals without reinforcing 'fat phobia'. Is there a way to support patients' weight loss goals but still promote fat acceptance and a belief that it is not necessary to possess a fat-free body to be attractive and healthy?

Patients vary in their risk tolerance for potentially health compromising behavior. Those with low risk tolerance will try to lose weight as preventative medicine especially if there is a history of family members suffering weight-related metabolic syndromes. Those with moderate risk tolerance may have a philosophy of 'if it isn't broke don't fix it'. For such moderate risk tolerance patients, the tipping point for losing weight may be when the biomarkers of a metabolic syndrome are elevated or when they have begun to suffer a metabolic syndrome. The highest risk tolerance patients who have acquired a metabolic syndrome may be willing to bet that medication is sufficient to manage their condition without having to change their eating habits. Psychotherapists are free to explore the pros and cons of different levels of risk tolerance. Ultimately, out of respect for patients' autonomy, therapists must accept patients' tolerance for risk, be it low or high, if conducting a methodical cost-benefit analysis doesn't change their calculations.

Ruptures to the therapeutic relationship are likely whenever patients feel pressured by their therapists to adopt strategies that seem riskier or more conservative than they feel comfortable adopting. Encouraging fat acceptance when patients aspire to lose weight can feel dangerous if patients' worry that fat acceptance will doom them to being unattractive, at least to the weight-normative majority, and unhealthy, someone who will eventually succumb to a metabolic syndrome with advancing age. Encouraging weight loss when patients accept their fat and believe they can be healthy at any size if supplemented with medication as needed will be resented. They will resist the therapeutic arm twisting and implicit fat shaming if they believe that dieting will dramatically decrease their quality of daily life without any substantial health pay off in the long-term to compensate for their daily privations. Patients who are two minds about this issue so remain undecided might believe that therapists have lost their objectivity if they come down too strongly on one side or the other of this complicated issue.

Intuitive and Mindful Eating

Instead of dieting, advocates of health at every size have developed an approach that they call 'intuitive eating' (Napolitano & Foster, 2012). Non-dieting or anti-dieting approaches emphasize education about the negative impact of dieting and the biological underpinnings of body size. Dietary restraint has been associated with eating disorders and loss of control of eating (Manasse, Lampe, Abber, Fitzpatrick, Srivastava, & Juarascio, 2023). What is encouraged is eating according to internal rather than external cues, balanced eating, acceptance of the body at any weight, and increased physical activity. Weight is not a target of intervention. Instead, there is encouragement to reduce or eliminate efforts to lose weight (Napolitano & Foster, 2012).

A perusal of the subscales of *The Intuitive Eating Scale* reveals the components of intuitive eating (Tylka & Kroon Van Diest, 2013). 1) The 'Eating for physical rather than emotional reasons' subscale has items such as 'I find myself eating when I'm lonely, even though I'm not physically hungry'. 2) The 'Unconditional permission to eat' subscale has items like 'If I'm craving a certain food, I allow myself to have it' or reverse scored 'I get mad at myself for eating something unhealthy'. 3) The 'Reliance on hunger and satiety cues to stop eating' subscale has items like 'I trust my body to tell me when to eat'. 4) The 'Body-food choice congruence' subscale has items like 'Most of the time, I desire to eat nutritious foods'.

Intuitive eating centers on overcoming emotional eating, lessen eating in response to external triggers, greater attention to physiological cues of hunger and satiety, reduce self-criticism for seeming to overeat or eat fattening foods, and finally to learn to trust one's intuitive food preferences. For the most part this is how 'normal' average weight individuals eat who are neither underweight nor overweight. Encouraging underweight individuals to eat more like average weight individuals is without controversy. Meta-analyses of intuitive eating suggest improvement in body image, self-esteem, well-being, and intuitive eating (Braun, Unick, Abrantes, Dalrymple, Conboy, Schifano, Park, C, & Lazar, 2022; Linardon, Tylka, & Fuller-Tyszkiewicz, 2021).

There is concern, though, that encouraging high weight individuals to eat like average weight individuals might be granting such individuals license to eat even more than they already do (Sainsbury & Hay, 2014). It might be perceived as license to relinquish all self-restraint when it comes to portion size and/ or preferentially eating calorie-dense foods. Nevertheless, studies of intuitive eating suggest that while it doesn't result in weight loss, it doesn't appear to result in weight gain either so may help with weight maintenance if not weight loss (Linardon, Tylka, & Fuller-Tyszkiewicz, 2021).

Mindful eating has been suggested as an alternative to or supplement to behavioral approaches to weight loss that require more cognitive skills like meal planning, keeping a food log, counting calories, and portion-control. Mindful eating has been given this definition: 'When considered in the context of nutrition, "mindful eating" can be used to describe a nonjudgmental awareness of physical and emotional sensations while eating or in a food-related environment' (Framson, Kristal, Schenk, Littman, Zeliadt, & Benitez, 2009). If 'mindless eating' accounts for weight gain and the poor long-term success of many weight loss interventions than mindful eating might be the antidote.

A perusal of the subscales of the Mindful Eating Questionnaire provides the components of mindful eating: 1) The 'disinhibition' subscale consists of items like: 'When I eat at "all you can eat" buffets, I tend to overeat'. 2) The 'awareness' subscale has items like 'I taste every bite that I eat'. 3) The 'external cues' subscale has items like 'I recognize when food advertisements make me want to eat'. 4) The 'emotional response' subscale has items like 'When I'm sad I eat to feel better'.

There is overlap between the concepts of intuitive eating and mindful eating as both try to overcome eating for emotional reasons rather than for physiological hunger and both try to overcome eating in response to external cues rather than inner states. What mindfulness adds is that in encouraging individuals to savor every bite, it slows down the process of eating and provides more time for the digestive process to send signals to the brain to stop eating. When individuals 'wolf down' their food, they may have already overeaten prior to the brain receiving signals to stop eating. A meta-analysis of mindful-based interventions (MBI) for problematic eating behavior suggested that MBI groups showed significant reduction in emotional eating, external eating, binge eating, and weight and shape concern (Yu, Song, Zhang, & Wei, 2020).

Many aspects of both intuitive and mindful eating would be helpful for those trying to lose weight as well as for those striving for fat acceptance rather than weight loss. Overcoming emotional eating, overcoming eating driven by external cues, savoring every bite while paying greater attention to feelings of satiety, and refraining from panic and self-flagellation for violating dietary rules are worthy goals regardless of one's ultimate weight management strategy.

The controversy resides in whether 'unconditional permission to eat' paired with fat acceptance without weight loss is preferable to dietary restrictions that might facilitate weight loss. Advocates of health at every size believe that the research literature suggests that dieting only has negative effects and part of their educational messaging is making individuals aware of the negative effects of dieting to dissuade high weight individuals from dieting or trying to lose weight (Watkins, Clifford, & Souza, 2018). Advocates of behavioral weight loss interventions believe that the research literature suggests that not all the initial weight lost is regained, that some of the weight lost is maintained in long-term follow-up, that small but significant sustained weight loss has health benefits, and that certain individuals are able to utilize behavioral principles to sustain their weight loss in the long-term (Gomez-Rubalcava, Stabbert, & Phelan, 2018).

The dichotomy between dieting and nondieting may be a false dichotomy. The question that is rarely asked and answered is what are reasonable or unreasonable dietary restrictions. Unreasonably restrictive diets, like starvation diets, are most likely to generate the negative effects of which advocates of health at any size are legitimately concerned. Perhaps more reasonable restrictions might be more sustainable and might not feel like 'dieting' but might be experienced instead as a healthful lifelong approach to eating that is eventually preferred to one's old way of eating.

Dietary guidelines could be experienced as useful goalposts towards which to aim rather than as hard and fast rules that demand perfectionistic compliance. What is reasonably restrictive might have to be determined on a case-by-case basis as universal guidelines on this issue are lacking and individuals vary on the extent to which they may need an externally imposed structure to achieve their goals. There should be no shame if some individuals are dependent on an external structure to which they voluntarily surrender to achieve their goals, whatever those goals may be (i.e., like 12 step programs for various addictions).

Diane was a single 50-year-old affluent lawyer who enjoyed going out to eat frequently with her friends. She had put on considerable weight and found that she no longer fit into her expensive wardrobe. Diane wanted to lose weight rather than buy new clothes and she wanted to lose weight quickly. Diane discovered a diet that promised to do just that; a very low 800 calorie a day liquid diet she had read about that her family doctor would supervise. Diane excitedly told me about it and sought my validation. Diane became annoyed with me when I raised questions about the sustainability of such a diet. Diane decided she would give it a try despite my skepticism and quickly began to lose weight.

After several months it became apparent that she could not sustain what appeared to be a "starvation diet" and demoralized returned to her old eating habits regaining all the lost weight. Diane found it difficult to choose between fat acceptance which would require buying a new wardrobe or adopting a more viable long-term approach to weight loss that wouldn't be a quick fix and might require permanent lifestyle adjustments in terms of her frequency of eating out. Only a mild rupture ensued due to my skepticism as I showed respect for her autonomy by not trying to obstruct her attempt to discover what worked through trial and error or to perhaps decide that she would just have to buy new clothes at a larger size.

Orthorexia Nervosa

Bratman (1997) coined the term Orthorexia Nervosa to refer to a kind of disordered eating characterized by excessive concern about eating healthy food with specific nutritional properties chosen to eat healthily but also to prevent and manage diseases by facilitating weight loss. Concern with eating healthfully can turn into a neurotic obsession. Foods are dichotomized into good and bad foods based on calorie density, fat content, carbohydrate content, fiber content, and degree processed. Anxiety aroused by the temptation to eat bad foods and self-flagellation after having succumbed to that temptation characterize this condition. Individuals that score high on a measure of Orthorexia Nervosa also score high on measures of eating disorders, perfectionism, anxiety, and depression (Novara, Pardini, Maggio, Mattioli, & Piasentin, 2022).

Among low weight individuals, orthorexia nervosa may contribute to self-starvation, among average weight individuals it may contribute to binging and purging, and among high weight individuals it may contribute to emotional eating (Dawson, Strodl, & Kitamura, 2022). Among high weight individuals, orthorexia nervosa could be exacerbated by various dietary recommendations like weighing oneself regularly, counting calories, limiting portion size, limiting consumption of calorie-dense foods, limiting consumption of highly processed foods, foods with added sugar, etc. Individuals with orthorexia nervosa experience dietary guidelines or rules as rigid authoritarian demands that require absolute compliance less dire consequences accrue.

Health at any size recommends eliminating diets and dieting since diets may trigger and exacerbate Orthorexia Nervosa. Yet for individuals who discover that they can't be healthy at any size Orthorexia Nervosa may become an impediment to successful dieting as it triggers patients' perfectionism and catastrophizing when dietary compliance is less than perfect. High weight patients may rebel against externally imposed perfectionistic demands if 'policing' their eating habits and weight diminishes their sense of autonomy. Or high weight patients may internalize perfectionistic demands and suffer self-hatred, depression, and anxiety when they cannot live up to them. The principles of mindfulness could be applied to this situation if patients can learn to look at their weight or their calorie count without judgment but with self-compassion when the numbers are 'bad'.

The extent to which high weight individuals can learn to accept their less than perfect compliance with dietary guidelines has yet to be thoroughly investigated. Can high weight individuals learn to be satisfied with 'good-enough' compliance yet assume responsibility without defensiveness or self-flagellation when compliance is insufficient to achieve reasonable weight loss goals? 'Responsibility without blame' (Pickard, 2017) is a difficult state of mind to achieve when trying to overcome addictive or compulsive behavior as overeating could be considered from the perspective of food addiction (Schulte, Joyner, Potenza, Grilo, & Gearhardt, 2015).

References

Adame, A. L. (2022). Self-in-relation: Martin Buber and D. W. Winnicott in dialogue. *The Humanistic Psychologist*, 50(3), 376–388. https://doiorg/10.1037/hum0000203

Adams, C., Stears, A., Savage, D., & Deaton, C. (2018). "We're stuck with what we've got": The impact of lipodystrophy on body image. *Journal of Clinical Nursing*, 27(9–10), 1958–1968. https://doi-org/10.1111/jocn.14342

Bacon, J. G., Scheltema, K. E., & Robinson, B. E. (2001). Fat phobia scale revisited: The short form. *International Journal of Obesity and Related Metabolic Disorders: Journal of the International Association for the Study of Obesity*, 25(2), 252–257. https://doi.org/10.1038/sj.ijo.0801537

Braden, A., & O'Brien, W. (2021). Pilot study of a treatment using dialectical behavioral therapy skills for adults with overweight/obesity and emotional eating. *Journal of Contemporary Psychotherapy: On the Cutting Edge of Modern Developments in Psychotherapy*, 51(1), 21–29. https://doi-org/10.1007/s10879-020-09477-1

Bratman, S. (1997). The health food eating disorder. *Yoga Journal*, 42–50. Retrieved from http://www.orthorexia.com.

Braun, T. D., Unick, J. L., Abrantes, A. M., Dalrymple, K., Conboy, L. A., Schifano, E., Park, C. L., & Lazar, S. W. (2022). Intuitive eating buffers the link between internalized weight stigma and body mass index in stressed adults. *Appetite*, 169, 105810. https://doi.org/10.1016/j.appet.2021.105810

Burgard, D. (2009). What is "Health At Every Size"? In E. Rothblum & S. Solovay (Eds.), *The fat studies reader* (pp. 41–53). New York: NYU Press.

Campos, P. (2004) *The obesity myth: Why America's obsession with weight is hazardous to your health.* New York: Gotham Books.

Cardoso, B.L.A., Paim, K., Catelan, R.F., Liebross, E. H. (2022). Minority stress and the inner critic/oppressive sociocultural schema mode among sexual and gender minorities. *Current Psychology* (2022). https://doi.org/10.1007/s12144-022-03086-y

Colditz, G. A., & Dart, H. (2018). Epidemiology and health and economic consequences of obesity. In T. A. Wadden & G. A. Bray (Eds.), *Handbook of Obesity Treatment* (pp. 3–23). The Guilford Press.

Dawson, D., Strodl, E., & Kitamura, H. (2022). Childhood maltreatment and disordered eating: The mediating role of emotion regulation. *Appetite*, 172, 105952. https://doi.org/10.1016/j.appet.2022.105952

deVos, K. (2018). The problem with body positivity. *The New York Times*. https://www.nytimes.com/2018/05/29/opinion/body-positivity-fat-acceptance.html

Dion, K., Berscheid, E., & Walster, E. (1972). What is beautiful is good. *Journal of Personality and Social Psychology*, 24(3), 285–290. https:// doi.org/10.1037/h003373

Framson, C., Kristal, A. R., Schenk, J. M., Littman, A. J., Zeliadt, S., & Benitez, D. (2009). Development and validation of the Mindful Eating Questionnaire. *Journal of the American Dietetic Association*, 109(8), 1439–1444. https://doi.org/10.1016/j.jada.2009.05.006

Freud, S. (1911). *Psycho-analytic notes on an autobiographical account of a case of paranoia (dementia paranoides).* S. E., 12, 3–82.

Gomez-Rubalcava, S., Stabbert, K., & Phelan, S. (2018). Behavioral treatment of obesity. In T. Wadden & G. A. Bray (Eds.), *Handbook of obesity treatment* (pp. 336–348). The Guilford Press.

Irby, S. (2023). Samantha Irby says it's OK to hate your body. *New York Times.* June 16, 2023.

Jensen, M. D., Ryan, D. H., Apovian, C. M., Ard, J. D., Comuzzie, A. G., Donato, K. A., Hu, F. B., Hubbard, V. S., Jakicic, J. M., Kushner, R. F., Loria, C. M., Millen, B. E., Nonas, C. A., Pi-Sunyer, F. X., Stevens, J., Stevens, V. J., Wadden, T. A., Wolfe, B.M., & Yanovski, S. Z. (2014). 2013 AHA/ACC/TOS guideline for the management of overweight and obesity in adults: A report of the American College of Cardiology/American Heart Association task force on practice guidelines and The Obesity Society. *Journal of the American College of Cardiology*, 63(25 Pt. B), 2985–3023. https://doi.org/10.1016/j.jacc.2013.11.004

Linardon, J., Tylka, T. L., & Fuller-Tyszkiewicz, M. (2021). Intuitive eating and its psychological correlates: A meta-analysis. *The International Journal of Eating Disorders*, 54(7), 1073–1098. https://doi.org/10.1002/eat.23509

Manasse, S. M., Lampe, E. W., Abber, S. R., Fitzpatrick, B., Srivastava, P., & Juarascio, A. S. (2023). Differentiating types of dietary restraint and their momentary relations with loss-of-control eating. *International Journal of Eating Disorders*. https://doi-org/10.1002/eat.23896

Merkin, D. (2010). My life in therapy. *New York Times Magazine.* August 8, 2010.

Merkin, D. (2014). I'm at fat camp. But I'm not here to make friends. *Elle.* October 16, 2014.

Miller, W. R., & Moyers, T. B. (2017). Motivational interviewing and the clinical science of Carl Rogers. *Journal of Consulting and Clinical Psychology*, 85(8), 757–766. https://doi.org/10.1037/ccp0000179

Mizock, L. (2015). The double stigma of obesity and serious mental illnesses: Promoting health and recovery. *Stigma and Health*, 1, 86–91. https://doi.org/10.1037/2376-6972.1.S.86

Meulman, M. A. (2019). Sizeism in therapy: Fat shaming in supervision. *Women & Therapy*, 42(1–2), 156–163. https://doi.org/10.1080/02703149.2018.1524072

Napolitano, M. A., & Foster, G. D. (2012). Non-dieting approaches to the treatment of obesity. In S. R. Akabas, S. A. Lederman, & B. J. Moore (Eds.). *Textbook of obesity: Biological, psychological, and cultural influences* (pp. 273–294). Ames, Iowa: John Wiley & Sons.

Novara, C., Pardini, S., Maggio, E., Mattioli, S., & Piasentin, S. (2022). Orthorexia Nervosa: Over concern or obsession about healthy food? *Eating and Weight Disorders*, 26(8), 2577–2588. https://doi-org/10.1007/s40519-021-01110-x

O'Hara, L., Ahmed, H., & Elashie, S. (2021). Evaluating the impact of a brief Health at Every Size®-informed health promotion activity on body positivity and internalized weight-based oppression. *Body Image*, 37, 225–237. https://doi.org/10.1016/j.bodyim.2021.02.006

Pearl, R. L., & Puhl, R. M. (2018). Weight bias internalization and health: A systematic review. *Obesity Reviews: An Official Journal of the International Association for the Study of Obesity*, 19(8), 1141–1163. https://doi.org/10.1111/obr.12701

Pickard, H. (2017). Responsibility without blame for addiction. *Neuroethics*, 10(1), 169–180. https://doi-org.adelphi.idm.oclc.org/10.1007/s12152-016-9295-2

Puhl, R., & Brownell, K. D. (2001). Bias, discrimination, and obesity. *Obesity Research*, 9(12), 788–805. https://doi.org/10.1038/oby.2001.108

Puhl, R. M., & Brownell, K. D. (2006). Confronting and coping with weight stigma: An investigation of overweight and obese adults. *Obesity (Silver Spring, Md.)*, 14(10), 1802–1815. https://doi.org/10.1038/oby.2006.208

Puhl, R. M., Himmelstein, M. S., & Pearl, R. L. (2020). Weight stigma as a psychosocial contributor to obesity. *The American Psychologist*, 75(2), 274–289. https://doi.org/10.1037/amp0000538

Robison, J. I. (1999). Weight, health and culture: Shifting the paradigm for alternative health care. *Alternative Health Practitioner*, 5(1), 45–69. https://doi.org/10.1177/153321019900500107

Rodney A. (2018). Pathogenic or health-promoting? How food is framed in healthy living media for women. *Social Science & Medicine*, 213, 37–44. https://doi.org/10.1016/j.socscimed.2018.07.034

Sainsbury, A., & Hay, P. (2014). Call for an urgent rethink of the 'health at every size' concept. *Journal of Eating Disorders*, 2, 8. https://doi.org/10.1186/2050-2974-2-8

Schnepper, R., Richard, A., Wilhelm, F. H., & Blechert, J. (2019). A combined mindfulness–prolonged chewing intervention reduces body weight, food craving, and emotional eating. *Journal of Consulting and Clinical Psychology*, 87(1), 106–111. https://doi-org/10.1037/ccp0000361

Schulte, E. M., Joyner, M. A., Potenza, M. N., Grilo, C. M., & Gearhardt, A. N. (2015). Current considerations regarding food addiction. *Current Psychiatry Reports*, 17(4), 563. https://doi.org/10.1007/s11920-015-0563-3

Tylka, T. L., & Kroon Van Diest, A. M. (2013). The Intuitive Eating Scale–2: Item refinement and psychometric evaluation with college women and men. *Journal of Counseling Psychology*, 60(1), 137–153. https://doi-org/10.1037/a0030893

Tylka, T. L., & Wood-Barcalow, N. L. (2015). What is and what is not positive body image? Conceptual foundations and construct definition. *Body Image*, 14, 118–129. https://doi.org/10.1016/j.bodyim.2015.04.001

Valenzuela, P. L., Santos-Lozano, A., Barrán, A. T., Fernández-Navarro, P., Castillo-García, A., Ruilope, L. M., Ríos Insua, D., Ordovas, J. M., Ley, V., & Lucia, A. (2022). Joint association of physical activity and body mass index with cardiovascular risk: A nationwide population-based cross-sectional study. *European Journal of Preventive Cardiology*, 29(2), e50–e52. https://doi.org/10.1093/eurjpc/zwaa151

Watkins, P. L., Clifford, D., & Souza, B. (2018). The Health At Every Size® paradigm: Promoting body positivity for all bodies. In E. A. Daniels, M. M. Gillen, & C. H. Markey (Eds.), *Body positive: Understanding and improving body image in science and practice* (pp. 160–187). Cambridge University Press. https://doi-org.adelphi.idm.oclc.org/10.1017/9781108297653.008

Wing, R. R., Lang, W., Wadden, T. A., Safford, M., Knowler, W. C., Bertoni, A. G., Hill, J. O., Brancati, F. L., Peters, A., Wagenknecht, L., & the Look AHEAD Research Group. (2011). Benefits of modest weight loss in improving cardiovascular risk factors in overweight and obese individuals with Type 2 diabetes. *Diabetes Care*, 34(7), 1481–1486. https://doi.org/10.2337/dc10-2415

Yu, J., Song, P., Zhang, Y., & Wei, Z. (2020). Effects of mindfulness-based intervention on the treatment of problematic eating behaviors: A systematic review. *Journal of Alternative and Complementary Medicine*, 26(8), 666–679. https://doi.org/10.1089/acm.2019.0163

Behavioral Weight Loss Intervention and the Consumer Culture

2

Whereas advocates of health at any size assume that body size is largely a function of a genetic predisposition towards an endomorphic body type (Rodney, 2018), behavioral psychology assumes that how much one eats is a learned behavior determined by environmental conditioning (Stuart, 1967). Overeating is therefore learned behavior that can be unlearned through cognitive-behavioral intervention. Cognitive-behavioral approaches to weight management assume that if certain learned eating habits result in excessive weight gain that unlearning those maladaptive eating habits and learning more constructive alternatives can result in weight loss. Since behaviorists believe that learned habits, bad as well as good, are sustained by environmental contingencies, the key to successful weight loss is the extent to which environmental contingencies can be controlled and altered in ways that reinforce and sustain eating in moderation rather than overeating.

In contrast to the advocates of health at any size, advocates of cognitive-behavioral approaches assume based on the available evidence that being overweight constitutes a significant medical risk to be reduced (Tronieri, 2021). Despite differences in attitudes towards dietary restrictions and weight loss, there are areas of overlap between the two approaches. Though the cognitive-behavioral approach believes that eating behavior is learned there is acknowledgement that different individuals due to differences in genetic predisposition will respond differently to similar food environments (Tronieri & Wadden, 2018). Some will have more difficulty managing portion size than others when calorie-dense foods are available in abundance.

In terms of treatment, both approaches believe that healthy eating means eating that is less triggered by external cues (i.e., conditioned responses) and/or by internal cues that do not constitute physiological hunger (i.e., emotional eating). From a cognitive perspective, both would advocate reduction of internalized weight stigma and fat phobia. Behavioral weight loss interventions, even when weight loss is maintained in the long-term, do not routinely result in fat-free bodies so fat acceptance becomes a necessity. Individuals trying to lose weight may become disappointed and demoralized if they do not achieve unrealistic weight loss goals and then regain the lost weight for lack of motivation to stick with the diet (Cooper & Fairburn, 2001). Both approaches view regular exercise as part of a healthful lifestyle.

Whereas advocates of health at every size and intuitive eating reject dietary restriction, the essence of cognitive-behavioral approaches to weight loss are to teach individuals trying to lose weight a wide repertoire of coping strategies to help high weight individuals stick to a reduced calorie diet and maintain a regular exercise routine. Behavioral coping strategies include: 1) setting realistic goals for weight loss, daily caloric intake, and exercise,

DOI: 10.4324/9781003402336-5

2) self-monitoring of weight (at least weekly), daily caloric intake, and one's exercise routine (i.e., calories burned), 3) finding ways to avoid external and internal cues that trigger overeating as well as learn to reduce reactivity to such cues, and 4) acquiring cognitive coping strategies that center on replacing maladaptive food beliefs (i.e., I went over my daily calorie count for the day so I may as well stop counting calories) with more adaptive ones (i.e., If I keep counting calories despite exceeding my daily budget it will curtail the extent to which I go above my daily calorie budget).

Outcome research has suggested that such approaches can result in 4–5% sustained weight loss (Gomez-Rubalcava, Stabbert, & Phelan, 2018). In addition, individuals who maintain their weight loss in the long-term appear to do so by applying various self-monitoring strategies (Santos, Vieira, Silva, Sardinha, & Teixeira, 2017). Thus, successful weight loss maintainers do not grant themselves 'unconditional permission to eat' but rather consistently apply a variety of coping strategies, of which enhanced self-monitoring is crucial. Despite the proven effectiveness of this approach, such lifelong self-monitoring for weight loss maintenance can be experienced as an arduous never-ending chore of which individuals may be ambivalent.

Sustaining such a structured approach in an unsupportive environment adds to the challenge. Such individuals may be subject to divergent weight management stigma (Romo, 2018). They might not be perceived as eating 'normally' or 'intuitively' like everybody else if they do things like keep a daily food log or weigh their food to maintain an accurate calorie count. That kind of self-monitoring could be perceived by others, even some clinicians, as pathologically rigid, perfectionistic, and obsessive (Novara, Pardini, Maggio, Mattioli, & Piasentin, 2022).

Learning Theory and Overeating

Behavioral psychology began with an insight into the psychology of eating with Pavlov's discovery of classical conditioning (Weir, 2012). Pavlov found that if he paired the sound of a bell with feeding his dogs that his dogs would begin to salivate at the sound of the bell. Likewise, human eating behavior can be a learned behavior, a conditioned response to a conditioned stimulus. The sight of food, the smell of food, the waking up ritual, the bedtime ritual, the work break ritual, the holiday ritual, the vacation ritual, the movie theater ritual, the work meeting ritual, the after work meet up with colleagues for drinks ritual, weekend brunch with friends, etc. can all become conditioned stimuli once they have been paired with eating. Those situations can become triggers of eating as a conditioned response regardless of whether one is hungry or not.

Weight gain occurs as more and more life situations are paired with eating and especially when paired with eating generous portions of highly palatable calorie-dense foods to make those everyday life situations more rewarding. Eating, whether one is hungry or not, is a natural reinforcer when food tastes good, smells good, and possesses a comforting stomach feel. Eating calorie-dense foods like ice cream is generally more pleasurable than eating low calorie foods like celery. Eating will be an intrinsically rewarding experience until the point in time that one is sick to one's stomach from overeating. Yet even without binge eating, one could gain weight by simply eating for pleasure throughout the day without ever getting to the point that eating becomes aversive by virtue of eating until one is sick to one's stomach.

The principles of operant conditioning suggest that behavior that is reinforced will increase in frequency (Epstein, Leddy, Temple, & Faith, 2007). Thus, eating tasty and filling calorie-dense food is inherently pleasurable (i.e., rewarding) so eating such food increases in frequency as do the associated behaviors like going to the places (i.e., the ice cream parlor) that offer the most rewarding culinary experiences. Eating highly palatable food increases in frequency when it increases positive emotions (i.e., positive reinforcement) or alleviates negative emotions (i.e., negative reinforcement).

The pleasure that food provides can make the good times even better, more celebratory like weddings, and make the bad times more tolerable (i.e., eating comfort food in response to loss). Behavioral weight loss interventions provide strategies to alter these enduring patterns of eating behavior and provide constructive alternatives. These strategies aim at altering the environmental contingencies that reinforce overeating calorie-dense food by replacing them with environmental contingencies that reward eating in a way that will help one achieve and maintain one's weight loss goals.

When behavioral weight loss interventions fail or obtain only modest results, it may not be that the strategies are misguided or that patients' lack motivation and willpower, or that their genetic predisposition is determinative. It may be because the environmental contingencies that reinforce overeating are so culturally entrenched that not even the most creative problem solving, like cue avoidance, is sufficient to alter environmental control of eating behavior.

Behavioral Weight Loss Intervention

The standard behavioral weight loss intervention is a structured time-limited treatment to be administered by clinicians specifically trained in this approach. The approach is a psychoeducational approach administered individually or in groups that is delivered sequentially in modules that address specific topics like barriers to weight loss or body image (Tronieri, 2021). Behavioral weight loss treatment can be more flexibly delivered and individually tailored. The research findings on this approach are based on highly structured time-limited treatments delivered at research centers.

Psychotherapy patients working with therapists who are not trained weight-loss specialists may resist referral to such structured time-limited symptom targeted behavioral programs for a variety of reasons:

1. They want to work on weight loss with their current therapist who is helping them with multiple interrelated issues and don't want to be referred to another clinician in addition to or instead of their current therapist.
2. A structured program has too many rules and is too demanding. They want a more flexible approach that is more individually tailored, like Noom, a commercial online behavioral weight loss program that patients can use in their own way at their own pace.
3. They may want something more programmatic to supplement their individual psychotherapy, but they prefer a more open-ended 12-step type program like Overeaters Anonymous or Food Addicts in Recovery Anonymous that provides guidelines and social support while letting them apply the 'steps' at their own pace without a timetable.

4. They would accept a referral to a nutritionist or dietician but want their current therapist to address the behavioral dimensions of their weight concerns without being the one who helps them with meal planning or who monitors their daily calorie count online.

Despite reservations about the need to enter an intensive behavioral weight loss program, high weight patients may still be open to and solicitous of their psychotherapists coaching them on the application of behavioral principles like goal setting, self-monitoring, and cognitive reappraisal in an individually tailored way that respects their readiness to apply such principles at their own time and pace. Ruptures to the therapeutic relationship are likely when patients feel pressured to adopt such behavioral principles prior to their readiness to do so. Ruptures can also occur when therapists fail to supply the coaching patients' desire.

Dialectical Behavior Therapy's recommendation for clinicians to try to maintain the dialectic between acceptance and change is especially pertinent when patients want to lose weight but aren't yet emotionally prepared to implement an approach that has a proven track record but seems unreasonably demanding (Robins, Zerubavel, Ivanoff, & Linehan, 2018). Psychotherapists may have to accept patients' unreadiness to adopt behavioral strategies for long periods of time or their willingness to adopt only certain strategies but not others. Thus, integrative psychotherapists could prepare themselves to coach patients on various behavioral strategies at the points in treatment when patients become open to using them.

Dan was an affluent retired gay man and frequently traveled to exotic places with his husband for long periods of time. His favorite activity was to enjoy the local cuisine by going out for breakfast, lunch, and dinner and experiencing a new taste treat. Dan had gained weight since retiring which had not been problematic to him until his doctor said he was prediabetic and needed to lose weight. Dan wanted to lose weight, but Dan didn't want to count calories, he didn't want to eat out less frequently while traveling, and he didn't want to abstain from calorie-dense foods. What he wanted was to learn to control his portion size without making any other lifestyle changes.

Dan wanted me to validate his weight loss strategy. He was annoyed and disappointed with me when I expressed some concern about whether his strategy would be sufficient without making other lifestyle changes as well like eating out less frequently. I said it's hard to learn self-restraint when you are constantly around temptation, and you want to eat what everybody else is eating. Nevertheless, I said that I wanted to support his self-determination to discover an approach that worked for him and my guesstimate of what might work for him could be erroneous.

Dan spent six months trying out his own approach and finally conceded that it wasn't working for him. We then started discussing what lifestyle changes he would be willing to make. We decided that when on vacation he wouldn't eat breakfast or lunch out. He would stay in places with a kitchenette where he could prepare his own food for those meals which he would keep low-calorie. While Dan was on vacation, I started getting texts from him with photographs of perfectly plated dishes consisting of local freshly caught simply prepared fish with a salad on the side. Dan had a flair for making attractive food plates when entertaining. Dan could live with this compromise as it still allowed him to taste the local cuisine without many dietary restrictions when he went out for dinner in the evenings. Ironically, once he got used to preparing his own low-calorie meals for breakfast and lunch, he started skipping some evening meals out preferring to eat a lighter meal that he prepared himself.

Goal Setting

Behavioral weight loss strategies involve setting realistic goals for weight loss, daily calorie consumption, and regular exercise. Realistic goal setting is not simply about establishing the endpoint one hopes to reach but also about how quickly one can realistically aspire to arrive at the destination. The question, though, is whether rapid substantial weight loss may be as sustainable as slow incremental weight loss. Some initial research suggests that it might be.

Standard behavioral weight loss intervention recommends low-calorie diets of 1200 to 1500 calories a day for individuals below 250 pounds and diets of 1500 to 1800 calories a day for individuals above 250 pounds (Wadden et al, 2020). Very low-calorie diets of fewer than 800 calories per day with high protein to prevent muscle loss achieve the most rapid weight loss, 15–25% in four months, but with weight regain do not do better or worse than the daily calorie budget recommended in standard behavioral weight loss intervention (Tsai & Wadden, 2006). Research has discovered that slow and steady does not necessarily win the race (Nackers, Ross, & Perri, 2010) and more recently that the rapidity of the initial weight loss did not predict percentage of weight regain (Vink, Roumans, Arkenbosch, Mariman, & van Baak, 2016).

Nevertheless, it was found that long-term weight loss maintainers were able to maintain their weight loss on an average of 2199 calories per day (Santos, Vieira, Silva, Sardinha, & Teixeira, 2017). It has yet to be thoroughly researched the extent to which higher daily calorie budgets that are still significantly below patients' daily calorie count at their highest weight might still result in sustainable weight loss among patients who refuse to try the low and very low-calorie diets that have been better studied. Some patients who refuse adoption of low or very low-calorie diets might be more open to adopting more average or above average calorie diets that would still be significantly below their current daily calorie count.

Weight loss applications that patients can download onto their smart phones can help patients calculate the daily calorie budget for losing different amounts of weight per week or for weight maintenance given their current weight, height, gender, and weight loss goal. Thus, psychotherapy patients could exercise a high degree of autonomy in selecting a target weight loss goal, determining the daily calorie allowance based upon how quickly they aspire to achieve that goal, and adjusting those goals through a process of trial and error to discover what is most sustainable. Patients who don't stick to low or very low-calorie diets can see if they have better success with average or above average calorie diets.

A self-determination approach to psychotherapy suggests that therapist support of client's autonomy is associated with positive outcomes to treatment (Ryan & Deci, 2008). Individuals high in self-determination have better diet quality than those low on that dimension (Carbonneau et al., 2021). In addition, autonomy support has been associated with weight loss success (Gorin, Powers, Koestner, Wing, & Raynor, 2014).

The advocates of behavioral weight loss treatment assume that a realistic weight loss goal is what has been achievable on average through that specific approach and to date there are no other evidence-based approaches that yield comparable or better results. Thus, a realistic weight loss goal from this perspective would be 10% initial weight loss but then maintaining 5% in the long-term (Gomez-Rubalcava, Stabbert, & Phelan, 2018). Patients can set themselves up for disappointment if they set unrealistic weight loss goals. Feeling demoralized they might not be motivated to continue deploying the behavioral strategies that are sustaining the 5% long-term weight loss.

It might not be so easy to determine in advance what is a realistically attainable goal for an individual patient. Supporting patients' self-determination may mean providing them the time, space, and social support to determine what are realistic weight loss goals through trial and error. That doesn't mean the therapist can't offer an opinion as to what are overly ambitious or insufficiently ambitious goals. It means that patients' autonomous decision making is supported after some discussion. Goal consensus doesn't have to be agreeing on a particular target weight in advance but rather agreeing to a process of discovering a realistic weight loss goal through a process of trial and error.

Al Sharpton, the civil rights activist, weighed 305 pounds and sustained a weight loss of 176 pounds (Olya, 2022). At five-feet-ten-inches and 129 pounds some might view Sharpton as underweight for his height and as possessing an eating disorder. Sharpton maintains his weight by just eating salads with balsamic vinaigrette, a few slices of whole wheat bread, green vegetables juices, fish, and hard-boiled eggs. He walks for 20 to 30 minutes five days a week on a treadmill. He attributes his success to self-determination but also says he no longer misses the foods he no longer eats like fried chicken. Not everyone will have that level of self-determination, can tolerate such a low-calorie diet, or will reconcile themselves to such a 'boring' diet. Nevertheless, individual cases such as these are suggestive of some general principles that might have wider applicability for those with more modest weight loss goals.

Sharpton's observation that he no longer craves the foods he no longer eats might have some generalizability but has yet to be adequately studied. Recovery from food addiction has been thought to require abstention from trigger foods like sugar and white flour (Blumenthal, DuPont, & Gold, 2012). The not adequately researched assumption is that cravings gradually subside for calorie-dense foods one no longer eats once an initial period has been surmounted of intensified craving induced by withdrawal.

Sharpton was high in self-reported self-determination. Effective psychotherapy can increase patients' self-determination by consistently supporting it (Ryan & Deci, 2008) and thereby increase the probability that patients can sustain certain dietary restrictions if they so choose (Gorin, Powers, Koestner, Wing, & Raynor, 2014). Possibly high self-determination is required only to tolerate withdrawal symptoms without relapsing after which less self-determination is required if the cravings subside for what one no longer eats. High levels of social support during the withdrawal phase could compensate for low self-determination sufficiently to endure withdrawal symptoms without relapsing.

Self-Monitoring Strategies

Behavioral weight loss interventions recommend self-monitoring weight at least weekly and daily calorie count through a food log that keeps track of the portion size of the various foods consumed during the day (Tronieri, 2021). Research suggests that individuals regularly underestimate their daily caloric intake (Lichtman et al., 1992). They may mistakenly believe they are following the diet but not losing any weight when their calorie count is not as low as they think it is. Consequently, it is recommended that the calorie count be as accurate as possible. That can be accomplished by eating prepared meals with a predetermined calorie count or by measuring portion size as precisely as possible. Review of the daily food log allows for adjusting the diet by discovering the places during the day where calorie-dense foods can be replaced with lower calorie foods, or their portion size reduced.

The available evidence suggests that individuals who engage in such self-monitoring are more successful with dieting than those that don't (Santos, Vieira, Silva, Sardinha, & Teixeira, 2017). Nevertheless, many high weight individuals possess a strong aversion to counting calories and refuse to do it. They may complain that it's too time consuming. Yet with the advent of weight loss applications on one's smart phone counting calories has been made much easier and quicker. There may be a perception that counting calories is what individuals with eating disorders do (Obeid, Hallit, Akel, & Brytek-Matera, 2022) or a belief that reducing the daily calorie count doesn't necessarily result in weight loss (Benton & Young, 2017).

Motivated reasoning (Gold, 2013) can lead to believing what one wishes was true for self-serving reasons. High weight individuals may not wish to see how far they exceed the permissible daily calorie allowance for achieving their weight loss goals. It's upsetting to see that they consume 3000 calories per day when they can only eat 2000 calories a day to achieve their weight loss goals. They must then figure out where to make painful cuts in their daily consumption. Some individuals will count calories on 'good' days but won't cut calories on 'bad' days. Or they count calories on what starts out to be a 'good' day but stop counting calories at the point they see they will go over their daily calorie budget and don't want to track how far they will exceed their calorie budget by the end of the day.

High weight patients may need help looking at 'bad' numbers, be it their daily calorie count or their weight, without judgment and with self-compassion when the numbers are perceived as 'bad'. Patients may not be able utilize self-monitoring as a coping strategy until they can tolerate and then down-regulate the emotional distress triggered by 'bad' numbers. The challenge is to achieve a belief in 'responsibility without blame' (Pickard, 2017).

Self-monitoring may work when patients are ready to be honest with themselves and hold themselves accountable when failing to comply with a particular weight loss or weight maintenance strategy. Such honesty and accountability will be avoided when facing 'bad numbers' is just too upsetting and makes them feel too badly about themselves. Therapists who believe in counting calories may have to learn to patiently wait until patients are prepared to tolerate the distress of 'bad' numbers. Ruptures to the therapeutic relationship will arise if therapists are perceived as pressing on the benefits of counting calories in a way that is felt to undermine patients' self-determination and autonomy.

Kamala was an immigrant from India whose doctor told her she needed to lose weight because she was prediabetic. Her diet was high in fat from ghee, a type of clarified butter often utilized in Indian cooking and high in white rice, potatoes, and white flour used to make various Indian breads. She didn't binge eat but if she just ate her traditional Indian cuisine until she was reasonably full, she ended up overweight and now prediabetic. The therapist suggested that if she counted calories, she could lose weight by simply reducing the portion size of her favorite foods sufficiently to stay within her daily calorie budget. Kamala said that counting calories would drive her crazy and she knew she would be hungry all the time if she reduced her portion size.

Kamala decided that she didn't need to lose a lot of weight. She didn't mind her body size nor did her husband with whom she had a good sex life. She just wanted to lose enough weight so that her blood sugar would go back into the normal range. Kamala decided that since she did all the home cooking, she could reduce the fat content of all the dishes and in addition she would only use whole grain from now on, either brown rice or whole wheat flour, or use chickpeas instead of potatoes substantially increasing the fiber content of her diet.

Kamala lost about ten pounds using this approach. It didn't change her obese BMI, but her blood glucose returned to the normal range without medication. Kamala found a way to lose weight her way, had modest weight loss goals, and was able to achieve her weight loss goal without having to count calories or restrict her portion size. A shift in the macronutrient composition of her food that made it less calorie-dense but increased the fiber content, made the portion sizes she was used to eating sufficiently filling that she felt no need to increase the portion size to compensate for the lost calories.

Problem Solving

Behavior chain analysis is the procedure that behaviorists utilize to track the environmental contingencies that control eating behavior (Gomez-Rubalcava, Stabbert, & Phelan, 2018). These contingencies cue or trigger eating behavior. Eating behavior can be changed by teaching patients to either avoid those triggers entirely or to become less reactive to those triggers if such triggers prove unavoidable. The presence and ready availability of tasty and filling calorie-dense food is a trigger to eating such foods. If it looks good and smells good, one might begin salivating at the sight or even at the very thought of eating such foods. In such situations eating is a conditioned response regardless of how hungry one is. Nevertheless, the hungrier one is the more powerful will be one's response to the sight, smell, and taste of calorie-dense food as food will carry a higher reward value when self-reported hunger is high (Banica, Allison, Racine, Foti, & Weinberg, 2023). The power to resist temptation declines as hunger increases. Willpower is a limited resource that can rapidly decline with cognitive load or other forms of stress (Metcalfe & Mischel, 1999).

Social and emotional circumstances can also serve as triggers to eating calorie-dense food. Most social eating centers on eating calorie-dense foods as consumption of tasty and filling foods cements social bonds (i.e., bagels and donuts at work meetings, after work drinks with nachos with colleagues, romantic dinners at French bistros eating foie gras, pizza, and cake at children's birthday parties, etc.). To avoid such social situations entirely or to attend such events but not eat what everybody else is eating can result in feelings of social marginalization and alienation. Feelings of loneliness, alienation, and depression in response to social marginalization might then trigger the desire to eat comfort food to make oneself feel better. Consequently, creative problem solving is required to find ways to avoid or decrease reactivity to the innumerable social and solitary situations that trigger overeating calorie-dense foods when one is not that hungry and made only worse when one is hungry.

General coping strategies would be to not keep calorie-dense foods at home to avoid temptation, to eat out less frequently, to order salads and lean sources of protein when eating out, to bring one's own food to social situations in which low calorie food would not be served, and to not let oneself get too hungry prior to being in the presence of tempting calorie-dense food. Alternatives to emotional eating in response to negative emotional cues would be to use alternative forms of emotion regulation and stress management like exercise, meditation, distraction techniques, and social support from others. And if one must eat something to make oneself feel better then eat a low-calorie food instead of a high calorie food for comfort. In terms of social eating to make the good times even better one might try having just a small taste of what everybody else is eating but still fill up on the lower calorie alternatives or if one is abstaining just pretend to eat what everybody else is eating. Or just tell others that one is on a special diet and hope they respect one's dietary restrictions without trying to get one to relax those restrictions for a special occasion.

Psychotherapy patients may acknowledge that in general that these are eminently reasonable and practical coping strategies but might argue that in their unique circumstances that these are not viable solutions. They must keep junk food at home because their children eat those foods, and it wouldn't be fair to impose one's own dietary restrictions on them. One doesn't want to tell work colleagues about one's dietary restrictions because that's private and none of their business. They can't eat out less because they travel for work and must attend frequent business lunches and dinners. They don't have the time to prepare their own healthy food on a regular basis or the prepared foods with predetermined calorie counts are too expensive or too bland.

Are these excuses or rationalizations to avoid responsibility for learning how to manage the cues that trigger overeating or perhaps legitimate reasons that such coping strategies are misguided in certain circumstances? Ruptures to the therapeutic relationship are likely when patients and therapists begin debating the viability of applying these coping strategies in patients' unique circumstances. Therapists can certainly try to use creative problem solving to find ways of applying these coping strategies to patients' unique circumstances that patients might not think of on their own. Yet the therapeutic relationship becomes one-sided, less than fully collaborative, if therapists are doing all the creative problem solving and patients become the perennially skeptical audience who remain unconvinced and unwilling to give therapists' recommendations a trial run to see how it goes. Therapists can only go so far in campaigning for the applicability of a particular coping strategy in patients' unique circumstances without undermining patients' autonomous self-determination. Patients may become defensive in the face of threats to their autonomous self-determination.

Molly, a married social worker, had made good progress keeping off 20 pounds utilizing self-monitoring and the strategies recommended for managing her triggers. Then Molly became pregnant and decided that if she was eating for two, she would need to relax her dietary restrictions. By the time it came to give birth Molly realized she had gained considerably more weight than necessitated by her pregnancy and her fat phobia kicked in. Molly planned to breast feed for one year and didn't think she would be able to resume her old diet until she was finished breast feeding. She suffered internalized weight stigma even though her husband told her she was beautiful and was always eager for sexual intimacy. In addition, her overweight father who she looked like suffered diabetes and had to have quadruple heart bypass surgery. Molly didn't want to follow in her father's footsteps.

Whenever we contemplated the possibility of resuming dieting even in some attenuated form, Molly seemed close to bursting into tears. It was all too overwhelming as a working mother who had too much to juggle despite her husband's help. Instead, we worked on fat acceptance, despite her skepticism, with the working assumption that at a future point when her childcare responsibilities were reduced, she would reinstitute her prior dietary approach in sufficient time to avert her father's medical fate. And that is what she ultimately did.

Cognitive Strategies

Behavioral weight loss interventions also attempt to alter maladaptive beliefs that may contribute to overeating. The idea is that overweight individuals possess beliefs that justify or rationalize their maladaptive eating habits. Cognitive reappraisal can be utilized to replace maladaptive dietary beliefs with more adaptive ones that would support implementing and sticking with the behavioral weight loss strategy. Part of behavioral weight loss intervention is nutritional counseling (Tronieri, 2021) on the presumption that some individuals might not appreciate the calorie density of different foods they eat, the macronutrient composition of the foods they eat (i.e., carbohydrates, fat, protein, fiber, degree of food processing, added sugar, etc.), or the importance of monitoring the calories consumed and expended over the course of the day in order to remain within a certain daily calorie allowance for one's height. Such knowledge contributes to 'mindful eating' as opposed to 'mindless' eating (Framson, Kristal, Schenk, Littman, Zeliadt, & Benitez, 2009).

A greater clinical challenge for cognitive reappraisal arises when overweight individuals know how they 'should' eat (i.e., they are well informed about nutrition) but they don't eat the way they know they should eat and then castigate themselves after the fact. Such individuals might obtain a low score on an intuitive eating scale (Tylka & Kroon Van Diest, 2013) because they are quite cognizant of what are so-called 'good' foods (i.e., low calorie, low processed carbohydrate, low saturated fat, high fiber) and 'bad' foods (i.e., calorie-dense, high processed carbohydrates like sugar, high fructose corn syrup, white flour, high saturated fat, low fiber). Nevertheless, they eat the bad foods anyway and then become upset with themselves for so doing and then failing to lose weight. Part of cognitive reappraisal in such situations is to discover the automatic maladaptive beliefs that are activated in the face of temptation that maintain this self-defeating pattern. The clinical challenge is helping patients identify these maladaptive beliefs as they arise in the face of temptation and replace them with the more constructive alternatives.

Scales have been developed that capture the maladaptive beliefs that are associated with difficulties losing weight. The *Irrational Food Belief Scale* (Osberg, Poland, Aguayo, & MacDougall, 2008) possesses four major dimensions: 1) that food can help manage dysfunctional emotions such as anxiety and depression, 2) that food can substitute for things missing in one's life such as support, relationships, sex, 3) that it is impossible to live without certain favored foods, 4) that food choice is unrelated to health outcomes (p. 26)

The *Irrational Food Beliefs Scale* includes items such as 'I can't possibly live without my favorite food'. An irrational food belief is a belief that ignores or dismisses substantial evidence to the contrary. To believe that one couldn't possibly live without one's favorite foods overlooks the fact that many individuals do learn to live without if they believe they must; be it diabetics who give up added sugar, the gluten-intolerant who give up wheat products with gluten, those with gastric reflux who give up fried foods, or those with arteriosclerosis who give up saturated fats.

The *Compensatory Health Beliefs Scale* (Knäuper, Rabiau, Cohen, & Patriciu, 2004) assesses beliefs to the effect that that the negative effects of an unhealthy behavior can be compensated for and/or neutralized by engaging in a healthy behavior. It includes items such as: 'Eating dessert can be made up for by skipping the main dish'. Individuals that score high on such a scale may know how they 'should' eat to lose weight. Yet they make a conscious choice to violate certain dietary principles believing that if they engage in a compensatory strategy there is no harm in the violation. For example, individuals might justify overeating today because tomorrow they will eat an even lower calorie diet than they otherwise would to compensate. Those compensatory strategies may seem sensible at the time, but they fail when there is lack of follow-through. Individuals may overestimate their capacity to follow-through on the compensatory strategy.

Maladaptive cognitions can be 'state dependent cognitions' (Nettle, 2019) that reflect motivated reasoning (Gold, 2013). In calm and contemplative frames of mind as might arise during a psychotherapy session one knows how one should eat and it seems like the sensible thing to do. There are no external or internal cues that arouse hunger in the face of temptation. The presence of external or internal cues that arouse hunger in the face of temptation may alter one's mindset. It may activate maladaptive cognitions that would justify ignoring or dismissing the dietary principles that made perfect sense during more contemplative frames of mind unperturbed by hunger.

Psychotherapy for weight loss may require helping patients cultivate high levels of self-reflective awareness and metacognitive processing (Woolrich, Cooper, & Turner, 2008) in high arousal moments to counter maladaptive beliefs with more adaptive beliefs. Thinking quickly on one's feet is not easy when external or internal cues arouse not only hunger but also the maladaptive cognitions that justify ignoring sensible dietary principles in the face of temptation.

Steven's BMI bordered on morbid obesity. He had a stressful job and always had to eat on the run. Fast food was always the most convenient choice. He hoped he would eventually lose weight because he walked a lot on his job and hoped to reduce snacking in between meals or at least eat healthier snacks. Steven was venting his frustration that he had not lost any weight yet despite thinking he was doing a good job implementing his weight loss strategy. Trying to engage him in problem solving this dieting dilemma, I suggested that perhaps he could bring fruit to work as a snack. That might make it less likely that he would snack on readily available but calorie-dense energy bars that he usually snacked on.

Steven snapped at me contemptuously: 'Everyone knows that fruit has a lot of sugar'. I countered that it is true that all the calorie in fruit comes from sugar but that the calories in a piece of fruit, like an apple, were lower than an energy bar. In addition, because the sugar is embedded in a lot of fiber that most fruits were low on the glycemic index so wouldn't spike his blood sugar. Steven looked annoyed that I made a point that he already knew was valid when he snapped at me as though I had shamed him for being ignorant of the obvious. He changed the topic. He wasn't ready to concede the point. Steven wasn't prepared to admit that the underlying reason he didn't want to snack on fruit even if he knew it was a healthier choice was because he didn't think it would be as filling as his preferred but more calorie-dense snack.

I didn't press further on this touchy issue out of respect for his self-determination. I knew he would only lash out in anger if I belabored the issue rather than let it drop. I had at least gotten him to briefly consider an alternative perspective at a moment of high emotional arousal. Being able to engage in metacognition in states of high emotional arousal is a skill that is only gradually acquired.

The Consumer Culture and Overconsumption

Weight control theorists have concluded that the 'toxic environment' in which individuals live in modern societies is a major barrier to individuals' weight control efforts (Wadden, Brownell, & Foster, 2002). Overeating and weight gain is difficult to avoid when there is an abundance of affordable foods that are calorie-dense, high in processed carbohydrates, and high in fat and when modern conveniences, like cars, discourage physical activity, like walking. The food industry uses food science to discover the 'bliss point' of various processed foods to increase sales, advertising is utilized to market foods that deliver the greatest 'bliss', and such marketing is often directed at children at an early age to get them 'hooked' on their products (Moss, 2014). Consequently, successfully applying behavioral weight loss strategies is challenging in obesogenic environments (King, 2013).

References

Banica, I., Allison, G., Racine, S. E., Foti, D., & Weinberg, A. (2023). All the Pringle ladies: Neural and behavioral responses to high-calorie food rewards in young adult women. *Psychophysiology*, 60(3), e14188. https://doi.org/10.1111/psyp.14188

Benton, D., & Young, H. A. (2017). Reducing calorie intake may not help you lose body weight. *Perspectives on Psychological Science: A Journal of the Association for Psychological Science*, 12(5), 703–714. https://doi.org/10.1177/1745691617690878

Blumenthal, K., DuPont, R. L., & Gold, M. S. (2012). Treatment of alcohol and drug dependence in 2011 and relevance to food addiction. In K. D. Brownell & M. S. Gold, *Food and addiction: A comprehensive handbook* (pp. 318–328). Oxford University Press. https://doiorg/10.1093/med:psych/9780199738168.003.0048

Carbonneau, E., Pelletier, L., Bégin, C., Lamarche, B., Bélanger, M., Provencher, V., Desroches, S., Robitaille, J., Vohl, M. C., Couillard, C., Bouchard, L., Houle, J., Langlois, M. F., Rabasa-Lhoret, R., Corneau, L., & Lemieux, S. (2021). Individuals with self-determined motivation for eating have better overall diet quality: Results from the PREDISE study. *Appetite*, 165, 105426. https://doi.org/10.1016/j.appet.2021.105426

Cooper, Z., & Fairburn, C. G. (2001). A new cognitive behavioural approach to the treatment of obesity. *Behaviour Research and Therapy*, 39(5), 499–511.

Epstein, L. H., Leddy, J. J., Temple, J. L., & Faith, M. S. (2007). Food reinforcement and eating: A multilevel analysis. *Psychological Bulletin*, 133(5), 884–906. https://doi.org/10.1037/0033-2909.133.5.884

Framson, C., Kristal, A. R., Schenk, J. M., Littman, A. J., Zeliadt, S., & Benitez, D. (2009). Development and validation of the Mindful Eating Questionnaire. *Journal of the American Dietetic Association*, 109(8), 1439–1444. https://doi.org/10.1016/j.jada.2009.05.006

Gold, R. S. (2013). Perceived likelihood of experiencing a desirable versus undesirable outcome. *Psychological Reports*, 113(2), 525–527. https://doi.org/10.2466/04.07.PR0.113x18z5

Gomez-Rubalcava, S., Stabbert, K., & Phelan, S. (2018). Behavioral treatment of obesity. In T. Wadden & G. A. Bray (Eds.), *Handbook of obesity treatment* (pp. 336–348). The Guilford Press.

Gorin, A. A., Powers, T. A., Koestner, R., Wing, R. R., & Raynor, H. A. (2014). Autonomy support, self-regulation, and weight loss. *Health Psychology*, 33(4), 332–339. https://doi-org/10.1037/a0032586

King B. M. (2013). The modern obesity epidemic, ancestral hunter-gatherers, and the sensory/reward control of food intake. *The American Psychologist*, 68(2), 88–96. https://doi.org/10.1037/a0030684

Knäuper, B., Rabiau, M., Cohen, O., & Patriciu, N. (2004). Compensatory health beliefs: Scale development and psychometric properties. *Psychology & Health*, 19(5), 607–624, https://doi.org/10.1080/0887044042000196737

Lichtman, S. W., Pisarska, K., Berman, E. R., Pestone, M., Dowling, H., Offenbacher, E., Weisel, H., Heshka, S., Matthews, D. E., & Heymsfield, S. B. (1992). Discrepancy between self-reported and actual caloric intake and exercise in obese subjects. *The New England Journal of Medicine*, 327(27), 1893–1898. https://doi.org/10.1056/NEJM199212313272701

Metcalfe, J., & Mischel, W. (1999). A hot/cool-system analysis of delay of gratification: Dynamics of willpower. *Psychological Review*, 106(1), 3–19. https://doi.org/10.1037/0033-295X.106.1.3

Moss, M. (2014). *Salt sugar fat: How the food giants hooked us*. New York: Random House.

Nackers, L. M., Ross, K. M., & Perri, M. G. (2010). The association between rate of initial weight loss and long-term success in obesity treatment: Does slow and steady win the race? *International Journal of Behavioral Medicine*, 17(3), 161–167. https://doi.org/10.1007/s12529-010-9092-y

Nettle D. (2019). State-dependent cognition and its relevance to cultural evolution. *Behavioural Processes*, 161, 101–107. https://doi.org/10.1016/j.beproc.2018.01.018

Novara, C., Pardini, S., Maggio, E., Mattioli, S., & Piasentin, S. (2022). Orthorexia Nervosa: Over concern or obsession about healthy food? *Eating and Weight Disorders*, 26(8), 2577–2588. https://doi-org/10.1007/s40519-021-01110-x

Obeid, S., Hallit, S., Akel, M., & Brytek-Matera, A. (2022). Orthorexia nervosa and its association with alexithymia, emotion dysregulation and disordered eating attitudes among Lebanese adults. *Eating and Weight Disorders*, 26(8), 2607–2616. https://doi-org/10.1007/s40519-021-01112-9

Olya, G. (2022) How Al Sharpton dropped an amazing 176 lbs. *People*. August 17, 2022.

Osberg, T. M., Poland, D., Aguayo, G., & MacDougall, S. (2008). The Irrational Food Beliefs Scale: Development and validation. *Eating Behaviors*, 9(1), 25–40. https://doi.org/10.1016/j.eatbeh.2007.02.001

Pickard, H. (2017). Responsibility without blame for addiction. *Neuroethics*, 10(1), 169–180. https://doi-org.adelphi.idm.oclc.org/10.1007/s12152-016-9295-2

Robins, C. J., Zerubavel, N., Ivanoff, A. M., & Linehan, M. M. (2018). Dialectical behavior therapy. In W. J. Livesley & R. Larstone (Eds.), *Handbook of personality disorders: Theory, research, and treatment* (pp. 527–540). The Guilford Press

Rodney A. (2018). Pathogenic or health-promoting? How food is framed in healthy living media for women. *Social Science & Medicine* (1982), 213, 37–44. https://doi.org/10.1016/j.socscimed.2018.07.034

Romo L. K. (2018). An examination of how people who have lost weight communicatively negotiate interpersonal challenges to weight management. *Health Communication*, 33(4), 469–477. https://doi.org/10.1080/10410236.2016.1278497

Ryan, R. M., & Deci, E. L. (2008). A self-determination theory approach to psychotherapy: The motivational basis for effective change. *Canadian Psychology / Psychologie canadienne*, 49(3), 186–193. https://doi.org/10.1037/a0012753

Santos, I., Vieira, P. N., Silva, M. N., Sardinha, L. B., & Teixeira, P. J. (2017). Weight control behaviors of highly successful weight loss maintainers: The Portuguese Weight Control Registry. *Journal of Behavioral Medicine*, 40(2), 366–371. https://doi.org/10.1007/s10865-016-9786-y

Stuart, R. B. (1967). Behavioral control of overeating. *Behaviour Research and Therapy*, 5(4), 357–365. https://doi.org/10.1016/0005-7967(67)90027-7

Tronieri, J. S. (2021). Cognitive and behavioral treatments for obesity. In A. Wenzel (Ed.), *Handbook of cognitive behavioral therapy: Applications* (pp. 453–476). American Psychological Association. https://doi-org/10.1037/0000219-014

Tronieri, J. S., & Wadden, T. A. (2018). Behavioral assessment of patients with obesity. In T. A. Wadden & G. A. Bray (Eds.), *Handbook of obesity treatment* (pp. 253–280). The Guilford Press.

Tsai, A. G., & Wadden, T. A. (2006). The evolution of very-low-calorie diets: An update and meta-analysis. *Obesity*, 14(8), 1283–1293. https://doi.org/10.1038/oby.2006.146

Tylka, T. L., & Kroon Van Diest, A. M. (2013). The Intuitive Eating Scale–2: Item refinement and psychometric evaluation with college women and men. *Journal of Counseling Psychology*, 60(1), 137–153. https://doi-org/10.1037/a0030893

Vink, R. G., Roumans, N. J., Arkenbosch, L. A., Mariman, E. C., & van Baak, M. A. (2016). The effect of rate of weight loss on long-term weight regain in adults with overweight and obesity. *Obesity (Silver Spring, Md.)*, 24(2), 321–327. https://doi.org/10.1002/oby.21346

Wadden, T. A., Brownell, K. D., & Foster, G. D. (2002). Obesity: Responding to the global epidemic. *Journal of Consulting and Clinical Psychology*, 70(3), 510–525. https://doi.org/10.1037//0022-006x.70.3.510

Wadden, T. A., Tronieri, J. S., & Butryn, M. L. (2020). Lifestyle modification approaches for the treatment of obesity in adults. *American Psychologist*, 75(2), 235–251. https://doi.org/10.1037/amp0000517

Weir, K. (2012). Overcoming temptation. *Monitor on Psychology*, 43(9), 52–55. https://doi-org.adelphi.idm.oclc.org/10.1037/e652132012-014

Woolrich, R. A., Cooper, M. J., & Turner, H. M. (2008). Metacognition in patients with anorexia nervosa, dieting and non-dieting women: A preliminary study. *European Eating Disorders Review: The Journal of the Eating Disorders Association*, 16(1), 11–20. https://doi.org/10.1002/erv.802

When Food is Love and Food Choice is Autonomy

The Relational Dynamics of Emotional Eating

3

Chapters 1 and 2 examined the relational dimension of weight management from the cultural perspective. The culture expects us to be able to eat calorie-dense food in moderation though it constantly tempts us with such 'fattening' food by making it so readily available. We are subject to weight stigma if we gain weight in such a food rich environment. We are subject to divergent weight management stigma if we then try to lose weight and maintain our weight loss by subjecting ourselves to dietary restrictions that others find objectionable. Those cultural prejudices can play out in the therapeutic situation when patients feel shamed by therapists for either their weight or their eating habits if their eating habits strike their therapists as either excessively self-indulgent or excessively self-denying.

Another and equally important relational dimension of weight management derives from formative developmental experiences in relation to food beginning in the first years of life. Infants and toddlers may have little conception of what the culture or their parents for that matter deem too fat or too thin. The self-conscious emotions like shame, guilt, and embarrassment begin to emerge in the second year of life as children acquire a reflective self (Lewis & Minar, 2022). Also, in the second year of life children learn to recognize themselves in the mirror, acquire an image of their own body, and can begin to make social comparisons with others (Meltzoff, 1990). These developmental achievements set the stage for children becoming self-conscious about their bodies. At that point being criticized, teased, or ostracized for one's body appearance can leave lasting emotional scars and such teasing appears to peak during middle childhood (Guardabassi & Tomasetto, 2022).

Infants and toddlers know if they are hungry or sated and what tastes good or bad. There appears to be an innate preference for sweet and salty tastes that makes young children vulnerable to preferring nutrient poor but highly palatable foods (Mennella, Forestell, Ventura, & Fisher, 2020). Infants and toddlers may refuse to eat or spit out food when they aren't hungry, when it tastes bad, or when it is unfamiliar as food neophobia may hinder the acceptance of healthy foods (Momin, Hughes, Elias, Papaioannou, Phan, Vides, & Wood, 2018). As children acquire food preferences they may try to hold out for their preferred foods, like dessert, rather than consume the healthier option currently offered, like fruits and vegetables, or may refuse to eat healthier options entirely (Volkert, Patel, & Peterson, 2016). Considerable research has been conducted on the individual and social factors that contribute to healthy or unhealthy eating habits among children (Cook-Cottone, Tribole, & Tylka, 2013).

DOI: 10.4324/9781003402336-6

During earliest childhood, children's relationship with their parents revolves around children's dependence on their parents for basic human needs like food, comfort, protection, companionship, and entertainment. Over the course of childhood development children transition from relative dependence to relative independence and autonomy (Boykin, McElhaney, & Allen, 2012). Being fed becomes equated with being loved (Hamburg, Finkenauer, & Schuengel, 2014) and how well loved you are becomes equated with how well fed you are. From the child's egocentric perspective, it seems more loving to be fed macaroni and cheese than carrot sticks or fed chocolate milk rather than plain milk given their innate food preference for sweet and salty. The more calorie dense the food (i.e., the more it's tasty and filling to a child's palette) the greater the love. Children don't know or care about what's healthy, what's fattening, or what will give them cavities until they acquire such health beliefs with cognitive development and socialization to a culture's food beliefs.

Being able to feed oneself and make one's own independent food choices becomes equated with autonomy (Bassett, Chapman, & Beagan, 2008) How autonomous one is becomes equated with how well one is able to feed oneself. Throughout the lifespan including old age, being free to choose to eat what one wants, how much one wants, and when one wants constitutes an assertion of autonomous self-determination (Wang, Everett, Brunero, Northall, Villarosa, & Salamonson, 2020). Thus, in the first years of life food becomes associated with two fundamental relational issues; love (i.e., how much people care about your welfare) and autonomy (i.e., how much people respect your preferences, choices, and individuality).

Self-determination theory suggests the humans have basic human needs for competence, autonomy, and relatedness (Ryan & Deci, 2008). Being loved by significant others who respect one's autonomy fosters secure attachment (Anderson, 2019). From an early age food becomes implicated in the dialectical tension between maintaining loving connections while asserting autonomous self-determination. Parents become aware of infants' strivings for autonomous self-determination when babies refuse to eat by turning their heads away when parents are determined to feed them or when children are fussy about their food preferences (Volkert, Patel, & Peterson, 2016).

Later in life the dialectical tension between loving connection/social conformity and autonomous self-determination plays out in our relationship to normative standards and cultural prejudices (Feldman, 2003). Do we conform to normative standards of food consumption and oppressive cultural prejudices regarding body appearance to fit in and be accepted at the price of living falsely or inauthentically? Or do we assert our autonomous self-determination by rejecting normative standards of 'healthy' eating and confront weight stigma as the cost of living authentically? Therapists must respect patients' autonomous self-determination as patients are struggling to find the optimum balance between conformity and nonconformity in their own lives.

These relational issues enter the therapeutic situation when patients engage in 'emotional eating' (Matz & Frankel, 2014) to comfort themselves that results in unwelcome weight gain. Yet such high weight emotional eaters may still resent and resist any dietary recommendations that appear to undermine or limit their autonomous self-determination to make their own independent food choices or their ability to autonomously self-regulate their emotions by eating. It becomes challenging to help patients overcome emotional eating and learn constructive alternatives yet do so in a way that respects patients' autonomous self-determination when it comes to what, how much, and when they eat. On the one hand, patients can feel 'unloved' (i.e., unsupported) if therapists seem to supply insufficient help in overcoming emotional eating. On the other hand, patients can feel that their autonomous self-determination is being undermined if they feel required to submit to dietary rules and regulations or newly prescribed ways of 'healthy' eating that seem to unreasonably limit their freedom to eat however they like and feel OK about it.

Emotional Eating and Emotion Regulation

Freud (1905) suggested that 'a child sucking at his mother's breast has become the prototype of every relation of love' (p. 221). Central to the psychodynamic approach to weight gain is the idea that being fed by others is symbolic of love, security, and comfort beginning in infancy (Slochower, 1987). Consequently, people who feel unloved may overeat to feel loved. More recently this has been called 'emotional eating'. Emotional eating has been defined as a kind of disordered eating in response to affective experiences rather than hunger and satiety cues (Frayn & Knauper, 2018). Those affective experiences can be positive or negative (Sultson, Kukk, & Akkermann, 2017). Emotional eating can be considered a form of emotion regulation (Macht & Simons, 2011) that down regulates negative emotions and up regulates positive emotions. Emotional eating makes the bad times more tolerable and the good times even better.

Freud (1905) noted that non-nutritive sucking is a form of self-soothing (i.e., sucking on a thumb or a pacifier). Thus, the connection between oral behavior and emotion regulation is readily observable in the first year of life. More recent research on attachment style, emotion regulation, and emotional eating makes the link between formative childhood experiences and emotional eating that Freud originally observed. By the end of the first year of life attachment style can be assessed using the *Strange Situation* to see if a toddler is securely or insecurely attached. Insecure attachment has been associated emotion regulation deficits (Shi, Wang, Shang, & Liang, 2017). Emotional eating has been associated with both insecure attachment and emotion regulation deficits (Taube-Schiff, Van Exan, Tanaka, Wnuk, Hawa, & Sockalingam, 2015).

Early psychoanalytic theorists linked overeating and gaining weight to a defensive response to feelings of loss, be it the loss of a loved one or the loss of self-esteem (Fenichel, 1945). Feelings of loneliness, longing, emptiness, boredom, and low self-esteem can be assuaged through eating. Eating fills an inner void that has been left by experiences of rejection, abandonment, and/ or failure.

More recent research has linked emotional eating to various types of childhood adversity that could contribute to insecure attachment. Adults who have experienced early parental loss are more prone towards emotional eating (Høeg et al., 2017). Adults who scored higher on a measure of childhood adversity were more likely to engage in emotional eating (Kazmierski, Borelli, & Rao, 2022). Adults who suffered childhood trauma were prone towards emotional dysregulation and emotional eating (Ansari, Shakiba, Mousavi, Mohammadkhani, Aminoroaya, & Poor, 2018). Maladaptive parental feeding behavior has been associated with emotional eating among adolescents (Romano & Heron, 2021).

Treating Emotional Eating as an Emotion Regulation Deficit

Various psychotherapeutic approaches have been developed to address emotion regulation deficits and those approaches can be applied to treating emotional eating as an emotion regulation deficit. Lower levels of emotional eating have been associated with weight loss (Braden, Flatt, Boutelle, Strong, Sherwood, & Rock, 2016). Emotion regulation without emotional eating could be treated as a skill that can be taught and cultivated through mindfulness (A & Anto, 2022), distress tolerance (Braden & O'Brien, 2021), and acceptance and commitment (Hill, Masuda, Moore, & Twohig, 2015).

Mindful eating focuses on the process of eating rather than the types of food eaten. It is not a diet. It consists of three steps: 1) Noticing the taste, textures, and smells of the food eaten, 2) Recognizing repetitive habits such as eating while multitasking or eating on autopilot without conscious awareness (i.e., mindless eating), 3) Becoming aware of what triggers initiation and cessation of eating (Albers, 2008). Dialectical Behavior Therapy incorporates mindfulness to address emotional eating but also teaches distress tolerance and interpersonal effectiveness to facilitate emotion regulation (Braden & O'Brien, 2021). Acceptance and commitment approaches try to alleviate emotional eating by facilitating awareness, full experience, and tolerance of distressing or challenging emotions and thoughts by fortifying behavioral commitment to activities that express a person's basic values and that are intrinsically reinforcing. (Hill, Masuda, Moore, & Twohig, 2015). Teaching emotion regulation skills to reduce emotional eating can be paired with either Health at Any Size where weight loss is not a treatment goal or with behavioral weight loss treatment in which weight loss is a goal of treatment.

Emotion regulation can be acquired not only as a skill that is explicitly taught but as a capacity that arises out of relationships in which emotions have been well regulated. Emotion regulation appears to be a natural outgrowth of a securely attached relationship in which others respond to one's feelings in attuned, sensitive, empathetic, and trustworthy ways, an interpersonal process that also constitutes the foundations of the therapeutic alliance (Pressley & Vanden Hoek, 2014). Attachment-based interventions try to facilitate securely attached relationships (Allen, 2023). Thus, there is a relational dimension to treating emotional eating as an emotion regulation deficit.

Teaching interpersonal effectiveness and communication skills can facilitate emotion regulation. Knowing how to deal with others in constructive ways that deescalate rather than escalate interpersonal conflict and negative emotional reciprocity is often key to maintaining emotional stability (Salazar, 2015). Constructive marital communication has been associated with secure attachment while maladaptive marital communication has been associated with insecure attachment and a demand-withdraw communication pattern (Fournier & Brassard, 2010). Ruptures to the therapeutic relationship can precipitate emotion dysregulation whereas repair of those ruptures promotes emotion regulation (Muran & Eubanks, 2020). How patient and therapist learn to negotiate strong negative emotions in the therapeutic relationship may be key to patients learning emotion regulation skills.

Zelda came for psychotherapy because of marital problems. Her husband had an alcohol problem and spent money recklessly. He was depressed, withdrawn and irritable. Zelda felt overwhelmed and enraged that raising their three rambunctious boys and managing the family's precarious finances was all on her shoulders. Part of her wanted a divorce and sometimes in anger she threatened divorce. Yet when push came to shove, she didn't want to break up the family. She felt trapped and desperate. In passing Zelda expressed disgust with her late-night emotional eating of junk food and attendant weight gain.

Zelda made it clear that she wasn't coming to therapy looking for help with emotional eating but with her marital crisis. If I made any tentative suggestions in relation to her emotional eating, she responded irritably that her emotional eating at this point in her life was a psychological necessity she was not prepared to relinquish though she knew she should. Having to learn to relinquish emotional eating would only add to her overburdened state. I got the message and backed off to avoid adding to her overburdened state of mind.

Zelda's attachment security was seriously threatened by the marital crisis which threw her into a state of emotional dysregulation that was at least temporarily alleviated by late-night emotional eating. She wanted to use therapy to vent her feelings to a sympathetic audience and to get some practical suggestions for addressing her marital problems. From an attachment-based perspective the challenge would be to see if there was a way to restore a more securely attached marital relationship to improve her emotional regulation and thereby decrease her need for emotional eating. Simply venting her feelings to a sympathetic therapist offered some short-term emotional relief from her overburdened state of mind but by itself didn't solve the underlying problem of emotional dysregulation due to insecure attachment to her husband.

A demand-withdraw communication pattern arose when Zelda would browbeat her husband and threaten divorce unless he quit drinking. He became defensive and withdrawn. Zelda was receptive to working on her marital communication skills and anger management issues if not on her emotional eating. She appreciated that it wasn't best for the children to overhear her screaming at their father with whom they had a good relationship.

Despite her openness to improving her marital communication skills Zelda often wanted to use sessions to simply vent her frustration with her husband to a sympathetic audience without reflecting on the interpersonal effectiveness of her way of dealing with her husband and see if there was room for improvement. Zelda became annoyed with me when I pointed that out and protested that the only way that she could get past her anger was to vent it to get it out of her system. I noted that such an emotion regulation strategy might make her feel better in the moment, but it made the marital situation worse as her husband became emotionally flooded by her anger and responded defensively or shut down. At that point Zelda could see that she might get through to her husband better if she expressed herself in a calm, measured, and less judgmental way despite feeling enraged.

Zelda defiantly refused to express empathy and compassion towards her husband as she felt he didn't deserve it and didn't care if that made her seem to me like a bad person. I clarified that my goal was not to make her into a 'good' person but to be an effective communicator. I noted that an effective communicator is authentic and doesn't fake expressing feelings that aren't really felt. I said I could understand why she might want to make him feel as badly about himself as he made her feel about herself to give him a taste of his own medicine but that wouldn't do anything to improve the situation. Those clarifications appeared to alleviate her fear that I thought she was a bad person for browbeating her husband for his alcohol abuse and reckless spending.

As her marital communication skills improved, her husband agreed to see a therapist for his marital unhappiness if not his alcoholism. The husband's therapist helped him understand that he was drinking and spending to treat his underlying depression and that his drinking and spending only made his underlying depression worse. That motivated her husband to go to AA for further help with his alcoholism. Zelda's attachment security and emotion regulation improved as she became more optimistic about the future of the marriage as her husband started attending AA meetings.

Zelda came in one session saying that she had read an article on intermittent fasting and decided to give it try. She just wouldn't eat anything after dinner as she felt ready to give up the late-night snacking. This strategy worked and she began to lose the weight she had gained while the marriage was in crisis. Now that she was in a securely attached marital situation, she no longer needed emotional eating to down regulate her negative affect at the end of the day so she could enjoy relaxing a bit before going to sleep without snacking.

Autonomous Self-Determination and Freedom of Food Choice

Emotions can be regulated by others as well as by oneself. At the beginning of life infants are relatively dependent on their caretakers for emotion regulation and stress reduction (Easterbrooks, Bartlett, Beeghly, & Thompson, 2013). When infants are distressed parents must figure out how to soothe them whether it's too feed them, comfort them, help them fall asleep, change a wet diaper, help them pass gas, or socially stimulate them. Infants do have a few options for comforting themselves to self-regulate their own emotions and alleviate their own stress like sucking their thumbs (Heron-Delaney, Kenardy, Brown, Jardine, Bogossian, Neuman, de Dassel, & Pritchard, 2016). As children become better at self-regulation of their emotional states, they become less dependent on their parents for emotion regulation and more autonomous in that regard, especially if parents support their autonomous development (Bernier Carlson, & Whipple, 2010). Being able to comfort oneself with food makes one less dependent on others for emotion regulation even if it might not always be the most health facilitating form of emotion regulation because of its association with weight gain (Ahlich & Rancourt, 2022).

Emotional eating is a form of self-regulation that can arise early in life well before more mature emotion regulation strategies arise like cognitive reappraisal (Bergmeier, Paxton, Milgrom, Anderson, Baur, Hill, Lim, Green, & Skouteris, 2020). Being able to feed oneself is a developmental achievement. Being able to choose to eat what one wants, how much one wants, and when one wants becomes an assertion of autonomous self-determination and independence that increases with age (Bassett, Chapman, & Beagan, 2008). From an early age, children and their parents can become embroiled in power struggles about what the child eats, how much they eat, and when they eat if parents find their children's eating habits objectionable (Fishman, 2016). Children can become defiant and throw temper tantrums if they don't get their way (Sjuts, 2015). Children may refuse to eat what parents provide to assert their autonomy (Lucarelli, Ammaniti, Porreca, & Simonelli, 2017). At later ages children may surreptitiously eat in ways of which their parents would disapprove if they knew (Schechter, 2010). Thus, food can become a locus of parent-offspring conflict.

Because emotional eating can be an assertion of autonomous self-determination, though not necessarily the most healthful assertion of autonomous self-determination, patients can be of two minds about relinquishing it. On the one hand, patients may appreciate that emotional eating leads to weight gain and may therefore wish to overcome it as an act of self-determination. Individuals with autonomy support are more likely to lose weight (Powers, Koestner, Denes, Cornelius, & Gorin, 2022). On the other hand, in situations in which the highest motivational priority is to down regulate negative affect (i.e., like after a stressful day at work) or to up regulate positive affect (i.e., a holiday feast with family), patients might choose to assert their right to autonomous self-determination by choosing to eat what they want, how much they want, and when they want to make themselves feel better.

This choice may still be made even though they might also believe that they shouldn't for reasons of weight gain and well appreciate that alternative and healthier forms of emotion regulation exist. It doesn't seem in the moment like overeating reflects a loss of self-control as often conceptualized in the literature. In the moment overeating is experienced as a choice, as a defiant form of self-assertion against external pressure to do otherwise. Only in retrospect does overeating seem like a shameful loss of self-control that is a cause for self-flagellation.

According to 'reactance theory' (Brehm & Brehm, 1981) anything that seems to undermine the right to autonomous self-determination and freedom of choice will be defied. There can be reactance to counting calories, limiting portion size, abstaining from certain calorie-dense foods, having to eat mindfully rather than wolf down one's food with carefree abandon, or having to think about the future consequences of one's current eating behavior despite just wanting to just live in and enjoy the moment. Such behavior may be justified by compensatory health beliefs (Knäuper, Bärbel, et al., 2004) such as believing that one will resume a diet or mindful eating the next day to compensate so there is no need to be unduly rigid in the current situation about one's mindless eating.

Reactance theory holds that individuals try to preserve established freedoms so react resistantly to messages that appear to threaten their freedom of choice, motivating them to defend their freedom and oppose the recommended behavior (Brehm & Brehm, 1981). Health communication that threatens freedom and autonomy can be angrily resisted (Staunton, Alvaro, & Rosenberg, 2022). Interestingly, those low in self-compassion respond the most resistantly to health messages that threaten autonomy while those high in self-compassion are more likely to listen to the health message despite the threat to autonomy (Genin, Vinson, Lagrange, & Le Barbenchon, 2022).

Respecting Patients' Autonomous Food Choices

Regardless of the weight management goal, therapeutic communication is communication that empowers patients' autonomous self-determination (Ryan & Deci, 2008) and decreases their reactance to health messages that might seem to threaten their autonomy and freedom of choice (Brehm & Brehm, 1981). Patients may angrily resist health messages that make them feel that they 'should' lose weight or that they 'should' accept their fat though they don't want to. Patients who choose to diet to lose weight may resent messages about how they 'should' diet (i.e., should they try Keto or Paleo?). Instead, such patients might stubbornly insist on dieting in their own way regardless of how misguided others might judge their dietary approach (i.e., skip breakfast, only drink liquids, never drink one's calories, never consume fatty foods, primarily consume fatty foods). Such patients do not want to be made to feel badly about themselves for their autonomous choices that they feel should be at least respected if not validated by their therapists.

Emotional eaters may become emotionally dysregulated by health messages that threaten their autonomy and then resort to emotional eating to assert their autonomous self-regulation. Therapy could be dysregulating and increase emotional eating if it devolves into a power struggle about what patients 'should' do for their own good. Does that mean therapists need to be assiduously neutral about goals for treatment, nondirective in treatment approach, and refrain from making any recommendations or expressing any personal opinions to avoid any potential infringement on patients' autonomy? Or should therapists simply monitor the impact of their interventions to assess to what degree they are experienced as threatening patients' autonomy and then intervene to try to alleviate the autonomy threat?

The tenets of self-determination theory (Ryan & Deci, 2008) suggest that psychotherapy will be more effective when therapists support patients' intrinsic motivations (i.e., what they really want) as opposed to extrinsic motivations (i.e., what they should do). Self-determination theory believes there are three basic intrinsic motivations: competence, autonomy, and relatedness. Individuals feel vital, positive, and emotionally stable when those needs are met and dysphoric and poorly regulated when those needs are frustrated.

The problem, though, is that patients can be of two minds and therefore ambivalent about what they truly want or should do. In addition, it is not always so clear what is a genuine want and what is a should. Do patients really want to lose weight and diet or is it that they just think they should for social acceptance? Do patients really want to accept their fat and give up on trying to restrain their overeating or does that just seem to be the path of least resistance because they are demoralized by and tired of failed attempts at dieting?

Motivational interviewing (Butryn, Schumacher, & Forman, 2018) as well as psychodynamic psychotherapy (Schwartz, Nickow, Arseneau, & Gisslow, 2015) for weight management recommend exploring patients' inner conflicts, ambivalence, and being of two minds. The basic treatment approach consists of articulating the two states of mind, empathizing with each state of mind, clarifying the distinctions between the two states, discover the external triggers of each state, explore the developmental history of each state, explore the extent to which each state expresses a true or false sense of self, explore the extent that the thinking expressed in each state of mind is wishful or realistic, and finally assess the cost and benefits of acting on each state of mind. Both approaches aim to support patients' autonomous decision-making rather than simply adopt their therapists' beliefs when it comes to healthy eating.

The premise is that patients' autonomous decision making is best supported through an approach that is primarily exploratory and clarifying until patients make up their own minds. Once patients make up their minds about their treatment goals, patients' autonomy may then be best supported by interventions that empower patients to achieve their goals. Yet patients can still be of two minds about how to best achieve those goals. Therapists may need to resume an approach that is more exploratory and clarifying rather than campaign for a particular approach to goal achievement be it counting calories or mindful eating.

Therapists who possess the flexibility to work in nondirective as well as directive ways might do better with autonomy support. They can provide direction when patients are looking for guidance but can also provide empathy and clarification when patients want the space and time to figures things out for themselves and manage their weight in their own way.

Patients can be of two minds about how much they really want to give up emotional eating if it seems to them like a very effective form of autonomous self-regulation that makes the bad times more tolerable and the good times even better. Patients can also be of two minds over the best way to overcome emotional eating once they decide to make that a goal for treatment. Most approaches to emotional eating are to help patients acquire more constructive forms of self-regulation like mindful eating or distress tolerance in the short-term. Yet many patients adopt a more long-term relational approach to overcoming emotional eating. The underlying but not always consciously articulated rationale is something like:

> For the time being I'm going to put all my focus and effort into improving my work, love, and family life. Once those goals are achieved my life will be sufficiently less stressful to focus on myself. At that point I'll have more time and energy to focus on healthy eating and exercise. Until then, I will sustain my emotional stability by venting my feelings to my therapist for other-regulation and utilizing emotional eating for self-regulation.

From the therapist's perspective it is not always clear to what extent this is a viable long-term gameplan or simply a rationalization for maintaining an unsatisfactory status quo into some indefinite future. For this reason, acquiring a metabolic syndrome that raises mortality salience makes it clear that one doesn't have all the time in the world to address one's weight management issues so may constitute a tipping point for behavior change. It doesn't seem as urgent to address a 'bad' habit as a preventative measure when the negative long-term consequences of that habit might not materialize until some distant future [i.e., delayed reward discounting (Amlung, Gray, & MacKillop, 2016)].

Reactance theory (Brehm & Brehm, 1981) proposes that health messages will be resisted that threaten patients' autonomy. Reactance theory also proposes that it's not always what you say but how you say it. Health messages are inherently prescriptive. Such messages, be it explicitly or implicitly, suggest what one 'must' or 'should' do to be healthy. Consequently, health messages threaten autonomy because they predict a negative health outcome unless one changes one's behavior in the prescribed way.

Health messages communicated in a dogmatic way generate more reactance (Zhang, 2020). Zhang (2020) noted that dogmatic communication uses controlling language making clear the sources desire to control behavior. It tries to forcefully pressure recipients to conform to the message by using vivid and graphic language of the dire consequences of failure to conform. Dogmatic language uses words like 'must' and 'should' so make recipients feel badly about themselves if they fail to conform to what they must or should do.

Therapists might refrain from explicit and authoritative health directives to try to avoid seeming dogmatic and authoritarian. Psychotherapy outcome tends to be better with high reactance patients when therapists adopt a more reflective and nondirective stance than a more directive and authoritative one (Beutler, Edwards, & Someah, 2018). Nevertheless, therapists' opinions and biases, such as weight stigma, can be communicated implicitly without therapists' self-awareness (Meulman, 2019).

There can be a downside of nondirective and exploratory approaches despite its reactance-reducing benefits. It has been found that health communication that is direct and explicit is easier to understand than health communication that is indirect and implicit (Staunton, Alvaro, & Rosenberg, 2022). The autonomy threat of explicit health communication can be mitigated using 'low-controlling' language (Staunton, Alvaro, & Rosenberg, 2022). Low-controlling language produces less reactance but may not be as persuasive because health opinions, though explicitly stated, are expressed more tentatively so the implications for action are more ambiguous or uncertain. Low-controlling language leaves room for alternative interpretations and uncertainty as to the source's true intentions or beliefs.

Therapists can articulate alternate points of view and options for going forward without seeming to take sides to let patients decide for themselves. Patients may then take the path of least resistance rather than the more challenging option that might be more likely to lead to sustainable results in the long-term. High-controlling language is direct, straight-forward, unambiguous, and easy to understand but unfortunately produces more reactance (Staunton, Alvaro, & Rosenberg, 2022). Yet research has discovered a health communication strategy that capitalizes on the benefits of high-controlling language while mitigating the risks (Staunton, Alvaro, and Rosenberg, 2022).

1. Health messages can be presented authoritatively but with a reminder that the decision is ultimately the recipient's own decision.
2. Embed the health message in an engaging narrative (i.e., story) to foster identification with the protagonist.
3. Note the beneficial impact of health promoting behavior change on significant others so one is changing for the benefit of others as much as for oneself.
4. Forewarn recipients that the health message will likely be autonomy threatening to inoculate recipients to the possibility that their openness to the health communication might be clouded by their own reactance.
5. Harness recipients' own reactance to motivate health promoting behavior change. For example, one could highlight how the food industry creates highly processed addictive foods to exploit consumers. Reactance might be to eat more whole foods to prove that one is not a puppet of Machiavellian corporate executives.

Beckett had high blood pressure and his doctor recommended that he lose weight. He also had high cholesterol for which his doctor had recommended a lower fat diet. His father had died of heart disease at age 59 so it appeared that there was a family history of heart disease. His doctor prescribed medication. Beckett also worked long hours at a demanding job in finance. He always ate on the run and mostly ate high fat and high carbohydrate foods that he bought on the run at food carts (i.e., hot dogs and pretzels) or take out that was delivered to the office (i.e., spare ribs and French fries). At the end of the day, he would treat himself to a craft beer to relax.

Beckett mostly used therapy to discuss his contentious relationship with his ex-wife, his increasingly estranged relationships with his two teenage daughters, and performance pressure at work. He claimed he was working on losing weight by reducing portion size and going to the gym at work. I took what he said at face value though somewhere in the back of my mind it registered that he was not losing weight and maybe he was even gaining weight. Weight became more central when he came in one day to say that his doctor told him that he was prediabetic and if he didn't lose weight, he was risking Type 2 diabetes.

At that point I noted that his approach to dieting didn't seem to be working. Beckett responded defensively that he was doing the best he could given the various stresses with which he had to contend. Feeling alarmed and frustrated that his health situation might be deteriorating, I responded reactively and dogmatically when attempting a confrontation that might break through his denial. I stated that given his family history he just might be slowly eating himself to death if he didn't start to turn things around sooner rather than later. Beckett responded: 'Damn Right!' with a tone of triumphant and smug self-satisfaction. I realized we were beginning to get into a power struggle as we both were responding with reactance under threats to our autonomy. I tried to repair the rupture to the therapeutic relationship by saying that I respected his right to diet in his own way but that we could have a respectful difference of opinion about what might be the most effective way to go about it. Beckett said he knew that I cared about his welfare, but he was still determined to find a way to lose weight in his own way.

Beckett's cardiologist also worried about Beckett's health status so ordered a CT scan to assess the status of Beckett's atrial arteries. It turned out that Beckett had a substantial plaque buildup in his 'widow maker' artery. That alarmed Beckett so he began working with a nutritionist who would monitor his daily calorie count online. This health scare constituted the tipping point that motivated Beckett to make the kind of lifestyle modifications that previously would have been experienced as serious infringements on his autonomy to be defied. Now he was proactively engaged in a fight to save his own life, an act of autonomous self-determination. I was greatly relieved that I didn't have to helplessly watch as he seemed to be 'eating himself to death'.

There is much variability in how individuals respond to such medical scares or crises. In the face of increased mortality threat, reactance may lead some individuals to choose to 'live free or die' while others might choose to 'live long and prosper' (Dimoff, Dao, Mitchell, & Olson, 2021). It may be the preceding therapeutic work that enables individuals to respond to such medical events as a wake-up call rather than continue to live in denial despite a deteriorating health situation.

References

Ahlich, E., & Rancourt, D. (2022). Boredom proneness, interoception, and emotional eating. *Appetite*, 178, 8. https://doi.org/10.1016/j.appet.2022.106167

Albers, S. (2008). *Eat, drink, and be mindful: How to end your struggle with mindless eating and start savoring food with intention and joy.* Oakland: New Harbinger Publications, Inc.

Allen, B. (2023). *The science and clinical practice of attachment theory: A guide from infancy to adulthood.* American Psychological Association. https://doi.org/10.1037/0000333-000

Amlung, M., Gray, J. C., & MacKillop, J. (2016). Delay discounting and addictive behavior: Review of the literature and identification of emerging priorities. In C. E. Kopetz & C. W. Lejuez (Eds.), Addictions: A social psychological perspective (pp. 15–46). Routledge/Taylor & Francis Group.

Anderson, J. R. (2019). Inviting autonomy back to the table: The importance of autonomy for healthy relationship functioning. *Journal of Marital and Family Therapy*, 46(1), 3–14. http://doi.org/10.1111/jmft.12413

Ansari, N., Shakiba, S., Mousavi, M. E., Mohammadkhani, P., Aminoroaya, S., & Poor, N. S. (2018). Role of emotional dysregulation and childhood trauma in emotional eating behavior. *Journal of Practice in Clinical Psychology*, 6(1), 21–28. https://doi.org/10.29252/nirp.jpcp.6.1.21

Bassett, R., Chapman, G. E., & Beagan, B. L. (2008). Autonomy and control: The co-construction of adolescent food choice. *Appetite*, 50(2–3), 325–332. https://doi.org/10.1016/j.appet.2007.08.009

Bergmeier, H., Paxton, S. J., Milgrom, J., Anderson, S. E., Baur, L., Hill, B., Lim, S., Green, R., & Skouteris, H. (2020). Early mother-child dyadic pathways to childhood obesity risk: A conceptual model. *Appetite*, 144, 104459. https://doi.org/10.1016/j.ap pet.2019.104459

Bernier, A., Carlson, S. M., & Whipple, N. (2010). From external regulation to self-regulation: Early parenting precursors of young children's executive functioning. *Child Development*, 81(1), 326–339. https://doi.org/10.1111/j.1467-8624.2009.01397.x

Beutler, L. E., Edwards, C., & Someah, K. (2018). Adapting psychotherapy to patient reactance level: A meta-analytic review. *Journal of Clinical Psychology*, 74(11), 1952–1963. https://doi.org/10.1002/jclp.22682

Boykin McElhaney, K., & Allen, J. P. (2012). Sociocultural perspectives on adolescent autonomy. In P. K. Kerig, M. S. Schulz, & S. T. Hauser (Eds.), *Adolescence and beyond: Family processes and development* (pp. 161–176). Oxford University Press. https://doi-org/10.1093/acprof:oso/9780199736546.003.0011

Braden, A., Flatt, S. W., Boutelle, K. N., Strong, D., Sherwood, N. E., & Rock, C. L. (2016). Emotional eating is associated with weight loss success among adults enrolled in a weight loss program. *Journal of Behavioral Medicine*, 39(4), 727–732. https://doi.org/10.1007/s10865-016-9728-8

Braden, A., & O'Brien, W. (2021). Pilot study of a treatment using dialectical behavioral therapy skills for adults with overweight/obesity and emotional eating. *Journal of Contemporary Psychotherapy: On the Cutting Edge of Modern Developments in Psychotherapy*, 51(1), 21–29. https://doi-org/10.1007/s10879-020-09477-1

Brehm, S. S., & Brehm, J. W. (1981). *Psychological reactance: A theory of freedom and control*. San Diego, CA: Academic Press.

Butryn, M. L., Schumacher, L. M., & Forman, E. M. (2018). Alternative behavioral weight loss approaches: Acceptance and commitment therapy and motivational interviewing. In T. A. Wadden & G. A. Bray (Eds.), *Handbook of obesity treatment* (pp. 508–521). The Guilford Press.

Cook-Cottone, C. P., Tribole, E., & Tylka, T. L. (2013). Why we eat the way we do: The role of personal and external factors. In C. P. Cook-Cottone, E. Tribole, & T. L. Tylka, *Healthy eating in schools: Evidence-based interventions to help kids thrive* (pp. 45–65). American Psychological Association. https://doi.org/10.1037/14180-003

Dimoff, J. D., Dao, A. N., Mitchell, J., & Olson, A. (2021). Live free and die: Expanding the terror management health model for pandemics to account for psychological reactance. *Social and Personality Psychology Compass*, 15(3), Article e12585. https://doi.org/10.1111/spc3.12585

Easterbrooks, M. A., Bartlett, J. D., Beeghly, M., & Thompson, R. A. (2013). Social and emotional development in infancy. In R. M. Lerner, M. A. Easterbrooks, J. Mistry, & I. B. Weiner (Eds.), *Handbook of psychology: Developmental psychology* (pp. 91–120). John Wiley & Sons, Inc.

Fathima, F. M., & Anto, M. M. (2022). Mindful eating: A novel therapeutic tool. In S. K. Gupta (Ed.), *Handbook of research on clinical applications of meditation and mindfulness-based interventions in mental health* (pp. 55–67). Medical Information Science Reference/IGI Global. 10.4018/978-1-7998-8682-2.ch004

Feldman, S. (2003). Enforcing social conformity: A theory of authoritarianism. *Political Psychology*, 24(1), 41–74. https://doi.org/10.1111/0162-895X.00316

Fenichel, O. (1945). Nature and classification of the so-called psychosomatic phenomena. *Psychoanalytic Quarterly*, 14, 287–312. https://doi.org/10.1080/21674086.1945.11925606

Fishman, L. (2016). Review of Helping your child with extremely picky eating: A step-by-step guide for overcoming selective eating, food aversion, and feeding disorders [Review of the book Helping your child with extremely picky eating: A step-by-step guide for overcoming selective eating, food aversion, and feeding disorders, by J. Rowell & J. McGlothlin]. *Journal of Nutrition Education and Behavior*, 48(1), e3. https://doi-org/10.1016/j.jneb.2015.08.013

Fournier, B., & Brassard, A. (2010). Éclairage du fonctionnement conjugal: Attachement, communication, demande-retrait, violence et satisfaction conjugales [Couple functioning: Attachment, demand/withdraw communication pattern, intimate violence and relationship satisfaction]. *Revue Québécoise de Psychologie*, 31(1), 155–169.

Frayn, M., & Knauper, B. (2018). Emotional eating and weight in adults: A review. *Current Psychology*, 37(4), 924–933. https://doi.org/10.1007/s12144-017-9577-9

Freud, S. (1905). Three essays on the theory of sexuality. *The Standard Edition of the complete psychological works of Sigmund Freud*, 7, 123–246.

Genin, M., Vinson, E., Lagrange, A., & Le Barbenchon, E. (2022). Self-compassion and resistance to persuasion. *Psychology & Health*, 37(10), 1241–1252. https://doi.org/10.1080/08870446.2021.1941959

Guardabassi, V., & Tomasetto, C. (2022). Weight-based teasing, body dissatisfaction, and eating restraint: Multilevel investigation among primary schoolchildren. *Health Psychology*, 41(8), 527–537. https://doi.org/10.1037/hea0001213

Hamburg, M. E., Finkenauer, C., & Schuengel, C. (2014). Food for love: The role of food offering in empathic emotion regulation. *Frontiers in Psychology*, 5, 32. https://doi.org/10.3389/fpsyg.2014.00032

Heron-Delaney, M., Kenardy, J. A., Brown, E. A., Jardine, C., Bogossian, F., Neuman, L., de Dassel, T., & Pritchard, M. (2016). Early maternal reflective functioning and infant emotional regulation in a preterm infant sample at 6 months corrected age. *Journal of Pediatric Psychology*, 41(8), 906–914. https://doi.org/10.1093/jpepsy/jsv169

Hill, M. L., Masuda, A., Moore, M., & Twohig, M. P. (2015). Acceptance and Commitment Therapy for individuals with problematic emotional eating: A case-series study. *Clinical Case Studies*, 14(2), 141–154. https://doi.org/10.1177/1534650114547429

Høeg, B. L., Appel, C. W., von Heymann-Horan, A. B., Frederiksen, K., Johansen, C., Bøge, P., Dencker, A., Dyregrov, A., Mathiesen, B. B., & Bidstrup, P. E. (2017). Maladaptive coping in adults who have experienced early parental loss and grief counseling. *Journal of Health Psychology*, 22(14), 1851–1861. https://doi.org/10.1177/1359105316638550

Kazmierski, K. F. M., Borelli, J. L., & Rao, U. (2022). Negative affect, childhood adversity, and adolescents' eating following stress. *Appetite*, 168, 105766. https://doi-org/10.1016/j.appet.2021.105766

Knäuper, B., Rabiau, M., Cohen, O., & Patriciu, N. (2004). Compensatory health beliefs: Scale development and psychometric properties. *Psychology & Health*, 19(5), 607–624, https://doi.org/10.1080/0887044042000196737

Lewis, M., & Minar, N. J. (2022). Self-recognition and emotional knowledge. *European Journal of Developmental Psychology*, 19(3), 319–342. https://doi-org/10.1080/17405629.2021.1890578

Lucarelli, L., Ammaniti, M., Porreca, A., & Simonelli, A. (2017). Infantile anorexia and co-parenting: A pilot study on mother-father-child triadic interactions during feeding and play. *Frontiers in Psychology*, 8, 376. https://doi.org/10.3389/fpsyg.2017.00376

Macht, M., & Simons, G. (2011). Emotional eating. In I. Nykliček, A. Vingerhoets, & M. Zeelenberg (Eds.), *Emotion regulation and well-being* (pp. 281–295). Springer Science + Business Media. https://doi.org/10.1007/978-1-4419-6953-8_17

Matz, J., & Frankel, E. (2014). *Beyond a shadow of a diet: The comprehensive guide to treating binge eating disorder, compulsive eating, and emotional overeating* (2nd ed.). Routledge/Taylor & Francis Group.

Meltzoff, A. N. (1990). Foundations for developing a concept of self: The role of imitation in relating self to other and the value of social mirroring, social modeling, and self practice in infancy. In D. Cicchetti & M. Beeghly (Eds.), *The self in transition: Infancy to childhood* (pp. 139–164). University of Chicago Press.

Mennella, J. A., Forestell, C. A., Ventura, A. K., & Fisher, J. O. (2020). The development of infant feeding. In J. J. Lockman & C. S. Tamis-LeMonda (Eds.), *The Cambridge handbook of infant development: Brain, behavior, and cultural context* (pp. 263–302). Cambridge University Press.

Meulman, M. A. (2019). Sizeism in therapy: Fat shaming in supervision. *Women & Therapy*, 42(1–2), 156–163. https://doi.org/10.1080/02703149.2018.1524072

Momin, S. R., Hughes, S. O., Elias, C., Papaioannou, M. A., Phan, M., Vides, D., & Wood, A. C. (2018). Observations of toddlers' sensory-based exploratory behaviors with a novel food. *Appetite*, 131, 108–116. https://doi.org/10.1016/j.appet.2018.08.035

Muran, J. C., & Eubanks, C. F. (2020). From emotion to repair. In J. C. Muran & C. F. Eubanks, *Therapist performance under pressure: Negotiating emotion, difference, and rupture* (pp. 73–101). American Psychological Association. https://doi-org/10.1037/0000 182-005

Powers, T. A., Koestner, R., Denes, A., Cornelius, T., & Gorin, A. A. (2022). Autonomy support in a couples weight loss trial: Helping yourself while helping others. *Families, Systems, & Health*, 40(1), 70–78. https://doi-org/10.1037/fsh0000663

Pressley, J. D., & Vanden Hoek, K. K. (2014). Psychodynamic and attachment-based approaches to treatment. In K. S. Flanagan & S. E. Hall (Eds.), *Christianity and developmental psychopathology: Foundations and approaches* (pp. 247–281). InterVarsity Press.

Romano, K. A., & Heron, K. E. (2021). Regulatory parental feeding behaviors, emotion suppression, and emotional eating in the absence of hunger: Examining parent-adolescent dyadic associations. *Appetite*, 167, 105603. https://doi-org.adelphi.idm.oclc.org/10.1016/j.appet.2021.105603

Ryan, R. M., & Deci, E. L. (2008). A self-determination theory approach to psychotherapy: The motivational basis for effective change. *Canadian Psychology/Psychologie canadienne*, 49(3), 186–193. https://doi.org/10.1037/a0012753

Salazar, L. R. (2015). The negative reciprocity process in marital relationships: A literature review. *Aggression and Violent Behavior*, 24, 113–119. https://doi.org/10.1016/j.avb.2015.05.008

Schechter, L. R. (2010). *My big fat secret: How Jenna takes control of her emotions and eating. (J. Chin, Illustrator)*. Magination Press/American Psychological Association.

Schwartz, D. C., Nickow, M. S., Arseneau, R., & Gisslow, M. T. (2015). A substance called food: Long-term psychodynamic group treatment for compulsive overeating. *International Journal of Group Psychotherapy*, 65(3), 386–409. https://doi.org/10.1521/ijgp.2015.65.3.386

Shi, H., Wang, Y., Shang, X., & Liang, X. (2017). Toddlers' attachment style and development of emotion regulation strategies: A longitudinal study. *Chinese Journal of Clinical Psychology*, 25(4), 603–607.

Sjuts, T. M. (2015). Supporting positive parent-toddler relationships and reducing toddler tantrums: Evaluation of PCAT-E. *Dissertation Abstracts International Section A: Humanities and Social Sciences*, 75(12-A(E)).

Slochower, J. (1987). The psychodynamics of obesity: A review. *Psychoanalytic Psychology*, 4(2), 145–159. https://doi.org/10.1037/h0079130

Staunton, T. V., Alvaro, E. M., & Rosenberg, B. D. (2022). A case for directives: Strategies for enhancing clarity while mitigating reactance. *Current Psychology: A Journal for Diverse Perspectives on Diverse Psychological Issues*, 41(2), 611–621. https://doi.org/10.1007/s12144-019-00588-0

Sultson, H., Kukk, K., & Akkermann, K. (2017). Positive and negative emotional eating have different associations with overeating and binge eating: Construction and validation of the Positive-Negative Emotional Eating Scale. *Appetite*, 116, 423–430. https://doi.org/10.1016/j.appet.2017.05.035

Taube-Schiff, M., Van Exan, J., Tanaka, R., Wnuk, S., Hawa, R., & Sockalingam, S. (2015). Attachment style and emotional eating in bariatric surgery candidates: The mediating role of difficulties in emotion regulation. *Eating Behaviors*, 18, 36–40. https://doi.org/10.1016/j.eatbeh.2015.03.011

Volkert, V. M., Patel, M. R., & Peterson, K. M. (2016). Food refusal and selective eating. In J. K. Luiselli (Ed.), *Behavioral health promotion and intervention in intellectual and developmental disabilities* (pp. 137–161). Springer International Publishing/Springer Nature.

Wang, D., Everett, B., Brunero, S., Northall, T., Villarosa, A. R., & Salamonson, Y. (2020). Perspectives of residents and staff regarding food choice in residential aged care: A qualitative study. *Journal of Clinical Nursing*, 29(3–4), 626–637. https://doi.org/10.1111/jocn.15115

Zhang X. (2020). Effects of freedom restoration, language variety, and issue type on psychological reactance. *Health Communication*, 35(11), 1316–1327. https://doi.org/10.1080/10410236.2019.1631565

Food Addiction and Divergent Weight Management Stigma

The relational dimensions of weight management are conceived differently depending upon one's theory of weight gain. From the perspective of Health at Any Size weight is largely a function of genetic predisposition. The relational problem is therefore weight stigma, a cultural prejudice against individuals for their body appearance when their body appearance is simply a product of their genetic predisposition. From the perspective of behavioral weight loss treatment, eating habits are a product of social learning that can be unlearned. The relational problem is therefore the social reinforcement of overeating as well as the lack of social support for dieting in a consumer culture that provides a food rich environment. From the perspective of emotional eating the underlying relational problem is one of emotional dysregulation due to insecure attachment. The relational solution is therefore the facilitation of secure attachment and the improved emotional regulation that comes with secure attachment.

Another relational perspective comes with conceptualizing weight gain as a function of food addiction (Vasiliu, 2022). The premise of food addiction is that certain foods, especially processed foods like sugar and white flour, have addictive properties so that the more those foods are consumed the more one needs to consume such foods (Ahmed, 2012). Consumption of such foods increases rather than decreases craving so it can become difficult to feel sated on such foods without overconsumption. It may not be possible for some food addicted individuals to learn to eat such foods in moderation as consumption of small portions may increase craving for more. Like any addiction, abstention from the most addictive foods precipitate withdrawal symptoms so that at a certain point in the progression of the disorder one is eating foods with addictive properties to alleviate withdrawal symptoms despite wishing that one could resist that impulse without giving in to temptation (Blumenthal, DuPont, & Gold, 2012).

Some period of painful withdrawal must be tolerated until a time when cravings begin to subside for the 'trigger' foods that one no longer eats at all or only rarely. The relational problem is that some individuals may be perceived as barriers to healthful weight management while others are perceived as facilitators of it (Greaney, Less, White, Dayton, Riebe, Blissmer, Shoff, Walsh, & Greene, 2009).

Individuals who self-identify as "food addicts" and who subscribe to a 12-step approach like Overeaters Anonymous that advocates abstinence will not be eating like everyone else (Rodríguez-Martín & Gallego-Arjiz, 2018). They will be abstaining from their 'trigger foods' as well as engaging in other forms of self-monitoring like counting calories making them vulnerable to divergent weight management stigma (Romo, 2018). Others might believe that

DOI: 10.4324/9781003402336-7

abstinence from foods like pizza or ice cream is an excessive, if not unhealthy, dietary practice if they believe that food addiction is a fictitious illness. Self-identified food addicts might
be met with skepticism if they admit that there are foods that they haven't eaten in years, and
they don't miss it. Thus, their recovery is based in part on their ability to insulate themselves
from and resist conformist pressure to eat like everybody else.

Is Food Addiction Real?

Terms like 'foodporn' and 'foodgasm' have been used to describe how food advertising
promises a peak orgasm-like experience from certain advertised foods (Ranteallo & Andilolo,
2017) that might be designed by the food industry to achieve one's 'bliss point' (Moss, 2014).
So, although food is not exactly a mind-altering drug in the same way that alcohol or marijuana are, certain foods can be used to achieve a 'high', a happy and contented state of mind
that brings a smile to one's face because it tastes so good. That is why emotional eating can
become a preferred mode of emotion regulation.

Foods vary in how much they generate 'foodgasms' and therefore how much they tend to
be overeaten. On one end of the continuum would be a low-calorie fat-free food like celery.
Very few people overeat celery or use celery to alter their mental state. On the other end of
the continuum would a calorie-dense food like ice cream that tends to be overeaten and is a
food favored for emotional eating to alter one's mental state.

The fact that calorie-dense foods can create a high-like state and therefore tend to be
overeaten has led to describing such foods as 'addictive'. The question is then whether such
foods are 'literally' addictive or only addictive in a metaphorical sense just as 'foodgasms'
may be a term to be taken more figuratively than literally. The concept of food addiction
is a controversial one but there is a growing body of literature that views food addiction
as a genuine eating disorder that should have its own diagnostic code in the *Diagnostic and
Statistical Manual of the American Psychiatric Association* (Vasiliu, 2022).

Food addiction is a controversial diagnostic concept for a variety of reasons. Given soci-
etal weight stigma, is it simply a manner of pathologizing individuals for their weight by
creating a new stigmatized identity (DePierre, Puhl, & Luedicke, 2013)? If food addiction is
to be understood to be an actual addiction, is it a behavioral addiction like sex or gambling
addiction (i.e., an eating addiction) or a substance abuse disorder like addiction to alcohol or
heroin because certain foods like sugar do possess chemically addictive properties (Schulte,
Schiestl, & Gearhardt, 2020)? And if food addiction is real, how best should it be treated?
Must there be abstinence from 'trigger foods' (i.e., the most addictive highly processed
carbohydrate/high saturated fat/low fiber foods like ice cream and pizza) or might a 'harm
reduction model' (i.e., learning to eat the most addictive foods in moderation) be more sustainable (Storbjörk, 2017)?

To establish food addiction as a diagnostic entity the Yale Food Addiction Scale
(YAFS) was originally constructed to match DSM IV criteria for substance dependence
(Gearhardt, Corbin, & Brownell, 2009). Elevated scores on the YFAS were associated with
obesity, binge eating, impulsivity, craving, and medical conditions like diabetes (Meule &
Gearhardt, 2014; Pursey, Stanwell, Gearhardt, Collins, & Burrows, 2014). More recently
a YAFS 2.0 was developed to match DSM V criteria for substance-related and addictive
disorders (Gearhardt, Corbin, & Brownell, 2016). The YAFS 2.0 captures important features

of addiction such as tolerance, withdrawal, and craving. It assesses important features of addiction such as consumed more than planned, unable to cut down or stop, important activities given up, use despite the physical/emotional consequences, failure in role obligation, use despite interpersonal/social consequences, use in physically hazardous situations, and impairment or distress.

Tolerance, withdrawal, and craving are essential features of addictions but not features of the DSM criteria for other eating disorders such as binge eating. Food addiction as assessed by the YAFS 2.0 is a related but distinct construct from other eating disorders such as binge eating disorder (Gearhardt, Corbin, & Brownell, 2016). Not everyone with a food addiction binge eats and not everyone who binge eats possesses a food addiction though some individuals meet the criteria for both disorders.

Elevated scores on YAFS 2.0 were not associated with dietary restraint (Gearhardt, Corbin, & Brownell, 2016) though more recent research has associated food addiction with dietary restraint (Wiedemann, Carr, Ivezaj, & Barnes, 2021). Individuals with food addiction do tend to suffer weight cycling as well as obesity. Individuals who suffer food addiction, like any other addiction, are highly vulnerable to relapse as they search for a sustainable approach to recovery (Parylak, Koob, & Zorrilla, 2011). Addictive-like eating behavior, elevated BMI, and weight cycling is also associated with a processed food withdrawal scale. That scale was constructed to be consistent with scales assessing drug withdrawal. Withdrawal was reported to be most intense during two to five days of trying to cut down (Schulte, Smeal, Lewis, & Gearhardt, 2018).

As addictions are diseases of denial (Kearney, 1996) not all overweight individuals with food addiction attempt to diet and lose weight and that's why it may not be consistently associated with dietary restraint for everyone who suffers from it. Living in denial of the nature of the problem individuals with food addiction may not feel there is anything problematic about their weight or their eating habits even if they appreciate that other people do think it is problematic. Addicted individuals in general may deny, rationalize, or normalize their addictive behavior as their free choice to minimize the extent to which it has become a compulsion that has gotten out of control. Individuals who feel that their autonomous self-determination is threatened are more likely to respond with defensive behavior like denial (Knee & Zuckerman, 1998).

Addicted individuals may temporarily reduce or refrain from their addictive behavior just to prove to themselves or others that they can do it if they so choose but then resume their addictive behavior once they believe that they have proven that their behavior is not out of control. A food addiction may not be acknowledged until a medical condition like diabetes or heart disease necessitates weight loss (i.e., hitting bottom). At that point it is discovered that sustainable long-term weight loss is not possible without having to suffer through withdrawal symptoms and intensified cravings for the calorie-dense foods whose consumption must be greatly reduced or eliminated to treat a life-threatening medical condition.

There is greater acceptance of food addiction as a diagnostic entity since the advent of the YAFS 2.0 as hundreds of studies have been conducted with this measure (Schulte, Schiestl, & Gearhardt, 2020; Vasiliu, 2022). Yet controversy remains as to the extent that food addiction is a behavioral addiction like sex addiction or a substance abuse disorder like alcoholism. The current consensus appears to be that there is suggestive but not conclusive evidence supporting the idea that certain calorie-dense foods possess addictive properties (Schulte, Schiestl, & Gearhardt, 2020). Natural whole foods like fruits, vegetables, lean meats, and whole grains have not been associated with food addiction. The consumption of foods that are high in sugar and fat is highly associated with food addiction (Schulte, Schiestl, & Gearhardt, 2020).

Intriguingly, foods that are high in sugar as well as in fat do not occur in any naturally occurring food. Plant foods are generally fat-free except for plant foods like nuts or seeds. Animal foods outside of dairy are carbohydrate/sugar-free. Addictive foods as products of human culinary invention may possess a supra-additive rewarding effect (DiFeliceantonio, Coppin, Rigoux, Edwin Thanarajah, Dagher, Tittgemeyer, & Small, 2018). There is some research that suggests that foods such as sugar do function like addictive substances and that having a small taste of an addictive food has a priming effect that increases the craving for that food (Ahmed, 2012).

Initial studies of prevalence rates of food addiction utilizing the YAFS 2.0 found prevalence rates of 14.6% and 15.8% (Gearhardt, Corbin, & Brownell, 2016). Food addiction predicts level of obesity and of insulin resistance (Stojek, Maples-Keller, Dixon, Umpierrez, Gillespie, & Michopoulos, 2019). Just as BMI resides on a continuum from underweight to morbidly obese, food addiction also rests on a continuum that can be absent, mild, moderate, or severe that roughly parallels BMI.

Conceptualizing weight gain due to overeating as the manifestation of an addictive process has important implications for treatment:

1. The concept of tolerance suggests that increasingly greater quantities of the addictive foods are required to achieve satiety and increasingly greater quantities of addictive foods can be consumed before feeling sick to one's stomach. Satiety cues may not be entirely trustworthy if tolerance means that such cues are not activated until after one has already overeaten. The clinical challenge would be finding a way to lower the satiety set point (i.e., to reduce tolerance). Elevated satiety set points may not be as powerfully defended as are the lower ones that prevent starvation. Elevated satiety set points may be amenable to various modulatory influences (Berthoud, 2012).

2. Withdrawal suggests that the body reacts not simply to the reduction of calories when dieting but also to the reduction or elimination of the most addictive foods in one's diet. Craving for addictive foods can remain even when the calorie count remains adequate or high. That is the phenomena of having room for a sweet dessert after having overeaten.

3. The concept of craving implies that even a small taste of an addictive food can activate the craving for more than a small taste. Thus, learning to eat addictive foods in moderation is a challenge if small portions increase rather than decrease craving among addicted individuals though not necessarily among non-addicted individuals (van Kleef, Shimizu, & Wansink, 2013). Craving may never entirely subside even after the withdrawal phase has passed and can be reactivated in the face of temptation and/ or while stressed precipitating stress-induced relapse (Hutchinson, 2011).

4. Through mindful attention one might learn to distinguish genuine hunger from craving (Sodus, 2014). Hunger may serve to insure sufficient caloric intake while craving may seek to find specific nutrients like sugar or fat. High energy density, high fat, low protein, and low fiber foods tend to be the most craved foods that tend to be overeaten and when hungry craved foods are preferred (Gilhooly et al., 2007) Craving, therefore, may be experienced as a nutritional deficit; a craving for something a little sweeter, more savory, or more filling in one's diet even when not particularly hungry.

5. Hunger will only intensify over time when there is a growing caloric insufficiency whereas elevated cravings can eventually pass with time if not satisfied if the distress can be tolerated. The challenge then is to learn how to fill up on the least addictive foods when hungry while waiting for the craving to pass for the most addictive foods.

6. The working assumption is that cravings will eventually subside for the foods that had been most craved when those foods are no longer eaten at all or only infrequently. Meule (2020) reported that experimental evidence suggests that in the short-term dieting increases food craving for the avoided foods but that long-term energy restriction results in reduced craving among overweight adults. A three-month diet reversed differences in brain activation between participants scoring high and low on a measure of food addiction (Guzzardi et al., 2018).

7. The idea that diets and dieting are part of the problem rather than the solution may only be a partial truth. A starvation diet with too few calories or a diet with serious nutritional deficits, too little fat or to little carbohydrates might be unsustainable as well as unhealthful. Nutritionally balanced diets (i.e., sufficient carbohydrates, sufficient fat, sufficient fiber, sufficient protein) with sufficient calories minus the typical trigger foods none of which are essential for a balanced diet could be sustainable if there is sufficient social support for enduring the withdrawal phase without relapsing until cravings finally begin to subside.

8. As tolerance declines smaller portions of calorie-dense trigger foods may cause indigestion or begin to taste too cloying or too rich providing further disincentive for returning to prior eating habits. There is some experimental evidence that overweight individuals found that ingesting something sweet tasted better to them before and after ingestion than for normal or underweight individuals (Gilbert & Hagen, 1980). Another study found that temptation for highly palatable food results in a decrease in wanting among normal weight women but not overweight women (Ouwehand & de Ridder, 2008). Possibly an extended abstinence from trigger foods eventually decreases the craving for trigger foods and lowers the satiety set points for those foods when ingesting such foods. That may increase the sustainability of a diet in which trigger foods are rarely or never eaten.

If addictions are diseases of denial (Kearney, 1996), then all approaches may have to spend time, sometimes a long time, helping patients learn to accept their affliction without judgment and with self-compassion (i.e., mindfully). Thinking of oneself and accepting oneself as a food addict in recovery may be a necessary ingredient for some individuals to be able to commit themselves to the substantial lifestyle changes that may be required to achieve a sustainable recovery from their addiction (Best et al., 2016).

Carla, a divorced working mother of two, came to therapy to work on relationship problems. Carla was a high weight person who wasn't particularly bothered by her weight, but she did mention having one 'bad' eating habit that she wished to change. Carla drank various fruit juices constantly all day long. Initially she thought it was a healthful thing to do but after doing some reading worried that it couldn't be healthy because of all the sugar she was consuming. She had consulted with a nutritionist to see if there were ways, she could learn to moderate her fruit juice consumption. The nutritionist suggested switching to eating whole fruit as well as reducing her portion sizes of fruit juice. Nevertheless, whole fruit didn't satisfy her craving for pulp-free fruit juice, and she didn't want to stop drinking fruit juice until she felt sated. She didn't know what to do.

I explained the concept of food addiction to her, that she had developed a high tolerance for drinking fruit juice, and that she couldn't reduce her fruit juice consumption without suffering withdrawal symptoms and increased cravings. I suggested that even reasonable portions of fruit juice might not be satiating if it activates the craving for more. Carla responded nondefensively that what I said made intuitive sense though she had never thought of it that way before. Carla conceded that she was most likely a 'fruit juice addict'. Nevertheless, at this point in her life she didn't think she could go 'cold turkey'. It might take some time for her to get her head around the idea of abstinence and having to endure a withdrawal phase. Carla expressed worry that I would think she was resistant if she didn't immediately embrace abstinence as a treatment goal.

To provide autonomy support, I noted that it might take some time to process thinking of herself as suffering from a food addiction and trying to figure out what might be the best way to deal with her affliction given that drinking fruit juice appeared to have become her go-to method of stress reduction. Autonomy support reduced her reactance to the thought of abstinence though she appreciated that would probably be the eventual treatment goal since she had already tried and failed with moderation.

Abstinence versus Moderation

An ongoing controversy in the treatment of substance use addictions are the relative benefits of moderation as compared to abstinence (Storbjörk, 2017). Moderation reduces the potential harm of excessive alcohol or drug use. Abstinence in contrast eliminates the potential harm of continued alcohol or substance abuse so in that sense should be the preferred approach. Despite the superior health benefits of abstinence from alcohol and drugs many individuals will refuse abstinence as a treatment goal or can't sustain it despite giving it their best efforts. Addicted individuals may respond with more reactance to abstinence health messaging than harm reduction (i.e., moderation) health messaging as abstinence may constitute a greater autonomy threat than moderation (Slavin & Earleywine, 2019). They may believe that a life without their preferred substance is too boring, too depressing, too deprived, too frustrating, and too difficult to be endured. They may believe that abstinence is not sustainable for them so they would rather not try at all then try and fail.

Individuals that reject abstinence as a treatment goal may be much more motivated to try to learn to how to moderate their alcohol or substance use rather than abstain from it completely. Yet because of the priming effect of the use of addictive substances like alcohol (Halsall, Jones, Roberts, Knibb, & Rose, 2022), that it may increase rather than decrease craving, moderation, like abstinence, may also be difficult to sustain without relapsing. Individuals may need to learn through trial and error whether abstinence or moderation is most sustainable if there is no single pathway to recovery from addiction that works for everybody.

Recent research has discovered that there can be multiple paths to recovery from alcohol and other drug problems – some involving moderation and some involving abstinence (Eddie, Bergman, Hoffman, & Kelly, 2022). Approximately half of participants who reported having resolved their alcohol or other drug problem accomplished that feat by moderating their usage. The other half were either continuously abstinent or currently abstinent. Though abstinence was not necessary to recover from an alcohol or other drug problem the authors of the study suggested that abstinence is likely to lead to better functioning and well-being.

Unfortunately, research on food addiction treatment has yet to explore the viability of various pathways to recovery. If food addiction is like other addictions, there is no reason to think the results would be different than for alcohol and other drug problems. There may be multiple pathways to recovery, some involving abstinence from the most addictive foods and some involving moderating the consumption of the most addictive foods. Many individuals will refuse to try any diet that requires them to abstain from their favorite calorie-dense foods, like pizza or ice cream, for the rest of their lives. That is too much of a threat to their autonomy regardless of the potential health benefits (i.e., live free or die). For such individuals, complete abstinence is intolerable.

Moderation as well as abstinence may have its limitations for certain individuals. Some food addicted individuals may discover that they are unable to sustain eating their favorite calorie-dense foods in moderation without incremental portion creep over time with its attendant weight regain (James, 2021). Some weight cycling may be a product of failed attempts to sustain eating the more addictive foods in moderation because small portions can increase rather than decrease the craving for more than a taste. Consuming a small portion of an addictive food may trigger a desire to fill up to satiety on the addictive food. Due to the elevated satiety set point that tolerance generates it becomes impossible to feel sated on the addictive food without weight gain.

Satiety set points for the non-addictive foods like fresh fruits, vegetables, and lean meats are more likely to be set more closely to where they would need to be set to achieve and sustain a normal BMI as those foods do not appear to be associated with food addiction (Schulte, Schiestl, & Gearhardt, 2020). This is not to say that one couldn't overeat carrots, bananas, or skinless turkey breast. Nevertheless, the calorie count after overeating non-addictive foods is likely to be less as the satiety set point for those foods will be lower than for the more addictive foods. Thus, if one must overeat something it's better to overeat a non-addictive low-calorie food than an addictive high calorie food as a damage control strategy.

For some individuals, hybrid approaches could be a viable alternative. Most days one abstains from the more addictive foods, but low frequency 'cheat' or 'vacation' days as a reward for the privations of abstinent days could be allowed in which addictive foods are eaten in moderation. Consumption of addictive foods on infrequent cheat/vacation days may make abstinence on most days more tolerable by giving one something to look forward to. If one only eats or overeats addictive foods on infrequent cheat/vacation days, the damages are limited.

Howard had lost substantial weight using a hybrid model that he sustained over a several year period. Most days of the week he only ate fruits, vegetables, and lean meats and rewarded himself eating out with his wife and children once a week on the weekend to eat his favorite foods. Howard counted calories and became upset with himself and assumed I would be upset with him as well for going about 200 calories a day over his daily calorie budget on his abstinent days. In reviewing his daily food log, we discovered that he was overeating cantaloupe, honeydew melon, watermelon, and pineapple, the highest glycemic index fruits, to get his daily sugar fix and not eating that many green vegetables.

To alleviate the perfectionistic self-criticism activated by his conscientious self-monitoring (i.e., a mild case of orthorexia nervosa), I noted that his current approach was proving sustainable as prior to his weight loss he was going 500 to 1000 calories a day above his daily caloric allowance. To alleviate his perfectionistic self-criticism, I noted that what he had already achieved could be seen as good enough, so he need not be so hard on himself. Yet to provide autonomy support, I also noted that setting his own weight loss goals was his prerogative. If he wished to lose more weight, he could try to eat fewer high glycemic index fruits for his daily sugar fix and more green vegetables if that might help him stay within his daily calorie budget. I wanted to help him overcome dichotomous thinking, that there is only one right way to diet, but that there might be multiple pathways to a sustainable recovery that were equally viable. Dichotomous thinking has been linked to overly rigid dietary restraint and weight regain (Palascha, van Kleef, & van Trijp, 2015).

Treatment of Food Addiction

It's not clear to what extent the concept of food addiction requires entirely new approaches to weight management. Behavioral weight loss treatment has been shown to reduce food addiction as measured by the YAFS (Chao et al., 2019). Mindful eating has also been shown to reduce food addiction as measured by the YAFS (Kaya Cebioğlu et al., 2022). An attachment-based approach to food addiction has been developed but outcome research has yet to be conducted on that approach (Pennock, 2022). An Acceptance and Commitment Therapy approach to food addiction has also been proposed but outcome research has yet to be conducted (Cattivelli et al., 2015). Any approach that significantly lowers BMI most likely lowers food addiction as BMI and food addiction are correlated among individuals with Type 2 diabetes (Raymond, Kannis-Dymand, & Lovell, 2018). Recently, developed weight loss drugs appear to reduce craving so may also reduce food addiction (Blum, 2023).

The only approach that has been developed over the years that is specifically designed to treat food addiction has been 12-step self-help approaches such as Overeaters Anonymous or Food Addicts in Recovery Anonymous. Overeaters Anonymous (OA) was founded in 1960 on the model of Alcoholics Anonymous to treat compulsive overeating as a disease, an addiction like alcoholism (Suler & Barthelomew, 1986). OA assumes that compulsive overeating is beyond volitional control so one must surrender to a higher power. There is no shame in this admission since the loss of volitional control of eating behavior is the function of a disease process rather than a moral failure. Adopting a social identity as a food addict in recovery without shame but with self-acceptance and self-compassion is an essential aspect of recovery. Letting go of perfectionistic needs for control with its attendant feelings of failure facilitate greater self-acceptance (Ronel & Libman, 2003). One's self-identity evolves from being an addict to being an addict in recovery (Best et al., 2016). Relinquishing denial about the nature of the problem is required to accept the difficult lifestyle changes that would need to be made if one is going to live one's life according to the 12-steps listed below.

1. Admitting powerlessness over the addiction.
2. Believing that a higher power (in whatever form) can help.
3. Deciding to turn control over to the higher power.
4. Taking a personal inventory.
5. Admitting to the higher power, oneself, and another person the wrongs done.
6. Being ready to have the higher power correct any shortcomings in one's character.

7. Asking the higher power to remove those shortcomings.
8. Making a list of wrongs done to others and being willing to make amends for those wrongs.
9. Contacting those who have been hurt, unless doing so would harm the person.
10. Continuing to take personal inventory and admitting when one is wrong.
11. Seeking enlightenment and connection with the higher power via prayer and meditation.
12. Carrying the message of the 12 Steps to others in need (Alcoholics Anonymous World Services, 1952).

Twelve-step programs offer unlimited opportunities for attending self-help support groups on an as needed basis. Twelve-step programs also provide sponsors on an as needed basis to provide round the clock individual support when needed. Addicts in recovery are also encouraged to provide sponsorship to others as part of their recovery. Research suggests that the high level of social support that OA provides appears to facilitate secure attachment, an important ingredient of improved emotion regulation (Hertz, Addad, & Ronel, 2012). The problems of craving and withdrawal are addressed when they become intolerable by providing unlimited social support on an as needed basis.

This provision of comprehensive and free social support contrasts with approaches that center on improving one's capacity for self-regulation through teaching skills like mindful eating or distress tolerance. The 12-step assumption is that self-regulation based on will-power will be unreliable in the face of intolerable craving and withdrawal symptoms. Research suggests that willpower (i.e., volitional control) is a limited resource under stress. Stress can generate states of ego depletion that leaves no energy left for exercising self-control (Baumeister, Tice, & Vohs, 2018).

Twelve-step programs support abstinence, but abstinence is based on discovering one's trigger foods. The assumption is that food addicts know which foods they are most likely and least likely to overeat. An honest personal inventory would reveal one's trigger foods. Abstinence is not absolute and not necessarily all or none when it comes to food addiction. It's best not to overly restrict caloric intake lest excessive hunger further weaken one's already impaired self-control (Wilcox, 2021). OA encourages the adoption of a food plan that outlines one's individualized approach to abstinence, and it appears that relapse is less frequent the better the adherence to the overall program (Kriz, 2002).

A 12-step approach is a long-term, if not lifelong approach, that allows one to go at one's own pace so may generate less reactance than programs that require individuals to progress through a sequence of steps on a set timetable. It assumes that relapse is common and provides ongoing social support in the face of relapse. Studies regarding the effectiveness of OA remain scarce (Schulte et al., 2015) and not everyone is willing to give it a try.

OA does appear to generate significant reactance as different aspects may constitute an autonomy threat to certain individuals. 1) High weight individuals might resent the implication that they are powerless over addiction when food addiction might be a fictitious concept that stigmatizes high weight individuals. 2) OA might seem cultlike if it requires certain spiritual beliefs. They don't want to attend a group with true believers who will judge them if they don't succumb to indoctrination. 3) Individuals who hope to learn to eat their favorite calorie-dense processed foods in moderation don't want to have to abstain from 'forbidden' or 'bad' foods because of their addictive and fattening properties.

4) Individuals don't want to be that dependent on others for social support in managing craving and withdrawal. 5) It's too time consuming to attend all those meetings. For these reasons psychotherapists who recommend OA as an adjunct to individual psychotherapy might be met with considerable skepticism and reactance from patients who aren't ready for something that programmatic.

Patients who do find 12-step type approaches useful in dealing with their addictive tendencies will want to work with psychotherapists who are knowledgeable and supportive of that approach to recovery. Ruptures to the therapeutic relationship may arise if patients committed to 12-step approaches sense therapists' implicit skepticism to an approach in which patients believe and which appears to be working for them.

Food Addiction and Stigma

A feminist critique of 12-step programs and Overeaters Anonymous suggested that the concepts of disease, powerlessness, codependency, and abstinence may be unsuitable for the treatment of women. Such concepts were originally developed to help white middle-class alcoholic men (van Wormer, 1994). Nevertheless, others have suggested that the Awareness/Acceptance/Action Model, used frequently in 12-step programs, is a means by which to take initial steps to become aware of privilege and address oppression (Crisp, 2014).

Research has been conducted to assess the degree that the concept of food addiction creates a new stigmatized identity that pathologizes high weight individuals or perhaps alleviates weight stigma by construing high body weight as a function of an unfortunate affliction for which the individual does not possess moral culpability. Severity of food addiction is indeed associated with weight stigma and weight-related self-devaluation (Meadows & Higgs, 2020). Yet correlation does not equal causation. Interventions targeting food addiction appear to reduce weight-related self-stigma (Ahorsu et al., 2020). Viewing high weight individuals as suffering from food addiction appears to decrease weight stigma, blame, and perceived psychopathology in comparison to a non-addiction model of body weight (Latner, Puhl, Murakami, & O'Brien, 2014).

Food addiction appears to be associated with childhood trauma and is mediated by emotional dysregulation (Hoover, Yu, Duval, & Gearhardt, 2022) and minority stress is associated with trauma (Charak, Cano-Gonzalez, Ronzón-Tirado, Ford, Byllesby, Shevlin, Karatzias, Hyland, & Cloitre, 2023). Consequently, minorities who have experienced traumatic levels of minority stress growing up or currently may gain weight due to food addiction and then suffer weight stigma because of their weight. Sexual minorities appear to suffer twice the prevalence rate of food addiction in comparison to heterosexuals and it appears to be associated with heterosexist harassment (Rainey, Furman, & Gearhardt, 2018). African American women with Type 2 diabetes suffer greater insulin resistance the greater their food addiction and their food addiction is associated with childhood trauma (Stojek, Maples-Keller, Dixon, Umpierrez, Gillespie, & Michopoulos, 2019). Consequently, it may be important to find treatment approaches that address minority stress, childhood trauma, food addiction, and weight stigma simultaneously and their complex inter-relationships.

James was a successful African American attorney who came for psychotherapy for help with marital conflicts. He also suffered considerable minority stress as the only black man at his law firm. His children were enrolled at an exclusive private school in which his children were the only black children. At school events James perceived himself as a 'black dot in a sea of white'. James was very health conscious as his overweight father dropped dead of a heart attack when he was 12 years old. It was a traumatic loss, and he didn't want to follow in his father's footsteps in that regard. He went to the gym regularly and was quite muscular.

One day his wife affectionately teased him that he was developing a gut though it wasn't particularly noticeable given his broad shoulders. James realized that he was compulsively eating calorie-dense energy bars to alleviate his minority stress. He thought of energy bars as a health food rather than as a highly palatable processed food with addictive qualities. Once James appreciated that for him energy bars had become a trigger food, he stopped eating them. I noted that he needn't succumb to fat phobia when his wife teased him about having a gut because he appeared to be a healthy individual who received good reports at his yearly physicals. James replied that when it came to his health, he'd rather be safe than sorry and err on the side of caution. Autonomy support meant supporting his weight loss effort though to some that effort might have seemed unduly perfectionistic due to internalized weight stigma.

Research suggests that the perfectionism associated with being a 'model minority' has positive as well as negative aspects (Yao, 2010). It may be a form of dichotomous thinking to assume that perfectionism and dietary restraint are always 'bad' as though there are not adaptive forms of perfectionism and inflexibility reflective of a certain type of stubborn determination to do one's best in the face of adversity.

Those who identify as food addicts in recovery and use a food plan that includes abstinence as well as other forms of self-monitoring may suffer divergent weight management stigma (Romo, 2018). Others might observe that food addicts in recovery don't necessarily eat more intuitively or more flexibly like everyone else as their eating appears rule bound. They might abstain from certain calorie-dense foods, they might count their calories, they might bring their own food to social occasions, they might take visibly small servings without going for seconds, they might eat on a schedule, and they might avoid situations where there would be too much temptation. Others might judge food addicts in recovery as being excessively rigid in their approach to eating.

If others realize that the self-identified food addict in recovery participates in a 12-step type program of recovery, they might be perceived as a brainwashed member of a cult who might try to impose their excessively self-denying dietary rules on others as they look for converts. If others believe that the food addict's food plan is excessively strict, they assume it will eventually backfire and they will regain lost weight if not more. Consequently, they may instill doubt in the long-term viability of an approach that appears to be working for the time being. They might believe that relapse necessarily means that the food plan isn't working rather than that relapse is a common occurrence in the process of recovery and that individuals can tweak their approach as they learn from their mistakes. Thus, self-identified food addicts must maintain their commitment to their approach in the face of judgment and skepticism from individuals who find their approach objectionable and assume that they know better.

Food addicts in recovery might feel a need to hide their divergent approach to eating because they don't want to be judged for their divergent eating habits. Self-identified food addicts in recovery may therefore suffer a form of minority stress for their non-normative weight management practices. This is not to say that 12-step approaches and abstinence works for everybody or to deny the fact that some people have negative experiences with 12-step type approaches. Rather it is to appreciate that there are multiple pathways to recovery from food addiction and some people can sustain significant weight loss over the long-term utilizing this outlook despite the social stigma to which they are subjected.

References

Ahorsu, D. K., Lin, C.-Y., Imani, V., Griffiths, M. D., Su, J.-A., Latner, J. D., Marshall, R. D., & Pakpour, A. H. (2020). A prospective study on the link between weight-related self- stigma and binge eating: Role of food addiction and psychological distress. *International Journal of Eating Disorders*, 53(3), 442–450. https://doi.org/10.1002/eat.2321

Ahmed, S. H. (2012). Is sugar as addictive as cocaine? In K. D. Brownell & M. S. Gold, *Food and addiction: A comprehensive handbook* (pp. 232–237). Oxford University Press. https://doi.org/10.1093/med:psych/9780199738168.003.003

Alcoholics Anonymous World Services (1952). *Twelve steps and twelve traditions*. New York, NY: Author.

Baumeister, R. F., Tice, D. M., & Vohs, K. D. (2018). The strength model of self-regulation: Conclusions from the second decade of willpower research. *Perspectives on Psychological Science*, 13(2), 141–145. https://doi.org/10.1177/1745691617716946

Berthoud, H.-R. (2012). Central regulation of hunger, satiety, and body weight. In K. D. Brownell & M. S. Gold, *Food and addiction: A comprehensive handbook* (pp. 97–102). Oxford University Press.

Best, D., Beckwith, M., Haslam, C., Haslam, S. A., Jetten, J., Mawson, E., & Lubman, D. I. (2016). Overcoming alcohol and other drug addiction as a process of social identity transition: The social identity model of recovery (SIMOR). *Addiction Research & Theory*, 24(2), 111–123. https://doi.org/10.3109/16066359.2015.107598024.

Blum, D. (2023). The diabetes drug that could overshadow Ozempic. *New York Times*. April 11, 2023.

Blumenthal, K., DuPont, R. L., & Gold, M. S. (2012). Treatment of alcohol and drug dependence in 2011 and relevance to food addiction. In K. D. Brownell & M. S. Gold (Eds.), *Food and addiction: A comprehensive handbook* (pp. 318–328). Oxford University Press. https://doiorg.1093/med:psych/9780199738168.003.0048

Cattivelli, R., Pietrabissa, G., Ceccarini, M., Spatola, C. A. M., Villa, V., Caretti, A., Gatti, A., Manzoni, G. M., & Castelnuovo, G. (2015). ACTonFOOD: Opportunities of ACT to address food addiction. *Frontiers in Psychology*, 6, Article 396. https://doi.org/10.3389/fpsyg.2015.00396

Chao, A. M., Wadden, T. A., Tronieri, J. S., Pearl, R. L., Alamuddin, N., Bakizada, Z. M., Pinkasavage, E., Leonard, S. M., Alfaris, N., & Berkowitz, R. I. (2019). Effects of addictive-like eating behaviors on weight loss with behavioral obesity treatment. *Journal of Behavioral Medicine*, 42(2), 246–255. https://doi.org/10.1007/s10865-018-9958-z

Charak, R., Cano-Gonzalez, I., Ronzón-Tirado, R., Ford, J. D., Byllesby, B. M., Shevlin, M., Karatzias, T., Hyland, P., & Cloitre, M. (2023). Factor structure of the international trauma questionnaire in trauma exposed LGBTQ+ adults: Role of cumulative traumatic events and minority stress heterosexist experiences. *Psychological Trauma: Theory, Research, Practice and Policy*, 10.1037/tra0001440. Advance online publication. https://doi.org/10.1037/tra0001440

Crisp, C. (2014). White and lesbian: Intersections of privilege and oppression. *Journal of Lesbian Studies*, 18(2), 106–117. https://doi.org/10.1080/10894160.2014.849161

DePierre, J. A., Puhl, R. M., & Luedicke, J. (2013). A new stigmatized identity? Comparisons of a "food addict" label with other stigmatized health conditions. *Basic and Applied Social Psychology*, 35(1), 10–21. https://doi.org/10.1080/01973533.2012.746148

DiFeliceantonio, A. G., Coppin, G., Rigoux, L., Edwin Thanarajah, S., Dagher, A., Tittgemeyer, M., & Small, D. M. (2018). Supra-additive effects of combining fat and carbohydrate on food reward. *Cell Metabolism*, 28(1), 33–44.e3. https://doi.org/10.1016/j.cmet.2018.05.018

Eddie, D., Bergman, B. G., Hoffman, L. A., & Kelly, J. F. (2022). Abstinence versus moderation recovery pathways following resolution of a substance use problem: Prevalence, predictors, and relationship to psychosocial well-being in a U.S. national sample. *Alcoholism: Clinical and Experimental Research*, 46(2), 312–325. https://doi-org/10.1111/acer.14765

Gearhardt, A. N., Corbin, W. R., & Brownell, K. D. (2009). Preliminary validation of the Yale Food Addiction Scale. *Appetite*, 52(2), 430–436. https://doi.org/10.1016/j.appet.2008.12.003

Gearhardt, A. N., Corbin, W. R., & Brownell, K. D. (2016). Development of the Yale Food Addiction Scale version 2.0. *Psychology of Addictive Behaviors*, 30(1), 113–121. https://doi.org/10.1037/adb0000136

Gilbert, D. G., & Hagen, R. L. (1980). Taste in underweight, overweight, and normal-weight subjects before, during, and after sucrose ingestion. *Addictive Behaviors*, 5(2), 137–142. https://doi.org/10.1016/0306-4603(80)90031-3

Gilhooly, C. H., Das, S. K., Golden, J. K., McCrory, M. A., Dallal, G. E., Saltzman, E., Kramer, F. M., & Roberts, S. B. (2007). Food cravings and energy regulation: The characteristics of craved foods and their relationship with eating behaviors and weight change during 6 months of dietary energy restriction. *International Journal of Obesity* (2005), 31(12), 1849–1858. https://doi.org/10.1038/sj.ijo.0803672

Greaney, M. L., Less, F. D., White, A. A., Dayton, S. F., Riebe, D., Blissmer, B., Shoff, S., Walsh, J. R., & Greene, G. W. (2009). College students' barriers and enablers for healthful weight management: A qualitative study. *Journal of Nutrition Education and Behavior*, 41(4), 281–286. https://doi.org/10.1016/j.jneb.2008.04.354

Guzzardi, M. A., Garelli, S., Agostini, A., Filidei, E., Fanelli, F., Giorgetti, A., Mezzullo, M., Fucci, S., Mazza, R., Vicennati, V., Iozzo, P., & Pagotto, U. (2018). Food addiction distinguishes an overweight phenotype that can be reversed by low calorie diet. *European Eating Disorders Review: The Journal of the Eating Disorders Association*, 26(6), 657–670. https://doi.org/10.1002/erv.2652

Halsall, L., Jones, A., Roberts, C., Knibb, G., & Rose, A. K. (2022). The impact of alcohol priming on craving and motivation to drink: A meta-analysis. *Addiction*, 117(12), 2986–3003. https://doi.org/10.1111/add.15962

Hertz, P., Addad, M., & Ronel, N. (2012). Attachment styles and changes among women members of overeaters anonymous who have recovered from binge-eating disorder. *Health & Social Work*, 37(2), 110–122. https://doi.org/10.1093/hsw/hls019

Hoover, L. V., Yu, H. P., Duval, E. R., & Gearhardt, A. N. (2022). Childhood trauma and food addiction: The role of emotion regulation difficulties and gender differences. *Appetite*, 177, 1–8. https://doi-org/10.1016/j.appet.2022.106137

Hutchinson E. (2011). Systems neuroscience: The stress of dieting. *Nature reviews Neuroscience*, 12(2), 65. https://doi.org/10.1038/nrn2985

James, B. L. (2021). Identifying early predictors of success and valid measures of eating behavior and diet satisfaction in a portion-control weight loss trial. *Dissertation Abstracts International: Section B: The Sciences and Engineering*, 82(5-B).

Kaya Cebioğlu, İ., Dumlu Bilgin, G., Kavsara, H. K., Gül Koyuncu, A., Sarioğlu, A., Aydin, S., & Keküllüoğlu, M. (2022). Food addiction among university students: The effect of mindful eating. *Appetite*, 177, 106133. https://doi.org/10.1016/j.appet.2022.106133

Kearney, R. J. (1996). *Within the wall of denial: Conquering addictive behaviors*. W. W. Norton & Co.

Knee, C. R., & Zuckerman, M. (1998). A nondefensive personality: Autonomy and control as moderators of defensive coping and self-handicapping. *Journal of Research in Personality*, 32(2), 115–130. https://doi.org/10.1006/jrpe.1997.2207

Kriz, M. (2002). The efficacy of Overeaters Anonymous in fostering abstinence in binge-eating disorder and bulimia nervosa. *PhD in Counselor Education, Virginia Polytechnic Institute and State University*.

Latner, J. D., Puhl, R. M., Murakami, J. M., & O'Brien, K. S. (2014). Food addiction as a causal model of obesity. Effects on stigma, blame, and perceived psychopathology. *Appetite*, 77, 77–82. https://doi.org/10.1016/j.appet.2014.03.004

Meadows, A., & Higgs, S. (2020). Internalized weight stigma and the progression of food addiction over time. *Body Image*, 34, 67–71. https://doi-org/10.1016/j.bodyim.2020.05.002

Meule, M. A. (2020). The psychology of food cravings: The role of food deprivation. *Current Nutrition Reports*, 9, 251–257. https://doi.org/10.1007/s13668-020-00326-0

Meule, A., & Gearhardt, A. N. (2014). Five years of the Yale Food Addiction Scale: Taking stock and moving forward. *Current Addiction Reports*, 1, 193–205. http://dx.doi.org/10.1007/s40429-014-0021-z

Moss, M. (2014). *Salt sugar fat: How the food giants hooked us*. New York: Random House.

Ouwehand, C., & de Ridder, D. T. (2008). Effects of temptation and weight on hedonics and motivation to eat in women. *Obesity (Silver Spring, Md.)*, 16(8), 1788–1793. https://doi.org/10.1038/oby.2008.316

Palascha, A., van Kleef, E., & van Trijp, H. C. (2015). How does thinking in black and white terms relate to eating behavior and weight regain? *Journal of Health Psychology*, 20(5), 638–648. https://doi.org/10.1177/1359105315573440

Parylak, S. L., Koob, G. F., & Zorrilla, E. P. (2011). The dark side of food addiction. *Physiology & Behavior*, 104(1), 149–156. https://doi.org/10.1016/j.physbeh.2011.04.063

Pennock, S. (2022). Dysfunctional eating in recovering addicts: A therapist's shift to an attachment-focused approach. In L. Cundy (Ed.), *Attachment, relationships and food: From cradle to kitchen* (pp. 96–115). Routledge/Taylor & Francis Group.

Pursey, K. M., Stanwell, P., Gearhardt, A. N., Collins, C. E., & Burrows, T. L. (2014). The prevalence of food addiction as assessed by the Yale Food Addiction Scale: A systematic review. *Nutrients*, 6, 4552–4590. http://dx.doi.org/10.3390/nu6104552

Rainey, J. C., Furman, C. R., & Gearhardt, A. N. (2018). Food addiction among sexual minorities. *Appetite*, 120, 16–22. https://doi.org/10.1016/j.appet.2017.08.019

Ranteallo, I. C., & Andilolo, I. R. (2017). Food representation and media: Experiencing culinary tourism through foodgasm and foodporn. In: Saufi, A., Andilolo, I., Othman, N., Lew, A. A. (Eds.), *Balancing development and sustainability in tourism destinations.* Springer, Singapore. https://doi.org/10.1007/978-981-10-1718-6_13

Raymond, K. L., Kannis-Dymand, L., & Lovell, G. P. (2018). A graduated food addiction classification approach significantly differentiates obesity among people with Type 2 diabetes. *Journal of Health Psychology*, 23(14), 1781–1789. https://doi.org/10.1177/1359105316672096

Rodríguez-Martín, B. C., & Gallego-Arjiz, B. (2018). Overeaters Anonymous: A mutual-help fellowship for food addiction recovery. *Frontiers in Psychology*, 9, 1491. https://doi.org/10.3389/fpsyg.2018.01491

Romo L. K. (2018). An examination of how people who have lost weight communicatively negotiate interpersonal challenges to weight management. *Health Communication*, 33(4), 469–477. https://doi.org/10.1080/10410236.2016.1278497

Ronel, N. & Libman, G. (2003). Eating disorders and recovery: Lessons from Overeaters Anonymous. *Clinical Social Work Journal*, 31, 155–171 (2003). https://doi.org/10.1023/A:1022962311073

Schulte, E. M., Joyner, M. A., Potenza, M. N., Grilo, C. M., & Gearhardt, A. N. (2015). Current considerations regarding food addiction. *Current Psychiatry Reports*, 17(4), 563. https://doi.org/10.1007/s11920-015-0563-3

Schulte, E. M., Schiestl, E. T., & Gearhardt, A. N. (2020). Food versus eating addictions. In S. Sussman (Ed.), *The Cambridge handbook of substance and behavioral addictions* (pp.340–351). Cambridge University Press. https://doi-org.adelphi.idm.oclc.org/10.1017/9781108632591.035

Schulte, E. M., Smeal, J. K., Lewis, J., & Gearhardt, A. N. (2018). Development of the Highly Processed Food Withdrawal Scale. *Appetite*, 131, 148–154. https://doi.org/10.1016/j.appet.2018.09.013

Slavin, M. N., & Earleywine, M. (2019). Effects of messaging and psychological reactance on marijuana craving. *Substance Use & Misuse*, 54(14), 2359–2367. https://doi.org/10.1080/10826084.2019.1650771

Sodus, M. B. (2014). A resource guide for mindful eating. *Bariatric Surgical Practice and Patient Care*, 9(1), 51–52. https://doi.org/10.1089/bari.2014.9962

Stojek, M. M., Maples-Keller, J. L., Dixon, H. D., Umpierrez, G. E., Gillespie, C. F., & Michopoulos, V. (2019). Associations of childhood trauma with food addiction and insulin resistance in African-American women with diabetes mellitus. *Appetite*, 141, 104317. https://doi.org/10.1016/j.appet.2019.104317

Storbjörk, J. (2017). Commentary on Witkiewitz et al. (2017): Abstinence or moderation—A choice for whom and why? *Addiction*, 112(12), 2122–2123. https://doi-org/10.1111/add.14042

Suler, J., & Barthelomew, E. (1986). The ideology of Overeaters Anonymous. *Social Policy*, 16, 48–53.

van Kleef, E., Shimizu, M., & Wansink, B. (2013). Just a bite: Considerably smaller snack portions satisfy delayed hunger and craving. *Food Quality and Preference*, 27(1), 96–100. https://doi.org/10.1016/j.foodqual.2012.06.008

van Wormer, K. (1994). "Hi, I'm Jane; I'm a compulsive overeater". In P. Fallon, M. A. Katzman, & S. C. Wooley (Eds.), *Feminist perspectives on eating disorders* (pp. 287–298). The Guilford Press.

Vasiliu, O. (2022). Current status of evidence for a new diagnosis: Food addiction—A literature review. *Frontiers in Psychiatry*, 12, 824936. https://doi-org/10.3389/fpsyt.2021.824936

Wiedemann, A. A., Carr, M. M., Ivezaj, V., & Barnes, R. D. (2021). Examining the construct validity of food addiction severity specifiers. *Eating and Weight Disorders*, 26(5), 1503–1509. https://doi-org/10.1007/s40519-020-00957-w

Wilcox, C. E. (2021). Food addiction, obesity, and disorders of overeating: An evidence-based assessment and clinical guide. *Springer Nature Switzerland AG*. https://doi-org/10.1007/978-3-030-83078-6

Yao, M. P. (2010). An exploration of multidimensional perfectionism, academic self-efficacy, procrastination frequency, and Asian American cultural values in Asian American university students. *Dissertation Abstracts International: Section B: The Sciences and Engineering*, 70(10-B), 6597.

The Evolution of Human Food Sharing and Feasting

5

Evolutionary psychology is not associated with any specific treatment approach, but evolutionary psychology does clarify what is adaptive or maladaptive behavior from an evolutionary perspective. From the psychotherapeutic perspective, supporting patients' autonomous self-determination is supporting adaptive behavior (Ford, 2021). Unwittingly supporting maladaptive behavior would be doing patients a disservice if such behavior is misguided or self-defeating and prevents patients from becoming their best selves. If dietary restraint is maladaptive behavior because it contributes to uncontrolled eating (Manasse, Lampe, Abber, Fitzpatrick, Srivastava, & Juarascio, 2023), it might be best to stop supporting dieting and start supporting an anti-diet philosophy. If overeating and attendant weight gain is maladaptive because it increases the risk of acquiring a metabolic syndrome and/or impedes successful mating in certain socioeconomic contexts, it might be better not to support it. It would be better to support lifestyle changes that would contribute to sustainable weight loss maintenance (Garcia-Silva, Borrego, Navarrete, Peralta-Ramirez, Águila, & Caballo, 2022).

Autonomy support, though, isn't necessarily about supporting what therapists believe is adaptive or maladaptive based on their training, clinical experiences, personal experiences, and cultural biases. Therapists are certainly entitled to entertain such opinions and to express such opinions if they aim to be authentic and transparent therapists. All the evidence-based psychotherapies focus on the development of a trusting treatment alliance and the need for transparency and authenticity in this alliance (New, Perez-Rodriguez, & Rosenberg, 2017). Autonomy support first requires looking at what appears adaptive from patients' internal frame of reference (Ryan & Deci, 2019). It is then supporting what patients believe upon reflection is most adaptive for them given their unique individuality in their specific circumstances at this point in their lives; albeit factoring in a consideration of what their therapists believe to be most adaptive and their therapists' rationale for those beliefs.

When patients are of two minds about what is most adaptive, autonomy support from the perspective of motivational interviewing is supporting patients' independent decision making until they make up their minds for themselves (Villarosa-Hurlocker, O'Sickey, Houck, & Moyers, 2019). Weight management specialists are free to practice their specialty from their own weight management philosophy and only work with patients who already subscribe to that philosophy or who might be readily converted to their philosophy with some psychoeducation. Generalist psychotherapists don't have that luxury as their task is to help clarify patients' weight management concerns, establish weight management goals, explore the pros and cons of various weight management strategies, and ultimately support

DOI: 10.4324/9781003402336-8

patients' independent decision making. Generalist psychotherapists may make a referral to a weight management specialist or program if needed as an adjunct to or sometimes instead of psychotherapy cognizant of the substantial differences in approach of the various weight management specialists.

When higher weight patients seek psychotherapy for reasons other than their weight, like relationship problems, it is quite possible that psychotherapy will run its course without weight ever becoming a central problem to be addressed though it might be raised in passing. Such patients may accept their current weight and have no desire to diet. Autonomy support is then respecting their independent decision making in that regard.

When higher weight patients make weight a central problem to be addressed, it is often because they wish to lose weight for reasons that seem perfectly valid to them (i.e., looking more attractive and/or being healthier) and are seeking psychotherapeutic support to reach their weight loss goals. Autonomy support for such patients usually means following patients' lead in making the sorts of changes they aspire to make, seeing to what extent patients want a traveling companion or a guide on their weight management journeys, and providing patients space to discover for themselves through trial and error what works for them. Trial and error learning is an essential part of a reflective practice when trying to avoid a one-size-fits-all approach (Price & Deveci, 2022). Ruptures to the therapeutic alliance will likely occur when patients feel therapists are insufficiently supportive of their autonomous efforts to manage their weights in their own way on their own timetable.

Autonomy support is not necessarily undermined when patients and therapists possess a different opinion about the optimal weight management strategy. It can be therapeutic when patients learn how to have a respectful difference of opinion with someone who is allowed to have a mind of their own. A therapist who always and only validates patients' viewpoints is not equipping patients to deal with the realities of close relationships in which learning to negotiate conflicting points of view is essential to relationship satisfaction (Girma Shifaw, 2022). Yet patients' autonomy is undermined when therapists appear to be imposing their own point of view on uninformed, confused, indecisive, suggestible, or skeptical patients.

Patients, therapists, researchers, and science journalists may think of what is adaptive or maladaptive in dichotomous black or white ways. Dichotomous thinking such as thinking in terms of good and bad carbs or good and bad fat has been associated with various psychopathologies as well as eating disorders (Antoniou, Bongers, & Jansen, 2017). A common factor of successful psychotherapy of eating disorders may be helping patients overcome dichotomous thinking about their weight management challenges (Alberts, Thewissen, & Raes, 2012).

Contemporary evolutionary psychology has developed a sophisticated way of thinking about adaptation in terms of trade-offs and cost-benefit analyses that make it clear that adaptations are never simply good or bad/healthy or unhealthy but always contain significant costs as well as benefits. Those trade-offs vary for different individuals, in different circumstances, during different points in their life histories (Kaplan & Gangestad, 2005).

The Adaptationist Perspective

The adaptationist perspective of evolutionary psychology can begin to clarify controversies about what are or aren't healthful eating habits. Adaptation is not just about survival of the fittest. Adaptation is also about reproductive success and proceeds through processes of sexual selection (Darwin, 1871). Organisms that are successful in passing on their genes to subsequent generations are the drivers of evolution. An adaptive trait confers a reproductive advantage (Ash & Gallup, 2008).

Organisms that engage in parenting must survive long enough until offspring can survive on their own. If humans have evolved to engage in grandparenting, humans may have to survive a little bit longer to help raise the grandchildren (Hawkes, O'Connell, & Jones, 2003). In humans, reproductive success is partly a function of attracting of partners of high mate value (Symons, 1987), hence the importance of physical attractiveness, and partly a functioning of one's success at biparental care and grandparenting, hence the importance of partially heritable personality characteristics like altruistic self-sacrifice for the sake of family (Figueredo, Vásquez, Brumbach, & Schneider, 2004).

Adaptations reflect implicit cost-benefit analyses (Kaplan & Gangestad, 2005). For example, growing a big body can be adaptive if it makes one better able to defend oneself or attack others, better able to engage in heavy lifting, or sufficiently tall to reach things that are higher up. Because a big body may be associated with these adaptive traits it could be construed as a 'sexually selected indicator of fitness' (Andersson, 1994) that makes one attractive to potential mates or intimidating to potential rivals. But growing a big body comes at a cost. One must consume more calories to maintain it. When those calories are hard to find, having to maintain a big body can be a liability. Growing a smaller body can be adaptive in an environment where food is scarce as a smaller body can be maintained with fewer calories and the fewer calories one consumes the more calories that remain available for one's offspring who might have a better chance of survival when food is scarce.

Cost-benefit analyses vary depending on the nature of the environment in which one must survive and reproduce. What is adaptive in one environment may be maladaptive in another environment. Aquatic mammals like whales accumulate quite a bit of body fat (i.e., blubber) that helps them stay warm in cold waters. Many mammals, like bears, accumulate quite a bit of body fat in warmer months to store the energy that will help them survive a long winter when food is scarce. Yet accumulation of body fat might be maladaptive for predators like a cheetah for whom speed is of the essence if excess body fat might slow them down. Species vary in how much body fat they tend to accumulate depending on how adaptive it would be to accumulate body fat in a particular ecological niche and there are individual differences within species. Natural selection works on individual variation within species as some individual differences are more adaptive in some environments than others (Darwin, 1871).

Animals that possess cognitive flexibility can be adaptable to a wide variety of ecological niches (Biolsi & Woo, 2022). Humans can survive where it's hot or where it's cold, where it's wet or where it's dry, where food is abundant or where it's scarce. The invention of highly palatable highly processed high carbohydrate/ high fat/ low fiber food is a recent product of human technological and culinary ingenuity. The question is then what is the cost-benefit analysis of consuming such highly processed calorie-dense foods for different people, in different environmental situations at different points in their lifespans. For example, as mortality looms with increasing age there may be an ultimately futile hope to 'cheat death' by living a healthful lifestyle or more realistically to slow down the aging process as much as humanly feasible (Kaeberlein, Rabinovitch, & Martin, 2015).

Body weight can be an indicator of social status depending on the sociocultural context. High body weight can signal high status under sociocultural conditions in which mostly poor people are thin and only the rich people can afford to fill themselves on calorie-dense food. The social benefits of signaling one's high social status through high body weight in food scarce environments might outweigh the potential costs of acquiring a metabolic syndrome later in life after one is done with mating and parenting. Low body weight can suggest high social status under sociocultural conditions in which poor people have ample access to cheap highly palatable food and only the rich people can afford an expensive year-round diet of fresh fruits, vegetables, and seafood as well as personal trainers. The social benefits of remaining thin in food rich environments might exceed the costs of all the time, money, and angst spent 'working' at remaining thin. There may be intersectionality between weight stigma and classism if high body weight makes one vulnerable to the stigma of being considered low class (Chrisler & Barney, 2017).

Autonomy support in psychotherapy may mean clarifying the cost-benefit analyses of being fat or thin in patients' particular circumstances given their unique individuality at this time in their life and then respecting their own assessment of whether the benefits exceed the costs given their values and priorities. These calculations may vary across the lifespan. Patients may want to be thin when they are young adults trying to attract a desirable life partner, allow themselves to acquire a 'dad bod' or 'mom bod' while stressed out raising a family and making a living, and then perhaps want to lose weight once again when the nest is empty to mitigate the risk of acquiring a metabolic syndrome as a senior citizen. Or perhaps individuals might want to spend their golden years eating whatever they like and let nature takes its course. From the point of view of autonomy support to each his own and different strokes for different folks.

A problem with one-size-fits-all approaches to weight management is that such approaches may overgeneralize a preferred conception of what is adaptive (i.e., healthful) eating as though it's a black or white issue and as though there is but one correct approach for everybody despite their unique individuality, unique circumstances, and time of life. Conscientiously counting calories may be significantly correlated with weight loss maintenance (Gold et al., 2020) but not for everybody as the correlations are far from perfect (i.e., $r < 1.0$). Dietary restraint may be significantly correlated with eating disorders (Manasse, Lampe, Abber, Fitzpatrick, Srivastava, & Juarascio, 2023) but not for everybody as for some people dietary restraint may be associated with recovery from food addiction. High weight may be associated with certain life-threatening metabolic syndromes but not for everyone. Nor should it be assumed that everyone can be healthy at any size if they just follow certain lifestyle prescriptions.

Certain evidence-based approaches may work on average but not for everybody and some people may have negative therapeutic reactions (Rozental, Kottorp, Forsström, Månsson, Boettcher, Andersson, Furmark, & Carlbring, 2019). Research demonstrates significant trends in large groups of people of what may be small, moderate, or large effect sizes but that does not yield results that are true for everybody in all circumstances at all points in the life cycle. Psychotherapists must deal with unique individuals who may not be reflective of the statistically significant group averages that research reveals not infrequently of small effect sizes.

One element of individual variability when it comes to weight management is genetic predisposition as body weight possesses a significant hereditability (Farooqi, 2018). A genetic predisposition to develop an endomorphic body is a genotype. The phenotype is how that genetic predisposition expresses itself in a particular environment. Many individual difference variables, like personality traits, have significant heritability (Zwir et al., 2020) but are not entirely determined by genetics as are physical traits like blue eyes. The field of behavioral ecology studies how anthropomorphic changes (i.e., human built environments) influence gene expression in humans and other species (Gabor, Lindström, & Macias Garcia, 2022).

In a high stress food rich human built environment, the emergent phenotype might be the following for those with an endomorphic genotype: 1) Childhood trauma or minority stress gives rise to emotional eating of highly processed calorie-dense food. 2) Emotional eating gives rise to food addiction. 3) Food addiction gives rise to weight gain. 4) Weight gain makes one a target of weight stigma. 5) Internalized weight stigma gives rise to perfectionistic obsessive approaches to dieting. 6) Orthorexia nervosa contributes to weight cycling. 7) High weight may then contribute to the development of metabolic syndromes when the endomorphic genotype is associated with genetic predispositions towards various metabolic syndromes.

An endomorphic genotype may lead to only a slightly huskier than average phenotype in a low stress natural environment devoid of processed foods that also facilitates secure attachment and an active lifestyle. That huskier body could be adaptive if it better withstands cold weather, stores energy for lean times, and can be used to throw one's weight around on an as needed basis. Anthropomorphic change may be why rates of obesity and metabolic syndromes increase when affordable American style processed food starts to replace indigenous cuisines more reliant on whole foods (Burnette, Ka'apu, Scarnato, & Liddell, 2020). The poor dietary quality that marginalized communities suffer may be a kind of environmental racism (Browne et al., 2022). Obesity as a phenotype as well as metabolic syndromes are rare among hunter gatherers (King, 2013) though the genotype for obesity and such syndromes is most likely common.

The results of individual psychotherapy can be constrained to the degree patients have limited ability to alter the 'obesogenic environment' (King, 2013) in which they live. Community psychology can try to change the unhealthy food environments in which children are raised despite the resistance of such social systems to structural change (Suarez-Balcazar, Redmond, Kouba, Hellwig, Davis, Martinez, & Jones, 2007). Until those social systems are changed individual psychotherapy remains a vital resource for autonomy support in challenging life circumstances.

The Evolution of Human Eating Habits

John Bowlby (1969), the founder of attachment theory, coined the term 'environment of evolutionary adaptedness'. The basic idea is that the human body and mind evolved to adapt to particular environments over millions of years of human evolution. Five to seven million years ago chimpanzees and humans possessed a common ancestor after which they went their separate ways (Lancaster & Kaplan, 2007). Chimpanzees are mostly vegetarian, preferring ripe fruit (Nelson & Hamilton, 2017), though the male chimpanzees do hunt small animals, like monkeys, and share the raw meat among themselves (John, Duguid, Tomasello, & Melis, 2019). Food sharing and begging for food has been observed among chimpanzees but food sharing among chimpanzees is not as common as it is among humans (Fröhlich, Müller, Zeiträg, Wittig, & Pika, 2020).

Humans evolved to be bipedal to walk around the African savannah, an open-country terrestrial terrain, searching for food (Turner, 2021). Around two million years ago *homo erectus* made simple stone tools that appear to have been used for hunting and/or butchering animal food (Hunt & Uomini, 2016). Between 600,000 and 250,000 humans started hunting big game with spears which was associated with a rapid expansion of human brain size (Mithen, 1999). Exactly when humans started using fire to roast meat or plants foods that would be more difficult to chew and digest raw is unknown. Evidence has been found of fire use in Europe dating from 300,000 to 400,000 years ago (Roebroeks & Villa, 2011). Some evolutionary anthropologists believe it could have been earlier. In comparison to chimpanzees, humans have small teeth and weak jaw muscles, and modern humans have difficulty surviving on a diet of raw wild foods (Wrangham, 2017). In comparison to chimpanzees, human diets have been much more oriented towards calorie-dense foods that are easy to chew and digest (Carmody, 2017).

Farming grain, the domestication of livestock for meat and dairy, domestication of fruits and vegetables, long-term food storage, cooking techniques like baking and boiling, and less nomadic lifestyles are inventions of modern civilization. Humans started to make such innovations approximately 10,000 years ago (Betzig, 2014). Human cognitive ingenuity allows humans to continue to innovate along these lines to this day. Humans continue to create and consume ever more calorie-dense/low fiber foods that are easy to chew and digest that can be consumed year-round from peanut butter and jelly sandwiches to premium ice cream. Progress in generating large quantities of calorie-dense foods that are easy to chew and digest has provided a bulwark against starvation. That bulwark has resulted in considerable population growth since the dawn of civilization (Betzig, 2014) as well as larger body size.

In the environment of evolutionary adaptedness, the preference for calorie-dense foods that are easy to chew and digest could have meant a feast of roasted wooly mammoth meat over roasted root vegetables dripping with wooly mammoth fat. Early humans could have topped off such a feast with a dessert of wild berries, nuts, seeds, and honey. The paleolithic diet could have sometimes been quite calorie-dense, as well as easy to chew and digest even without modern innovations like granulated sugar, white flour, cooking oil, butter, and deep frying.

Weight gain among early humans may have been constrained by the high number of calories that would have had to have been expended hunting and gathering to generate such a calorie-dense feast. Given the seasonal nature of access to such foods and the lack of food storage early humans might not have been able to eat this way all the or even most of the time. Other times, perhaps much of the time, they might have had to subsist on lower calorie/highly fibrous undomesticated plant foods that were chewy and difficult to digest or the lean meat of starving wild game that were only sporadically caught. Early humans may not have preferred to eat in this lower calorie/lower fat/higher fiber way, just like modern humans, but may have had to have frequently eaten this way out of necessity to avoid starvation. Modern hunter gatherers generally have low body weight as well as shorter stature because of the limited access to calorie-dense foods that are easy to chew and digest (King, 2013).

The diet that is currently considered most healthful is a high fiber diet of fresh fruits, vegetables, and lean meats, a diet that may have antidepressant effects (Francis, Stevenson, Chambers, Gupta, Newey, & Lim, 2019). Early humans may have frequently eaten this way but more out of necessity than preference. Possibly when they could, they held out for better if they anticipated a kill of a large well fed game animal or that a fruit tree would soon be bearing a cornucopia of sweet juicy ripe fruit to be quickly consumed before it was overly ripe. Consequently, the evolved human culinary predisposition that we might possess to this day might be something like this:

> Feast on calorie-dense food that is easy to chew and digest when you can, the more calorie-dense/ lower fiber and the greater the quantity the better, since you never know for sure when your next opportunity will be to eat so well. Fill up on low calorie foods that are chewy and hard to digest only if you must out of necessity. It's better than starving. Hold out for better if you anticipate that your next calorie-dense feast will be sooner rather than later.

Quite possibly dogs and cats have food preferences that are like human preferences as many pets gain more weight eating unlimited supplies human-made food than they would in the wild on a natural diet (Spence, 2022). Sedentary obese pets living in stressful environments are also at higher risk of cardiovascular disease (Cunha Silva & Fontes, 2019). Like humans, there appear to be genetic differences among pets as some gain weight because they are predisposed to eat whatever is available (Spence, 2022). Others will leave food in their bowls and remain thinner. Some pets become finicky eaters as they begin to reject pet food when they've had a taste of foods that humans eat. Like humans, dogs would prefer cooked meat over raw as it's easier to digest (Wrangham, 2017).

The modern problem with weight management from an evolutionary perspective is this: All weight management strategies require placing a conscious intentional curb of one sort or another on the evolved automatic tendency to mindlessly feast on calorie-dense foods that are easy to chew and digest when available. This dietary restraint must be exercised even though there has been very little selection pressure, if any, for almost the entirety of human evolution to evolve reliable dietary curbs to prevent overconsumption and weight gain. For almost the entirety of human evolution losing weight was neither a problem for survival (i.e., metabolic syndromes) or for reproduction (i.e., diminished sexual desirability due to weight stigma) that required the evolution of a prewired effective and reliable adaptive solution.

Humans have reliable prewired adaptations, a behavioral immune system, to spit out or vomit foods that will make us sick (Bradshaw & Gassen, 2021) but no prewired adaptations to prevent us from overeating if we are predisposed to do so in obesogenic environments. Sometimes the only surefire cue to stop eating is feeling sick to one's stomach because it activates the behavioral immune system. Unfortunately, by the time one feels sick from overeating an excessive number of calories have already been ingested. That's why mindful eating cultivates a heightened awareness of more subtle satiety cues that might otherwise go unnoticed. The point of mindful eating is to not let it get to the point of feeling sick to one's stomach as humans like dogs didn't evolve to eat mindfully but rather to 'wolf down' one's food while the supply lasts. Mindful eating would not have to be taught and effortfully practiced if it was something that developed effortlessly with maturation as a cross-cultural human universal like language acquisition.

Consequently, intentional weight management requires levels of self-control, like mindful eating, and levels of cognitive ingenuity, like cue avoidance (Bennett, 1986), that early humans would not have needed to deploy to remain thin. Modern humans must creatively jerry-rig novel adaptive solutions [i.e., an exaptation (Sol, 2015)] to a modern problem of adaptation with which our hunter gatherer forebears never had to contend. At present there is no jerry-rigged solution that reliably works for everybody though drug companies may eventually develop safe weight loss drugs without serious side effects that could work for everybody (Blum, 2023).

Modern food environments are obesogenic (King, 2013) though not necessarily for everybody. It may be obesogenic only for vulnerable individuals due to various combinations of genetic predisposition, insecure attachment, trauma, and minority stress compounded by food addiction and weight stigma. Individuals who are vulnerable to weight gain in modern contexts would not in the environment of evolutionary adaptedness have had to cultivate and exercise the kind of effortful cognitive restraints, like cue avoidance or mindful eating, that may be required for successful weight management in modern obesogenic environments. Individuals who are vulnerable in modern environments could have in the environment of evolutionary adaptedness mindlessly 'wolfed' down their favorite foods until they were 'stuffed' and still have remained reasonably thin.

In modern obesogenic food environments orthorexia nervosa might be activated by the emotionally taxing demands of having to cultivate and exercise such high levels of cognitive restraint to remain thin. Self-control as a weight management strategy is not necessary in food environments in which highly palatable calorie-dense foods are unavailable. That's the rationale among behavioral approaches that teach cue avoidance. Self-control is unnecessary if one can create a temptation-free environment for oneself. High levels of self-control are only a necessity when unlimited quantities of highly palatable calorie-dense foods are omnipresent.

Fears of loss of self-control are associated with obsessive-compulsive disorder (Denys, de Geus, van Megen, & Westenberg, 2004). High temptation food rich environments may trigger fears of loss of self-control of impulses to feast on calorie-dense foods which then activate perfectionistic and obsessive attempts to stick with a lower calorie diet to counter the fear of loss of control. Self-flagellation ensues when the perfectionistic effort to maintain self-control fails. Since volitional self-control is a limited resource in stressful circumstances (Baumeister, Tice, & Vohs, 2018) approaches to dieting primarily based on improved self-control may be doomed to fail in high temptation/high stress environments.

That loss of self-control will be difficult to accept if the maintenance of self-control in high temptation/high stress environments is construed as a reasonable self-expectation for a mature adult. From an evolutionary perspective that may not be a reasonable self-expectation for individuals with an endomorphic genotype and especially so when compounded by high levels of stress.

The Evolution of Pleasure in Feeding Others and Feasting with Others

What is notable about human cooperative behavior in comparison to other primates is the exceptionally high level of food sharing (Kaplan & Gurven, 2005). Humans not only share food with their offspring and hunting partners as do chimpanzees. Humans also share food with romantic partners, parents, friends, benign strangers, other people's children, pets, wild animals, the ill, the disabled, the elderly, the dying, prisoners, and enemies.

Pleasure in feeding others appears to be a cross-cultural human universal (Wang, Huang, & Wan, 2021). Eating by oneself can be a lonely enterprise. Elderly men living alone suffer poor diet quality (Hughes, Bennett, & Hetherington, 2004).

Feeding others low calorie food that is chewy and difficult to digest or withholding food from a hungry person is considered a form of mistreatment. One can seem less than human if one doesn't share food with those in need. Withholding food has been associated with child abuse (Zuilkowski, Thulin, McLean, Rogers, Akinsulure-Smith, & Betancourt, 2019). How we feed or don't feed others is a statement of who we love and who we hate or towards whom we feel indifferently. Dieting is difficult when it means partially excluding oneself from the social bonds forged by sharing calorie-dense food that is easy to chew and digest. It's not much of a birthday party, a romantic dinner, a holiday feast, or a wedding banquet if one is only serving carrot sticks, apples, and hard-boiled eggs to keep it low calorie.

Dieters can feel left out and alienated when everybody but them seems to be eating their fill of calorie-dense foods at social events. Overweight dieters often experience social isolation that can be ameliorated to some degree by support groups (English, 1993). It can feel rude to reject the offer of a tasty and filling calorie-dense food that has been made and offered with love when others don't approve of one's approach to dietary restraint (Romo, 2018). Dieters may feel that they are missing out on the party not unlike the way that alcoholics in recovery can feel when everybody seems to be enjoying an alcoholic beverage but them.

Programs like Overeaters Anonymous or Weight Watchers counter that social exclusion by creating a community of dieters who can support one another in the face of divergent weight management stigma as well as weight stigma. Dieters may see a psychotherapist or a weight loss specialist as much for the emotional support as for the psychoeducation about dieting as many individuals already know how they 'should' eat. The problem is not always the lack of nutritional knowledge but the inability to self-sufficiently exercise the self-control necessary to stick with any approach to weight management without sufficient social support.

The Costs and Benefits of Perfectionistic Weight Management

Orthorexia nervosa has been associated with maladaptive perfectionism (Novara, Pardini, Maggio, Mattioli, & Piasentin, 2022) and maladaptive perfectionism has been associated with a wide variety of pathological conditions including increased risk of suicide (Smith, 2023). In contrast, studies of adaptive perfectionism have found perfectionism associated with conscientiousness, endurance, active coping, and achievement despite it also being associated with obsessive-compulsiveness and rigidity (Stoeber & Rennert, 2008).

From the adaptationist perspective one would not necessarily conceptualize perfectionism in dichotomous ways as either adaptive or maladaptive. Instead, the idea would be that perfectionism always has costs and benefits and the relative costs and benefits vary for different people in different circumstances at different times of their lives. From the adaptationist perspective, psychotherapists would have to assess such costs and benefits on a case-by-case circumstance rather than risk overgeneralizing based on extant research findings.

Successful dieting may require conscientious task persistence (Gold et al., 2020). It would be preferable to be capable of being stubbornly persevering in a worthwhile endeavor without feeling as though one is always falling shamefully short of one's high self-expectations. A goal of psychotherapy is self-acceptance, helping patients feel that they are good enough as they are warts and all. Narratives of acceptance nourish traits such as grace, humility, and wisdom as well as intimacy and warmth (McAdams, Logan, & Reischer, 2022). Despite the benefits of self-acceptance, many patients believe that their perfectionistic beliefs motivate them to persevere in attaining long-term goals that are difficult to achieve. They worry that they wouldn't try as hard if they eased up on themselves. They believe that perfectionism is a good thing if it motivates them to devote themselves to succeeding at a challenging task.

The implicit cost-benefit calculation is that perfectionism is worth it if perfectionism will help them achieve their long-term weight management goals despite the emotional suffering it causes in the process of goal pursuit (i.e., no pain no gain). From the perfectionistic perspective the point of psychotherapy is not to lower one's standards or aspire to more readily attainable goals. The point is to assuage the self-doubts and insecurities activated by aspiring to ambitious goals sufficiently so that the dogged pursuit of ambitious goals won't be impeded by fears of failure.

The benefits of being rule-bound even if it strikes others as excessively rigid and fanatical are worth it if it's helping to achieve an ambitious weight management goal like maintaining a normal BMI or abstention from trigger foods. Efforts to help such patients achieve their weight management goals in more flexible, easy going, and less rule-bound ways might generate reactance because it is experienced as undermining their autonomous self-determination to achieve an ambitious goal despite the costs of rigid compliance with stringent dietary rules and restraints.

Ezra was diagnosed with Type 1 insulin dependent diabetes when he was 15 years old. He was put on a low glycemic index/low fat diet. Ezra pricked himself regularly to assess blood sugar levels and gave himself insulin injections accordingly. Occasionally he suffered insulin shock in which his blood sugar levels were dangerously low, and his cognitive functioning was seriously impaired. Friends and family always made sure there was something Ezra could eat given his dietary restrictions.

Over the years Ezra's blood sugar regulation became increasingly unstable. He subjected himself to ever more stringent dietary restrictions under the guidance of a diabetes specialist to try to get his blood sugar levels better under control. That meant he would bring his own meals when dining with others and stopped going out to eat at restaurants entirely. Ezra would sometimes be subject to divergent weight management stigma as when he put diet soda in his tuna broccoli casserole for flavor or when an irritated physician with whom he was consulting told him to just live his life when he was recounting the precise details of his dieting efforts.

At age 65, Ezra received Harvard University's Joslin Diabetes Center's 50-year bronze medal award for the remarkable achievement of living a successful life with insulin-dependent diabetes for half a century. Unfortunately, Ezra died in his sleep two years later from heart failure that resulted from the long-term complications of diabetes despite his best efforts to minimize those complications. For much of Ezra's adult life he worked with a psychotherapist who diagnosed him with obsessive compulsive personality disorder but offered considerable autonomy support when it came to Ezra's perfectionistic compliance with extremely exacting dietary restrictions (i.e., he weighed his portion sizes to be precise).

Some patients may develop a consistent routine be it counting calories, walking a certain number of miles per day, or meditating every day at a certain time for a certain length. They may feel better when they stick with these daily routines and feel discombobulated as well as self-flagellating whenever they stray from their established routines. Straying from such routines may be associated with relapse to prior out of control eating habits. Maintaining the strict routine is therefore perceived as an adaptive form of relapse prevention. Thus, psychotherapists may need to explore on a case-by-case basis in collaboration with their perfectionistic patients whether their perfectionistic approach to weight management is something to be supported despite the costs or something to be alleviated despite the benefits.

References

Alberts, H. J. E. M., Thewissen, R., & Raes, L. (2012). Dealing with problematic eating behaviour. The effects of a mindfulness-based intervention on eating behaviour, food cravings, dichotomous thinking and body image concern. *Appetite*, 58(3), 847–851. https://doi.org/10.1016/j.appet.2012.01.009.

Andersson, M. (1994). *Monographs in behavior and ecology: Sexual selection.* Princeton, NJ: Princeton University Press.

Antoniou, E. E., Bongers, P., & Jansen, A. (2017). The mediating role of dichotomous thinking and emotional eating in the relationship between depression and BMI. *Eating Behaviors*, 26, 55–60. https://doi.org/10.1016/j.eatbeh.2017.01.007

Ash, J., & Gallup, G. (2008). Brain size, intelligence, and Paleolithic variation. In G. Geher & G. Miller (Eds.), *Mating intelligence: Sex, relationships, and the mind's reproductive system* (pp. 313–336). Erlbaum. https://doi.org/10.1080/07481187.2017.1322644

Baumeister, R. F., Tice, D. M., & Vohs, K. D. (2018). The strength model of self-regulation: Conclusions from the second decade of willpower research. *Perspectives on Psychological Science*, 13(2), 141–145. https://doi.org/10.1177/1745691617716946

Bennett, G. A. (1986). Cognitive rehearsal in the treatment of obesity: A comparison against cue avoidance and social pressure. *Addictive Behaviors*, 11(3), 225–237. https://doi.org/10.1016/0306-4603(86)90051-1

Betzig, L. (2014). Eusociality in history. *Human Nature*, 25(1), 80–99. https://doi.org/10.1007/s12110-013-9186-8

Biolsi, K. L., & Woo, K. L. (2022). Equivalence classification, learning by exclusion, and long-term memory in pinnipeds: Cognitive mechanisms demonstrated through research with subjects under human care and in the field. *Animal Cognition*, 25(5), 1077–1090. https://doi.org/10.1007/s10071-022-01658-w

Blum, D. (2023). The diabetes drug that could overshadow Ozempic. *New York Times*. November 4, 2023.

Bowlby, J. (1969). *Attachment: Attachment and loss*, Vol. I. New York: Basic Books.

Bradshaw, H. K., & Gassen, J. (2021). The evolution of disgust, pathogens, and the behavioural immune system. In P. A. Powell & N. S. Consedine (Eds.), *The handbook of disgust research: Modern perspectives and applications* (pp. 31–51). Springer Nature Switzerland AG. https://doi-org/10.1007/978-3-030-84486-8_3

Browne, N. T., Hodges, E. A., Small, L., Snethen, J. A., Frenn, M., Irving, S. Y., Gance-Cleveland, B., & Greenberg, C. S. (2022). Childhood obesity within the lens of racism. *Pediatric Obesity*, 17(5), 1–9. https://doi.org/10.1111/ijpo.12878

Burnette, C. E., Ka'apu, K., Scarnato, J. M., & Liddell, J. (2020). Cardiovascular health among U.S. Indigenous peoples: A holistic and sex-specific systematic review. *Journal of Evidence-Based Social Work*, 17(1), 24–48. https://doi-org/10.1080/26408066.2019.1617817

Carmody, R. N. (2017). Evolution of the human dietary niche: Quest for high quality. In M. N. Muller, R. W. Wrangham, & D. R. Pilbeam (Eds.), *Chimpanzees and human evolution* (pp. 311–338). The Belknap Press of Harvard University Press. https://doi-org/10.4159/9780674982642-009

Chrisler, J. C., & Barney, A. (2017). Sizeism is a health hazard. *Fat Studies: An Interdisciplinary Journal of Body Weight and Society*, 6(1), 38–53. https://doi.org/10.1080/21604851.2016.12 13066

Cunha Silva, C., & Fontes, M. A. P. (2019). Cardiovascular reactivity to emotional stress: The hidden challenge for pets in the urbanized environment. *Physiology & Behavior*, 207, 151–158. https://doi.org/10.1016/j.physbeh.2019.05.014

Darwin, C. (1871). *The descent of man and selection in relation to sex*. London: Murray.

Denys, D., de Geus, F., van Megen, H. J., & Westenberg, H. G. (2004). Symptom dimensions in obsessive-compulsive disorder: Factor analysis on a clinician-rated scale and a self-report measure. *Psychopathology*, 37(4), 181–189. https://doi.org/10.1159/000079509

English, C. (1993). Gaining and losing weight: Identity transformations. *Deviant Behavior*, 14(3), 227–241. https://doi.org/10.1080/01639625.1993.9967941

Farooqi, I. S. (2018). Genetics of obesity. In T. A. Wadden & G. A. Bray (Eds.), *Handbook of obesity treatment* (pp. 64–74). The Guilford Press.

Figueredo, A. J., Vásquez, G., Brumbach, B. H., & Schneider, S. M. R. (2004). The heritability of life history strategy: The K-factor, covitality, and personality. *Biodemography and Social Biology*, 51(3–4), 121–143. doi: http://dx.doi.org/10.1080/19485565.2004.9989090

Ford, J. D. (2021). Essential psychotherapy principles and practices. In J. D. Ford, *Crises in the psychotherapy session: Transforming critical moments into turning points* (pp. 81–109). American Psychological Association. https://doi.org/10.1037/0000225-005

Francis, H. M., Stevenson, R. J., Chambers, J. R., Gupta, D., Newey, B., & Lim, C. K. (2019). A brief diet intervention can reduce symptoms of depression in young adults – A randomised controlled trial. *PloS ONE*, 14(10), e0222768. https://doi.org/10.1371/journal.pone.0222768

Fröhlich, M., Müller, G., Zeiträg, C., Wittig, R. M., & Pika, S. (2020). Begging and social tolerance: Food solicitation tactics in young chimpanzees (*Pan troglodytes*) in the wild. *Evolution and Human Behavior*, 41(2), 126–135. https://doi.org/10.1016/j.evolhumbehav.2019.11.002

Gabor, C., Lindström, J., & Macias Garcia, C. (2022). Using behavioural ecology to explore adaptive responses to anthropogenic change—Introduction. *Behavioral Ecology and Sociobiology*, 76(95). https://doi-org/10.1007/s00265-022-03204-7

Garcia-Silva, J., Borrego, I. R. S., Navarrete, N. N., Peralta-Ramirez, M. I., Águila, F. J., & Caballo, V. E. (2022). Efficacy of cognitive-behavioural therapy for lifestyle modification in metabolic syndrome A randomised controlled trial with a 18-months follow-up. *Psychology & Health*, 39(2), 195–215. https://doi-org./10.1080/08870446.2022.2055023

Girma Shifaw, Z. (2022). Marital communication as moderators of the relationship between marital conflict resolution and marital satisfaction. *American Journal of Family Therapy*. https://doiorg/10.1080/01926187.2022.2089404

Gold, J. M., Carr, L. J., Thomas, J. G., Burrus, J., O'Leary, K. C., Wing, R., & Bond, D. S. (2020). Conscientiousness in weight loss maintainers and regainers. *Health Psychology*, 39(5), 421–429. https://doi-org/10.1037/hea0000846

Hawkes, K., O'Connell, J. F., & Jones, N. G. B. (2003). Human life histories: Primate trade-offs, grandmothering socioecology, and the fossil record. In P. M. Kappeler & M. E. Pereira (Eds.), *Primate life histories and socioecology* (pp. 204–227). Chicago: University of Chicago Press.

Hughes, G., Bennett, K. M., & Hetherington, M. M. (2004). Old and alone: Barriers to healthy eating in older men living on their own. *Appetite*, 43(3), 269–276. https://doi.org/10.1016/j.appet.2004.06.002

Hunt, G. R., & Uomini, N. (2016). A complex adaptive system may be essential for cumulative modifications in tool design. *Japanese Journal of Animal Psychology*, 66(2), 141–159. https://doi.org/10.2502/janip.66.2.2

John, M., Duguid, S., Tomasello, M., & Melis, A. P. (2019). How chimpanzees (*Pan troglodytes*) share the spoils with collaborators and bystanders. *PloS ONE*, 14(9), e0222795. https://doi.org/10.1371/journal.pone.0222795

Kaeberlein, M., Rabinovitch, P. S., & Martin, G. M. (2015). Healthy aging: The ultimate preventative medicine. *Science*, 350(6265), 1191–1193. https://doi.org/10.1126/science.aad3267

Kaplan, H. S., & Gangestad, S. W. (2005). Life history theory and evolutionary psychology. In D. M. Buss (Ed.), *The handbook of evolutionary psychology* (pp. 68–95). John Wiley & Sons, Inc.

Kaplan, H., & Gurven, M. (2005). The natural history of human food sharing and cooperation: A review and a new multi-individual approach to the negotiation of norms. In H. Gintis, S. Bowles, R. Boyd, & E. Fehr (Eds.), *Moral sentiments and material interests: The foundations of cooperation in economic life* (pp. 75–113). MIT Press.

King, B. M. (2013). The modern obesity epidemic, ancestral hunter-gatherers, and the sensory/reward control of food intake. *The American Psychologist*, 68(2), 88–96. https://doi.org/10.1037/a0030684

Lancaster, J. B., & Kaplan, H. S. (2007). Chimpanzee and human intelligence: Life history, diet, and the mind. In S. W. Gangestad & J. A. Simpson (Eds.), *The evolution of mind: Fundamental questions and controversies* (pp. 111–118). The Guilford Press.

Manasse, S. M., Lampe, E. W., Abber, S. R., Fitzpatrick, B., Srivastava, P., & Juarascio, A. S. (2023). Differentiating types of dietary restraint and their momentary relations with loss-of-control eating. *International Journal of Eating Disorders*. https://doi-org/10.1002/eat.23896

McAdams, D. P., Logan, R. L., & Reischer, H. N. (2022). Beyond the redemptive self: Narratives of acceptance in later life (and in other contexts). *Journal of Research in Personality*, 100, 1–8. https://doi.org/10.1016/j.jrp.2022.104286

Mithen, S. (1999). The hunter–gatherer prehistory of human–animal interactions. *Anthrozoös*, 12(4), 195–204. https://doi.org/10.2752/089279399787000147

Nelson, S. V., & Hamilton, M. I. (2017). Evolution of the human dietary niche: Initial transitions. In M. N. Muller, R. W. Wrangham, & D. R. Pilbeam (Eds.), *Chimpanzees and human evolution* (pp. 286–310). The Belknap Press of Harvard University https://doi.org/10.4159/9780674982642-008

New, A. S., Perez-Rodriguez, M. M., & Rosenberg, J. (2017). Personality disorders: Assessment and treatment. In A. B. Simon, A. S. New, & W. K. Goodman (Eds.), *Psychiatry* (pp. 152–160). Wiley Blackwell.

Novara, C., Pardini, S., Maggio, E., Mattioli, S., & Piasentin, S. (2022). Orthorexia nervosa: Over concern or obsession about healthy food? *Eating and Weight Disorders*, 26(8), 2577–2588. https://doi-org/10.1007/s40519-021-01110-x

Price, H., & Deveci, Y. (2022). 'One size does not fit all': Understanding the situated nature of reflective practices. *Journal of Social Work Practice*, 36(2), 227–240. https://doi-org/10.1080/02650533.2022.2058920

Roebroeks, W., & Villa, P. (2011). On the earliest evidence for habitual use of fire in Europe. *Proceedings of the National Academy of Sciences of the United States of America*, 108(13), 5209–5214. https://doi.org/10.1073/pnas.1018116108

Romo L. K. (2018). An examination of how people who have lost weight communicatively negotiate interpersonal challenges to weight management. *Health Communication*, 33(4), 469–477. https://doi.org/10.1080/10410236.2016.1278497

Rozental, A., Kottorp, A., Forsström, D., Månsson, K., Boettcher, J., Andersson, G., Furmark, T., & Carlbring, P. (2019). The Negative Effects Questionnaire: Psychometric properties of an instrument for assessing negative effects in psychological treatments. *Behavioural and Cognitive Psychotherapy*, 47(5), 559–572. https://doi.org/10.1017/S1352465819000018

Ryan, R. M., & Deci, E. L. (2019). Supporting autonomy, competence, and relatedness: The coaching process from a self-determination theory perspective. In S. English, J. M. Sabatine, & P. Brownell (Eds.), *Professional coaching: Principles and practice* (pp. 231–245). Springer Publishing Company.

Smith, M. M. (2023). Perfectionistic strivings are neither adaptive, healthy, positive, functional, nor advisable: Findings from six peer-reviewed journal articles. *Dissertation Abstracts International Section A: Humanities and Social Sciences*, 84(3-A).

Sol, D. (2015). The evolution of innovativeness: Exaptation or specialized adaptation? In A. B. Kaufman & J. C. Kaufman (Eds.), *Animal creativity and innovation* (pp. 163–187). Elsevier Academic Press.

Spence, C. (2022). Gastrophysics for pets: Tackling the growing problem of overweight/obese dogs. *Applied Animal Behaviour Science*, 256, 1–9. https://doi.org/10.1016/j.applanim.2022.105765

Stoeber, J., & Rennert, D. (2008). Perfectionism in school teachers: Relations with stress appraisals, coping styles, and burnout. *Anxiety, Stress, and Coping*, 21(1), 37–53. https://doi.org/10.1080/10615800701742461

Suarez-Balcazar, Y., Redmond, L., Kouba, J., Hellwig, M., Davis, R., Martinez, L. I., & Jones, L. (2007). Introducing systems change in the schools: The case of school luncheons and vending machines. *American Journal of Community Psychology*, 39(3–4), 335–345. https://doi.org/10.1007/s10464-007-9102-7

Symons, D. (1987). Can Darwin's view of life shed light on human sexuality? In J. H. Geer & W. T. O'Donohue (Eds.), *Theories of human sexuality* (pp. 91–125). New York, NY: Plenum Press.

Turner, J. H. (2021). On human nature: *The biology and sociology of what made us human*. Routledge/Taylor & Francis Group.

Villarosa-Hurlocker, M. C., O'Sickey, A. J., Houck, J. M., & Moyers, T. B. (2019). Examining the influence of active ingredients of motivational interviewing on client change talk. *Journal of Substance Abuse Treatment*, 96, 39–45. https://doi.org/10.1016/j.jsat.2018.10.001

Wang, C., Huang, J., & Wan, X. (2021). A cross-cultural study of beliefs about the influence of food sharing on interpersonal relationships and food choices. *Appetite*, 161, 105129. https://doi.org/10.1016/j.appet.2021.105129

Wrangham, R. (2017). Control of fire in the Paleolithic: Evaluating the cooking hypothesis. *Current Anthropology*, 58(S16), S303–S313. https://10.1086/692113

Zuilkowski, S. S., Thulin, E. J., McLean, K., Rogers, T. M., Akinsulure-Smith, A. M., & Betancourt, T. S. (2019). Parenting and discipline in post-conflict Sierra Leone. *Child Abuse & Neglect*, 97, 104138. https://doi.org/10.1016/j.chiabu.2019.104138

Zwir, I., Arnedo, J., Del-Val, C., Pulkki-Råback, L., Konte, B., Yang, S. S., Romero-Zaliz, R., Hintsanen, M., Cloninger, K. M., Garcia, D., Svrakic, D. M., Rozsa, S., Martinez, M., Lyytikäinen, L. P., Giegling, I., Kähönen, M., Hernandez-Cuervo, H., Seppälä, I., Raitoharju, E., de Erausquin, G. A., Cloninger, C. R. (2020). Uncovering the complex genetics of human character. *Molecular Psychiatry*, 25(10), 2295–2312. https://doi. org/10.1038/s41380-018-0263-6

Who to Believe? The Confusing Nature of Dietary Reality and Epistemic Trust

The evolutionary framework suggests that the advocates of intuitive eating are correct that dieting is not a natural way to eat. Dieting is not eating intuitively and learning to diet does not come easily to humans. That may be why humans frequently fail at dieting no matter how determined the attempt. Humans, like most species, have not developed reliable species-wide adaptations to prevent excessive weight gain as starvation rather than overconsumption has been the adaptive challenge that has driven natural selection (Shively, Register, & Clarkson, 2009). Consequently, humans must develop jerry-rigged adaptations to the evolutionary novel problems of survival (i.e., metabolic syndromes) and reproduction (i.e., if high weight decreases one's mate value) in an obesogenic environment that our forebears rarely had to face.

Advice from multiple sources is not lacking for those with weight management concerns. There is a plethora of conflicting advice from commercial diets and exercise plans that promise quick and sustainable weight loss as well as conflicting advice from the scientific community that debates the relative merits of the extant evidence. Patients with weight management concerns may be bombarded with conflicting one-size-fits-all solutions with little guidance on how to discover a sustainable personalized solution.

Generalist psychotherapists who are not weight management experts may not feel entirely qualified to consult with patients on this controversial issue. They may feel that they should stay within their lanes to avoid practicing outside of their areas of expertise. The weight management experts might feel similarly. Nevertheless, psychotherapy patients will consult with their psychotherapists on this issue for the very reason that they are not specialists with a specific one-size-fits-all approach to weight management. Their lack of expertise in this regard is a plus rather than a minus.

Patients may prefer to seek consultation from their generalist psychotherapists because they have come to trust that their psychotherapists as all-purpose sounding boards who have already helped them with their original presenting problems like depression, anxiety, anger management, and relationship problems (Reich & Neenan, 1986). Patients trust that their generalist psychotherapists as all-purpose sounding boards will provide consistent autonomy support and empathy with their weight management concerns as well as they did with patients' other presenting problems. They don't want to have to see a separate specialist for each of their psychological problems. Nevertheless, it's a plus if their generalists psychotherapists have given some thought to weight management issues, have some knowledge of the pros and cons of different approaches, have some experience helping patients with this issue, and have some insight from struggling with this issue in their own personal lives.

DOI: 10.4324/9781003402336-9

Psychotherapy patients appreciate that their psychotherapists aren't nutritionists who will work out a specific food plan, personal trainers who will work out a specific exercise routine, or physicians who will prescribe a weight loss drug. Psychotherapy patients are primarily choosing psychotherapists with relatable personality styles and a general approach to psychotherapy (i.e., good listener, teaches coping skills, addresses childhood trauma and family dynamics, etc.) to be their general all-purpose sounding boards for the various psychological problems that confront them on their journeys through life (Wong, 2017). The hope is to find a psychotherapist who can be a trustworthy traveling companion and guide for a diverse array of psychological issues of which weight management is but one.

Utilizing psychotherapists as all-purpose sounding boards raises the issue of "epistemic trust" (Fonagy & Allison, 2014), who does one trust to provide an objective view of reality when one doesn't know what to think or do. Is the therapist experienced enough, smart enough, well-trained enough, knowledgeable enough, relatable enough, unbiased enough, and/or ethical enough to be trusted? Questions about therapeutic efficacy arise in all psychotherapies for all sorts of problems. Such questions are particularly salient when weight management concerns arise because of the confusing nature of dietary reality.

How much weight is too much weight? What are the risks of eventually acquiring a metabolic syndrome over time if one is of high weight but exercises regularly, eats whole foods, has normal blood pressure, normal blood cholesterol levels, and normal blood sugar levels? What is the best diet for losing weight and is it better to lose weight slowly or quickly? What diet is most sustainable for weight loss maintenance? And are the benefits of losing weight and keeping it off worth the costs in terms of time, money, and feeling deprived?

There are not definitive answers to any of these questions. Nevertheless, therapists who have been thoughtful about such questions and can see the pros and cons of different ways of answering such questions are likely to be better sounding boards when patients raise their weight management concerns. A good sounding board can appreciate the logic behind different ways of looking at things and might offer new perspectives patients might not have thought of on their own. Such a sounding board supports patients' autonomous decision making. It doesn't simply validate what patients already think nor does it tell patients what to think. It facilitates patients' capacity to be reflective by fostering the capacity to look at things from multiple perspectives and then integrate those perspectives. (Petersen, Brakoulias, & Langdon, 2016). As such it helps to overcome the dichotomous thinking that may be associated with patients' weight management problems (Antoniou, Bongers, & Jansen, 2017) Increasing reflective functioning may be a common factor in all successful approaches to psychotherapy (Fonagy & Allison, 2014).

Is There an Ideal Diet?

It appears that most calorie restricted diets can help individuals lose weight (Tronieri, 2021). What has been less well researched is the long-term sustainability of various diets. In addition, the various dietary recommendations have yet to be analyzed through the prism of addiction psychology and how various diets would impact the issues of tolerance, withdrawal, and craving that make recovery from any addiction challenging. From the perspective of weight loss, abstaining from trigger foods or learning to consume trigger foods in moderation, be it daily or only on infrequent 'cheat' days, is likely to lead to weight loss. One is less likely to overeat the less addictive foods. Yet some severely food addicted individuals might overeat carrot sticks, bananas, and skinless turkey breast to compensate for the lasagna, potato chips, and cookies that they are trying to refrain from overeating.

Most calorie restricted diets not only facilitate weight loss but also contribute to improvements in the metabolic markers of good health (Alamuddin & Wadden, 2016). Sustained weight loss maintenance of as little as 3–5% can produce clinically mean-ingful health benefits (Jensen et al., 2014) and the greater the weight loss the greater the health benefits (Wing et al., 2011). Some studies of intuitive eating suggest that intuitive eating, though it does not necessarily contribute to weight loss, can sometimes facilitate improvements in biomarkers of good health or at least not make it worse (Clifford, Ozier, Bundros, Moore, Kreiser, & Morris, 2015). Nevertheless, since stress-induced relapse is common (Hutchinson, 2011), it would also be important to assess to what degree some dietary approaches are more sustainable than others in the face of stressful circumstances.

From the addiction perspective there can be multiple pathways to recovery (Eddie, Bergman, Hoffman, & Kelly, 2022) so there may be individual variability in terms of the sus-tainability of different weight management approaches (i.e., abstinence versus moderation, intuitive versus rule-bound eating, etc.). Individual variability in sustainability is not well researched as it would require tracking individuals applying a specific weight management strategy over long periods of time (i.e., years rather than months) to assess if some weight management strategies are more sustainable than others for certain individuals. Periodic relapse is not uncommon in recovery from food addiction like any other addiction (Parylak, Koob, & Zorrilla, 2011). Are some weight management strategies easier to reinstate or tweak after relapse for certain individuals, in certain circumstances, at certain points in the life cycle? Such questions have yet to be systematically researched.

From the point of view of addiction psychology sustainability may be as much about the sufficiency and sustainability of the emotional support structure as it is about culti-vating a capacity to independently exercise better self-control. Are some weight manage-ment strategies easier to sustain on one's own than others? When patients relapse is the problem with their impaired self-control or with the deficient emotional support structure? What are the optimal support structures for different individuals regardless of the specific diet? Is open-ended weekly psychotherapy sufficient? Does weekly psychotherapy need to be supplemented by also seeing a nutritionist and/or attending a self-help support group?

Any dietary approach can result in weight loss if it creates an energy deficit (Marlatt & Ravussin, 2018). To create an energy deficit the number of calories consumed must be less than the number of calories burned during a day. In behavioral weight loss treatment, that typically means prescribing a low-calorie diet from 1200 to 1800 calories per day adjusted based on sex, height, and current weight as well as prescribing an exercise routine to increase calorie expenditure (Jensen et al., 2014). The macronutrient composition of the diet doesn't appear to have any advantage for weight loss (Larsen et al., 2010). Low carbohy-drate diets, high protein diets, low fat diets, vegetarian diets, low glycemic load diets, as well as Mediterranean diets that center on 'good' carbs from fresh fruits and vegetables and 'good' fats from olive oil and fish all can result in weight loss if they remain within the prescribed daily calorie budget (Jensen et al., 2014). In addition, weight loss on any of these diets is associated with improvements in markers of metabolic functioning (Jensen et al., 2014)).

Very low-calorie diets of fewer than 800 calories per day for 12 to 16 weeks have been used for rapid weight loss. Those diets are high protein to protect against muscle loss (Tsai & Wadden, 2006). Very low calorie as well as low calorie diets can be viable options for weight loss (Vink, Roumans, Arkenbosch, Mariman, & van Baak, 2016). Very low-calorie diets, though, need to be undertaken under careful medical supervision. Low calorie diets when associated with behavioral weight loss treatment do on average lead to 10% reduction in body weight with 5% regained in long-term follow-up (Gomez-Rubalcava, Stabbert, & Phelan, 2018). It is not entirely clear, though, who is or isn't willing to participate in such a rigorous structured program and who can tolerate it without dropping out.

Relapse rates over the long haul could be higher for individuals who start out with what might prove to be overly ambitious weight loss goals. Radical caloric restriction and a demanding exercise routine may not be sustainable in the long-term though it may achieve quick and dramatic results in the short-term when compliance motivation is high. A chronic struggle with hunger becomes a chronic strain that incrementally wears down one's capacity for self-control contributing to stress-induced relapse.

The relationship between perfectionistic/overly ambitious approaches to dieting and weight cycling and regain has not been well investigated. Dichotomous thinking has been associated with emotional eating (Antoniou, Bongers, & Jansen, 2017) and that might be associated with all or none approaches to dieting. It's possible that some weight cycling derives from food addicted individuals cycling between perfectionistic/overly ambitious approaches to dieting in the hopes of achieving rapid weight loss and then relapsing back into old eating habits as the chronic strain on one's capacity for self-control becomes too much to bear.

The macronutrient composition of the diet does not appear to affect weight loss when the calorie counts are equivalent (Jensen et al., 2014). It has yet to be researched if the macronutrient composition influences the sustainability of the diet in the long-term. To the extent that addictive foods prime craving (Ahmed, 2012), the presence of more addictive foods in a calorie restricted diet even in low amounts may activate craving for larger portions of those foods. Thus, the problem of increased hunger due to reduced calorie count may be compounded by increased craving if withdrawal symptoms result from a significant reduction or elimination of addictive foods consumed in a calorie restricted diet.

It's not clear how diets possessing different macronutrient compositions might activate the problem of withdrawal from the more addictive foods. Withdrawal may increase craving not simply for more calories but for the more addictive macronutrients (i.e., foods with added sugar or white flour). In the grip of withdrawal, the food addicted individual might not want another apple for a snack but a potato chip or not another portion of grilled skinless chicken breast with steamed broccoli for a dinner entree but chicken parmesan over pasta. The former could supply sufficient calories with large enough portion size but only the latter would satisfy the craving for the processed carbohydrate/ higher fat foods that are considered most addictive.

A brief review of various diets suggests the presence in most well-known diets of at least small portions of more addictive foods that could prime craving. For example, low-fat diets might still allow for consumption of processed carbohydrates like bread, pasta, and cereal, though it may no longer be served with significant amounts of butter, whole milk, cheese, oil, or fatty meats (Gardner et al., 2018). Some believe that the obesity epidemic may be due to the increased consumption of processed carbohydrates after the recommendation to eat a low-fat diet to reduce the risk of heart disease (Moss, 2014).

Foods high in processed carbohydrates (i.e., high in added sugar and high in white flour) could be trigger foods that are difficult to stop eating even if fat-free (Schulte, Smeal, Lewis, & Gearhardt, 2018). Processed carbohydrates would be even more addictive when combined with fat (i.e., ice cream) but do not necessarily lose their addictive properties with the fat removed (i.e., fat free sugar candies like gummy bears, pasta in fat-free tomato sauce, low-fat chocolate milk). In addition, it is not entirely clear at what point a low-fat diet might have too little fat creating a nutritional deficiency that intensifies craving for the missing nutrient.

High fat, moderate protein, and low carbohydrate diets have also shown promise [i.e., Atkins diet, ketogenic diet (Gardner et al., 2018)]. Such diets could be more sustainable because high fat and/or high protein may be perceived as more satiating as they are more calorie-dense than carbohydrates (Bilman, van Trijp, & Renes, 2010). On a high fat diet, one would not need to restrict the consumption of high fat foods like steak, bacon, and brie. It is not entirely clear at what point a low carbohydrate diet has too little carbohydrates creating a nutritional deficit that intensifies craving for the missing nutrient.

Fat is a calorie-dense nutrient, and one would be more predisposed to overeat steak than one would low-fat tuna in water from a can that is almost pure protein. Fatty meats appear to have more addictive properties than lean meats. That is why fat as well as carbohydrates are often added to lean meats like adding mayonnaise to tuna or breading and frying a low-fat fish like cod. Nevertheless, high fat diets would have none or very little added sugar or white flour, the most common trigger foods.

A low glycemic diet would also exclude the most common trigger foods as processed carbohydrates like added sugar and white flour tend to spike blood sugar levels. Nevertheless, high fat foods that are low on the glycemic index can still be calorie dense as well as relatively easy to chew and digest like steak, brie, creamy peanut butter, and avocado so might be overeaten. Raw animal fat is not so easy for humans to digest but cooked animal fat, dairy fat, and plant oils are much more digestible (Wrangham, 2017).

The Paleolithic diet is not entirely free of calorie-dense foods as humans appear to have evolved to consume a diet of calorie-dense foods that are easy to chew and digest (Carmody, 2017). A Paleolithic diet would be free of added sugar, processed grains, and dairy. Those are culinary innovations of modern civilization that can be used to create highly addictive trigger foods like ice cream and cake. Nonetheless, early humans who used fire could have periodically feasted on roasted fatty meat, nuts, seeds, honey, and starchy roasted root vegetables (Berbesque & Marlowe, 2009).

The diet that seems to most restrict the consumption of potentially addictive foods that are calorie dense and easy to chew and digest would be Weight Watchers' list of 'Zero Point Foods' (Winchester, 2023). Weight Watchers assigns points to foods based on how calorie dense (i.e., how fattening) they are. Zero-point foods are assigned zero points on the assumption that it's better to fill up on such foods as much as one can rather than consume foods that are more calorie dense. If one must consume a higher calorie food one must track the number of points, a proxy for calories, to avoid overeating the more calorie-dense foods. Zero-point foods would be all fresh fruits and vegetables, all lean sources of protein be it fish, seafood, hard boiled eggs, skinless chicken or turkey breast, and all no-fat dairy, and a few starchier plant foods like corn, lentils, or chickpeas. Some zero-point lists may include whole grains as well.

Not that one couldn't overeat zero-point foods, but the list does not contain any of the foods that are usually considered the most addictive or the most fattening. For this reason, many individuals would not want to fill up on such foods even with permission to eat such foods without restraint because of the problem of craving. Some individuals don't want to eat another baby carrot when they crave a cookie. Many individuals don't want to eat another hardboiled egg when they would prefer a cheese omelet.

The question is then to what degree can humans acclimate to eating a predominantly zero-point type diet if humans have evolved to prefer a diet of more calorie dense-foods. A zero-point type diet would have a very high fiber content as whole plant foods would be eaten either raw or with minimal processing such as steaming to make the fiber more digestible. High fiber may also contribute to satiety though it's zero calories (Reverri, Randolph, Kappagoda, Park, Edirisinghe, & Burton-Freeman, 2017).

A predominantly zero-point diet may approximate the way early humans may have eaten by necessity when the more calorie-dense foods that were easy to chew and digest (i.e., honey or roasted meat) were unavailable. Eating an exclusively zero-point diet forever would be the equivalent of completely abstaining from the addictive trigger foods forever. Weight Watchers would not necessarily recommend that. Instead, the Weight Watchers approach would be to control portion sizes of foods that are assigned points rather than to abstain from them entirely.

There have always been individuals who can successfully acclimate themselves to an ascetic lifestyle abstaining from things like sex, alcohol, drugs, or certain foods for life and find it spiritually uplifting to do so. Some may see an ascetic lifestyle as an antidote to many of the diseases of the modern consumer culture (Kuhn, 2021). That is often by choice rather than by necessity. Yet such an ascetic lifestyle may not be for everyone or even for most people even if such a lifestyle spares one from suffering the diseases of modern civilization.

From the point of view of addiction psychology (i.e., tolerance, withdrawal, craving) there may be no perfect diet. All diets would activate withdrawal symptoms and learning to manage craving for addictive foods that are either eaten not at all or in moderation despite the danger that small portions can intensify craving. Given that every diet imposes some sort of adversity, the challenge is discovering the most tolerable adversity given one's unique individuality, individual circumstances in terms of current life stresses and sources of emotional support, and time of life.

The dialectical challenge is this: The more one can abstain from the most addictive calorie-dense foods and fill up instead on the least addictive foods the more weight one is likely to lose and keep off. Over time the intensity of cravings for the more addictive foods may subside to more manageable levels. Yet there may be a limit to the extent that less ascetically inclined individuals can learn to live without ever consuming the more addictive calorie-dense foods in obesogenic environments given the human vulnerability to stress-induced relapse in high temptation environments. Craving for such foods may be part of our evolved human nature and sharing and feasting on such foods is a central way that humans form close bonds with one another. Psychotherapy may be helping patients discover some sustainable middle ground between the often-incompatible goals of maintaining a healthy weight so that one likes what one sees in the mirror while also enjoying the pleasures of eating one's favorite foods in the company of friends and family.

The Weight Watchers' approach to assigning points has implications for the controversy around counting calories. The more one abstains from high calorie trigger foods and fills up on the lower calorie alternatives the less the need to count calories as the lower calorie foods are less likely to be overeaten or overeaten by as much as the higher calorie foods. The more one attempts to consume the more addictive higher calorie trigger foods in moderation the more prudent it would be to count calories as a damage control/harm reduction strategy. It may be safer to trust one's intuition about when to stop eating the lower calorie foods than it is to trust one's intuition about when to stop eating the more addictive higher calorie foods.

Since the higher calorie foods may increase rather than reduce craving among addicted individuals it may be risky to consume such foods without monitoring the portion size and calorie count.

Awareness of the calorie count may put a break on one's consumption and that is why some individuals stop counting calories when surrendering to the temptation to have more than just a taste. Food addicted individuals may wish to eat unaware of the calorie count rather than mindfully aware of it as addictions are diseases of denial (Kearney, 1996). Aspiring calorie counters may need to learn to look at that number mindfully as useful objective information without moralistic judgment. Calorie counters would need to cultivate self-compassion rather than surrender to self-disgust when the numbers are 'bad'.

Epistemic Trust and the Therapeutic Relationship

Epistemic trust is the capacity to 'trust in the authenticity and personal relevance of inter-personally transmitted knowledge' (Fonagy & Allison, 2014, p. 372). Epistemic trust arises in the early attachment relationship with the primary caretakers. Securely attached children trust in the reliability of their primary caretakers to nurture them, to be attuned to their feelings, and comfort them in their distress. Consequently, children trust that their caretakers are authoritative representatives of objective reality whose views of reality can be trusted and safely adopted as their own. This allows for the cultural transmission of knowledge from one generation to the next. Epistemic vigilance is suspicion towards information coming from others, like strangers, that may be potentially damaging, deceptive, or inaccurate (Fonagy & Allison, 2014).

Interestingly, securely attached children trusted their own perceptions over their mothers' when their mothers' claims appeared implausible. In contrast more insecurely attached children, especially children with disorganized attachment, are less trusting of parental views of reality but also mistrust their own perceptions (Corriveau et al., 2009). Insecure attachment can lead to an endless search for validation and reassurance that one's own perceptions are accurate (Fonagy & Allison, 2014). Yet insecure attachment also makes it difficult to trust in the validity of that validation and reassurance. Such individuals have lower tolerance for ambiguity, a tendency towards dogmatic thinking, a tendency towards premature closure, and a tendency to defend existing knowledge structures even when incorrect (Mikulincer, 1997; Piero & Kuglanski, 2008). Such individuals may feel emotionally overwhelmed when their dogmatically held beliefs are challenged.

This perspective is relevant to patients' weight management concerns as both food addiction and emotional eating are associated with insecure attachment (Pennock, 2022; Taube-Schiff, Van Exan, Tanaka, Wnuk, Hawa, & Sockalingam, 2015). Consequently, food addicted individuals who engage in emotional eating are prone to also having problems with epistemic trust. They may possess serious doubts about their own approach to eating especially when they have yet to discover a sustainable approach to weight management. To assuage their doubts, they may seek validation and reassurance that their current approach is essentially correct. They may feel undermined by anyone who questions the wisdom of their current approach or suggests a viable alternative that leads them to question their own food beliefs. They may ask for weight management guidance but then reject that guidance unless they are told what they were hoping to hear validating what they wished was true for them rather than what is true.

Dick had lost weight eating a predominantly zero-point diet. While working out on the elliptical in the fitness room of his apartment building, Julie, a next-door neighbor, who also struggled to lose weight said: 'What happened to you? You used to be fat. How did you lose all that weight?' Ignoring the retroactive fat shaming, Dick calmly explained his zero-point approach. Julie looked disappointed and annoyed. She dismissively replied, 'that might work for you but that wouldn't work for me'. Though stung by the combination of weight stigma and divergent weight management stigma in quick succession, Dick thought it best to let it drop and get on with his workout. Initially, Julie was eager to be enlightened to a new approach to weight loss that might work for her but became dismissive when she wasn't told what she was hoping to hear.

Individuals such as Julie don't possess the inner emotional security and confidence that comes from finding a weight management approach that has withstood the test of time. They may respond judgmentally or dismissively when confronted with a threatening perspective. Successful weight managers such as Dick become more thick-skinned in the face of individuals who sow the seeds of doubt by questioning their approach to weight management, be it too rigid (i.e., a zero-point diet) or too permissive (i.e., zero restrictions).

The epistemic mistrust of insecure weight managers is exacerbated by the fact that there are a plethora of commercial as well as scientifically-based approaches to weight management from which to choose that offer conflicting recommendations (i.e., healthy at any size or achieve a normal BMI, count calories or intuitive eating, low carbohydrate or low fat dieting, moderation or abstinence from trigger foods, lose weight quickly or lose weight slowly, improve self-regulation skills to the point of self-sufficiency or rely on a permanent emotional support structure to compensate for the limits of human willpower, live in temptation free environments or cultivate sufficient self-control to live in high temptation environments without relapsing).

Insecure weight managers with low tolerance for ambiguity may have difficulty accepting that answers to such questions can't always be answered in simple either/or ways and may need to be decided on a case-by-case rather than on a one-size-fits-all basis. Julie made a good point that what worked for Dick might not work for her, but her response was still a defensive one as she didn't want to contemplate the possibility that maybe it could work for her if she were more open to giving it a fair hearing. Individuals who succeed with more ascetic approaches to dieting may constitute a silent reproach to those who have yet to succeed with less restrictive approaches. Individuals who succeed with less restrictive approaches may arouse the envy of those who've yet to succeed with more permissive approaches.

What generalist psychotherapists are uniquely qualified to offer is how to think about weight management issues in ways that are less black or white, less dogmatic, more open to ambiguity, more skeptical of one-size-fits-all claims, more open to individualized and hybrid solutions, more open to trial and error learning, more perspectivist in seeing the kernel of truth in contradictory viewpoints, more dialectical in being able to flexibly counterbalance thinking from opposing viewpoints, and better able to appreciate the difficulty of decision making when the costs and benefits of a course of action are roughly equivalent. Cultivating such cognitive capabilities may be a common therapeutic factor in all successful psychotherapeutic approaches. Such enhanced cognitive functioning may be helpful to patients with a wide variety of psychological problems, be it depression, anxiety, anger management, relationship problems, and/ or weight management concerns, by increasing patients' reflective functioning (Fonagy & Allison, 2014).

Greta was a 32-year-old single cisgendered heterosexual female who sought psychotherapy because of dissatisfaction with her love life. She was demoralized that she had a long series of boyfriends who did not treat her with consideration and were disinterested in commitment. Greta attributed the difficulty to her weight. She was five foot four and weighed over 200 pounds. She believed she only attracted men who possessed a 'fat fetish' who did not view her as life partner material.

We discussed the problem of weight stigma among cisgendered heterosexual men. I raised the possibility that perhaps some men for whom her weight would not be an issue would view her as life partner material. Yet because of her internalized weight stigma she did not hold out for such men but settled for less. Consequently, she wasted time in dead-end relationships rather than look for better. Greta conceded that was most likely the case, but she still wanted to lose weight anyway before resuming dating. She believed that she could date more confidently as a thin person who could attract a wider pool of men.

I supported her weight loss goals to support her autonomy. Yet I noted that her love life need not be held hostage to losing weight as I thought the problem was as much about settling for unsatisfactory partners as it might be about her weight. Her presenting problem need not be construed in either/or ways. I wanted to help her overcome the dogmatic conviction derived from internalized weight stigma that she couldn't have a satisfactory love life without losing weight. Yet it was still her choice if she felt her love life would go better as a thinner person.

Greta decided to consult with a nutritionist. Initially, her nutritionist advised her to eat out less and coached her on how to make healthier lower fat/lower calorie meals at home. Greta liked to cook and didn't want to count calories, so this approach was appealing to her. There were no dietary restrictions. Yet after nine months she hadn't lost any weight. Greta was upset because she was eating more healthy food than she had ever eaten in her entire life so did not understand what the problem was.

I suggested that Greta could keep a food diary to try to understand why she wasn't losing weight. Initially she balked at the suggestion because she didn't want her eating behavior to be policed. After all, the nutritionist who was a weight loss specialist didn't ask for that. My suggestion set up a good cop/bad cop dichotomy in which I was the bad cop, and the nutritionist was the good cop. I suggested that perhaps she didn't want to know what she ate each day because she would get mad at herself to see the full extent to which she was not following her nutritionist's recommendation to predominantly consume healthy home cooked meals in lieu of frequently eating calorie-dense foods when out of the house.

My recommendation to keep a food log triggered her own warded off self-criticism. Greta appreciated without my having to remind her that eating more healthy food by itself would not result in weight loss unless she simultaneously reduced the consumption of the processed calorie-dense foods she liked to eat at work or when out with friends. Greta tried to maintain a compensatory food belief that somehow eating significantly more healthy food by itself when home would compensate for eating only marginally less amounts of the calorie-dense processed foods she usually ate when out of the house.

Greta started keeping a food log and discovered that she was eating a healthy breakfast and dinner at home each day as her nutritionist recommended, but she was supplementing those healthy meals with most of the same calorie-dense foods she had always eaten while at work for lunch or out with friends on weekends. Consequently, there wasn't any change in her daily calorie count or any weight loss. At this point Greta conceded that she needed to count calories, or she would never lose weight.

The nutritionist was flexible in her approach and suggested a daily calorie allowance of 1500 calories a day that over time would enable her to achieve her weight loss goal of 140 pounds. Greta started counting calories but found it near impossible to have 1500 calories a day without feeling like she was starving by the end of the day. She would beat herself up for that failure. The nutritionist suggested trying for 1700 calories a day instead and Greta was able to stick with that without undue hardship. Greta discovered through trial and error the most sustainable approach for her. The first approach was too permissive while the second approach was too strict. The third approach discovered the sustainable middle ground between the two extremes.

Increasing Mentalization in the Face of Motivated Reasoning, Self-Serving Bias, Confirmation Bias, and Worldview Defense

Social psychologists have discovered several biases inherent in social cognition (i.e., how we think about our relationships with others). Reasoning about relationships can be motivated by basic human needs such as being close to others while maintaining autonomy (Gold, 2013; Ryan & Deci, 2019). Consequently, therapeutic communication as well as health messaging may be rejected if it appears to constitute an autonomy threat (Beutler, Edwards, & Someah, 2018).

Human reasoning is also guided by a self-serving bias to construe things in ways that implicitly serve a person's self-interest often by taking personal credit for good outcomes while deflecting blame for bad ones. The self-serving bias has been found to influence individuals' health beliefs and nutrition behaviors (Renner, Knoll, & Schwarzer, 2000).

Human reasoning possesses a confirmation bias as there is a tendency to search for information that validates what one already believes to be true. Confirmation bias may reinforce individuals' aversion towards eating more fruits and vegetables (Dibbets, Borger, & Nederkoorn, 2021). Human reasoning can also be motivated by a worldview defense when one's sense of safety and security in the world is threatened by the elevated possibility of dying from a life-threatening disease like a metabolic syndrome (Arrowood, Cox, Kersten, Routledge, Shelton, & Hood, 2017). The insecurely attached would appear to be under the influence of various cognitive biases more so than the securely attached (Doolan & Bryant, 2021).

Therapists who aspire to help patients think about their weight management concerns in more reflective ways will likely be met with varying levels of resistance due to these cognitive biases. The tension in the therapeutic relationship isn't simply about differences of opinion regarding whether the patient should or shouldn't lose weight, should eat in more intuitive or more rule-bound ways, should eat low carb or low fat, should aspire to abstinence or moderation, etc. The tension would also be around whether such issues will be thought about and discussed in dichotomous ways (i.e., patients' automatic and sometimes well-defended default position) or in the more dialectical/pros and cons ways that many therapists try to facilitate.

Patients may want the sense of surety that comes with a more black or white and dogmatic way of thinking about weight management than the uncertainty that arises when being invited to contemplate in an open-minded way the merits of alternative points of view. Patients can feel that their personal belief system (i.e., their worldview defense) is being undermined when therapists note that although their beliefs contain a kernel of truth their beliefs may also possess a tunnel vision that does not allow them to appreciate that there are two or more sides to any story. Processing their weight management concerns at that level of cognitive complexity and sophistication can seem overwhelming.

Epistemic vigilance means that any time a therapist suggests an alternative perspective the patient might experience the therapist as advocating that perspective and putting coercive pressure on the patient to adopt it. Patients' epistemic vigilance is not without its kernel of truth because therapists do have their biases and their favored viewpoints. Epistemic vigilance can reflect a healthy skepticism towards new points of view. It means putting new viewpoints to the test to see how well they withstand critical thought. Being overly gullible or suggestible can make one vulnerable to brainwashing. Consequently, therapists should welcome patients' epistemic vigilance and try to nondefensively tolerate having one's ideas and motives interrogated by skeptical patients. Epistemic trust is earned in part by therapists' welcoming response to patients' skepticism.

Mentalizing refers to the capacity to imagine ourselves from the outside looking in and to imagine others from the inside looking out (Fonagy, Campbell, & Luyten, 2023). As such mentalizing is a conjecture, an inference, an exercise of the human imagination. Mental states are opaque as we never know for sure what someone else thinks and feels. We only know what others say and do and make inferences about their mental states on that basis. Communication breakdown is an omnipresent possibility in human conversations as individuals may make faulty inferences about what others mean.

Human conversation involves a constant and ongoing process of correction and clarification such as 'what I meant to say', 'do you mean that', 'yes, that was exactly what I was saying', 'I agree', 'I don't agree', 'I partially agree', 'yes, but did you consider this', etc. (Fonagy, Campbell, & Luyten, 2023, p. 255). Human communication is jointly focusing attention on a topic of attention, like how to lose weight, with an appreciation that each person will be viewing that joint object of attention from their own unique perspective (Tomasello, 2016). There will always be a jostling of perspectives, differences of opinion, and misunderstandings about where others are coming from that require continual clarification and negotiation. According to Fonagy, Campbell, and Luyten (2023, p. 254) moments of misunderstanding are therapeutically advantageous precisely because they provide opportunities to recap and align perspectives, affording moments of joining for further shared exploration.

Patients high on epistemic vigilance, like those with borderline personality disorder, may perceive the process of clarifying and correcting as acts of aggression, rejection, hostility, and failure (Fonagy, Campbell, & Luyten, 2023). That may be accompanied by an unwillingness to invest the time, effort, and resources necessary to work on relationship repair after communication breakdown (Michael et al., 2021).

It falls on the therapist to repair the ruptures to the therapeutic relationship that arise when the inevitable clash of perspectives results in communication breakdown. The therapist must transcend the pull towards polarizing either/or debate rather than thoughtful nuanced discussion when patients engage in negative mind reading, like ascribing malevolent motives to the therapist, after therapists offer alternative but threatening perspectives.

It is easy to fall into power struggles with patients over the nature of dietary reality (i.e., Should fruit be avoided because it has too much sugar? Is counting calories too much work even with a smartphone app? Is a weight management approach proving ineffective or was the implementation faulty?) The self-serving bias motivates patients to blame the approach rather than their suboptimal implementation but also motivates therapists to blame patients for treatment failures rather than the limitations of their own approach.

When therapists feel attacked by patients and their own reflective functioning deteriorates, they might respond with the sort of maladaptive communicative responses that Gottman (2002) has found result in communication breakdown in close dyadic relationships. Therapists' defensive self-justification and countercomplaint deflects blame back on to the patient and can result in further confrontation ruptures. Stonewalling, a kind of hostile withdrawal that might masquerade as professional neutrality, may result in withdrawal ruptures. As therapists' reflective functioning recovers after communication breakdown, they may need to assume the initiative to repair the rupture to the therapeutic relationship caused in part by their lapse in reflective functioning and their concurrent regression to more defensive ways of responding.

Liam a married 40-year-old businessman with one child suffered Type 2 diabetes. His BMI was obese, and his physician recommended he lose weight. His blood sugar tended to be poorly controlled despite taking medication. When he went to the dentist to have his teeth cleaned, his gums bled profusely which was a symptom of his poorly controlled diabetes. During a discussion of his diet, I discovered that he rarely ate any fruits or vegetables and just filled up on bread, pasta, and fried foods. I suggested that he might try consuming more fruits and vegetables and eating less bread, pasta, and fried food. Liam sounded skeptical but in a tone of begrudging accommodation said he would give it a try.

The next session Liam came in to say that he voraciously filled himself up on watermelon, cantaloupe, and pineapple and then tested his blood sugar which went through the roof. He sounded triumphant to prove that I didn't know what I was talking about. I responded with defensive self-justification that he was overeating the fruits that were high on the glycemic index rather than eating in moderation the fruits that were low on the glycemic index as recommended by the American Diabetic Association. I could see that we were getting into a power struggle about the true nature of dietary reality.

To repair the rupture, I acknowledged his point that replacing bread and pasta that he overate with overeating fruit might not help him lose weight or better control his blood sugar. I suggested that he might need to work with a nutritionist who specialized in working with diabetics to figure out what might be the optimum diet for him. Liam appeared smugly self-satisfied that I conceded his point. Validating his viewpoint repaired the rupture to the therapeutic relationship. Yet he declined my recommendation to work with a nutritionist because he didn't have the time to consult with another professional and still believed he could figure out his diet on his own.

His contemptuous attitude towards me was off-putting and I responded with defensive self-justification in my attempt to clarify my initial dietary recommendation. In retrospect I appreciated that my intervention produced considerable reactance. Liam was feeling out of control and needed to buttress his shaky sense of autonomy. Yet he did so in a way that struck me as defiantly self-destructive. The performance pressure I felt to work through his defiant self-destructiveness before his poorly controlled diabetes wreaked further havoc with his health contributed to my defensiveness. To communicate more constructively I had to learn to better contain my worry about his deteriorating health situation as well as the shame triggered by his contemptuous dismissal of what I had thought of as helpful common-sense advice.

References

Ahmed, S. H. (2012). Is sugar as addictive as cocaine? In K. D. Brownell & M. S. Gold, *Food and addiction: A comprehensive handbook* (pp. 232–237). Oxford University Press. https://doi.org/10.1093/med:psych/9780199738168.003.0035

Alamuddin, N., & Wadden, T. A. (2016). Behavioral treatment of the patient with obesity. *Endocrinology and Metabolism Clinics of North America*, 45(3), 565–580. https://doi.org/10.1016/j.ecl.2016.04.008

Antoniou, E. E., Bongers, P., & Jansen, A. (2017). The mediating role of dichotomous thinking and emotional eating in the relationship between depression and BMI. *Eating Behaviors*, 26, 55–60. https://doi.org/10.1016/j.eatbeh.2017.01.007

Arrowood, R. B., Cox, C. R., Kersten, M., Routledge, C., Shelton, J. T., & Hood, R. W. (2017). Ebola salience, death-thought accessibility, and worldview defense: A terror management theory perspective. *Death Studies*, 41(9), 585–591. https://doi.org/10.1080/07481187.2017.1322644

Berbesque, J. C., & Marlowe, F. W. (2009). Sex differences in food preferences of Hadza hunter-gatherers. *Evolutionary Psychology*, 7(4), 601–616. https://doi.org/10.1177/147470490900700409

Beutler, L. E., Edwards, C., & Someah, K. (2018). Adapting psychotherapy to patient reactance level: A meta-analytic review. *Journal of Clinical Psychology*, 74(11), 1952–1963. https://doi.org/10.1002/jclp.22682

Bilman, E. M., van Trijp, J. C., & Renes, R. J. (2010). Consumer perceptions of satiety-related snack food decision making. *Appetite*, 55(3), 639–647. https://doi.org/10.1016/j.appet.2010.09.020

Carmody, R. N. (2017). Evolution of the human dietary niche: Quest for high quality. In M. N. Muller, R. W. Wrangham, & D. R. Pilbeam (Eds.), *Chimpanzees and human evolution* (pp. 311–338). The Belknap Press of Harvard University Press. https://doi-org/10.4159/9780674982642-009

Clifford, D., Ozier, A., Bundros, J., Moore, J., Kreiser, A., & Morris, M. N. (2015). Impact of non-diet approaches on attitudes, behaviors, and health outcomes: A systematic review. *Journal of Nutrition Education and Behavior*, 47(2), 143–155.e1. https://doi.org/10.1016/j.jneb.2014.12.002

Corriveau, K. H., Harris, P. L., Meins, E., Fernyhough, C., Arnott, B., Elliott, L., Liddle, B., Hearn, A., Vittorini, L., & de Rosnay, M. (2009). Young children's trust in their mother's claims: Longitudinal links with attachment security in infancy. *Child Development*, 80(3), 750–761. https://doi.org/10.1111/j.1467-8624.2009.01295.x

Dibbets, P., Borger, L., & Nederkoorn, C. (2021). Filthy fruit! Confirmation bias and novel food. *Appetite*, 167, 105607. https://doi.org/10.1016/j.appet.2021.105607

Doolan, E. L., & Bryant, R. A. (2021). Modifying insecure attachment style with cognitive bias modification. *Journal of Behavior Therapy and Experimental Psychiatry*, 73, 101664. https://doi.org/10.1016/j.jbtep.2021.101664

Eddie, D., Bergman, B. G., Hoffman, L. A., & Kelly, J. F. (2022). Abstinence versus moderation recovery pathways following resolution of a substance use problem: Prevalence, predictors, and relationship to psychosocial well-being in a U.S. national sample. *Alcoholism: Clinical and Experimental Research*, 46(2), 312–325. https://doi-org/10.1111/acer.14765

Fonagy, P., & Allison, E. (2014). The role of mentalizing and epistemic trust in the therapeutic relationship. *Psychotherapy*, 51(3), 372–380.

Fonagy, P., Campbell, C., & Luyten, P. (2023). Alliance rupture and repair in mentalization-based therapy. In C. F. Eubanks, L. W. Samstag, & J. C. Muran (Eds.), *Rupture and repair in psychotherapy: A critical process for change* (pp. 253–276). American Psychological Association. https://doi.org/10.1037/0000306-011

Gardner, C. D., Trepanowski, J. F., Del Gobbo, L. C., Hauser, M. E., Rigdon, J., Ioannidis, J. P. A., Desai, M., & King, A. C. (2018). Effect of low-Fat vs low-carbohydrate diet on 12-month weight loss in overweight adults and the association with genotype pattern or insulin secretion: The DIETFITS randomized clinical trial. *JAMA*, 319(7), 667–679. https://doi.org/10.1001/jama.2018.0245

Gold, R. S. (2013). Perceived likelihood of experiencing a desirable versus undesirable outcome. *Psychological Reports*, 113(2), 525–527. https://doi.org/10.2466/04.07.PR0.113x18z5

Gomez-Rubalcava, S., Stabbert, K., & Phelan, S. (2018). Behavioral treatment of obesity. In T. Wadden & G. A. Bray (Eds.), *Handbook of obesity treatment* (pp. 336–348). The Guilford Press.

Gottman, J. M. (2002). A multidimensional approach to couples. In F. W. Kaslow & T. Patterson (Eds.), *Comprehensive handbook of psychotherapy: Cognitive-behavioral approaches*, Vol. 2 (pp. 355–372). John Wiley & Sons, Inc.

Hutchinson E. (2011). Systems neuroscience: the stress of dieting. *Nature Reviews Neuroscience*, 12(2), 65. https://doi.org/10.1038/nrn2985

Jensen, M. D., Ryan, D. H., Apovian, C. M., Ard, J. D., Comuzzie, A. G., Donato, K. A., Hu, F. B., Hubbard, V. S., Jakicic, J. M., Kushner, R. F., Loria, C. M., Millen, B. E., Nonas, C. A., Pi-Sunyer, F. X., Stevens, J., Stevens, V. J., Wadden, T. A., Wolfe, B.M., & Yanovski, S. Z. (2014). 2013 AHA/ACC/TOS guideline for the management of overweight and obesity in adults: A report of the American College of Cardiology/American Heart Association task force on practice guidelines and The Obesity Society. *Journal of the American College of Cardiology*, 63(25 Pt. B), 2985–3023. https://doi.org/10.1016/j.jacc.2013.11.004

Kearney, R. J. (1996). *Within the wall of denial: Conquering addictive behaviors*. W. W. Norton & Co.

Kuhn, M. (2021). Fasting and prayer: Can it help in the resolution of modern diseases of culture? *Dissertation Abstracts International: Section B: The Sciences and Engineering*, 82(7-B).

Larsen, T. M., Dalskov, S. M., van Baak, M., Jebb, S. A., Papadaki, A., Pfeiffer, A. F., Martinez, J. A., Handjieva-Darlenska, T., Kunešov., M., Pihlsg.rd, M., Stender, S., Holst, C., Saris, W. H., Astrup, A., & the Diet, Obesity, and Genes (Diogenes) Project. (2010). Diets with high or low protein content and glycemic index for weight-loss maintenance. *New England Journal of Medicine*, 363(22), 2102–2113. https://doi.org/10.1056/NEJMoa1007137.

Marlatt, K. L., & Ravussin, E. (2018). Energy expenditure and obesity. In T. A. Wadden & G. A. Bray (Eds.), *Handbook of obesity treatment* (pp. 38–63). The Guilford Press.

Michael, J., Chennells, M., Nolte, T., Ooi, J., Griem, J., Christensen, W., Feigenbaum, J., King-Casas, B., Fonagy, P., Montague, P. R., & the London Personality and Mood Disorder Research Network. (2021). Probing commitment in individuals with borderline personality disorder. *Journal of Psychiatric Research*, 137, 335–341. https://doi. org/10.1016/j.jpsychires.2021.02.062

Mikulincer, M. (1997). Adult attachment style and information processing: Individual differences in curiosity and cognitive closure. *Journal of Personality and Social Psychology*, 72, 1217–1230. https:// doi.org/10.1037/0022-3514.72.5.1217

Moss, M. (2014). *Salt sugar fat: How the food giants hooked us.* New York: Random House.

Parylak, S. L., Koob, G. F., & Zorrilla, E. P. (2011). The dark side of food addiction. *Physiology & Behavior*, 104(1), 149–156. https://doi.org/10.1016/j.physbeh.2011.04.063

Pennock, S. (2022). Dysfunctional eating in recovering addicts: A therapist's shift to an attachment-focused approach. In L. Cundy (Ed.), *Attachment, relationships and food: From cradle to kitchen* (pp. 96–115). Routledge/Taylor & Francis Group.

Petersen, R., Brakoulias, V., & Langdon, R. (2016). An experimental investigation of mentalization ability in borderline personality disorder. *Comprehensive Psychiatry*, 64, 12–21. https://doi.org/10.1016/j.comppsych.2015.10.004

Reich, J., & Neenan, P. (1986). Principles common to different short-term psychotherapies. *American Journal of Psychotherapy*, 40(1), 62–69. https://doi.org/10.1176/appi. psychotherapy.1986.40.1.62

Renner, B., Knoll, N., & Schwarzer, R. (2000). Age and body make a difference in optimistic health beliefs and nutrition behaviors. *International Journal of Behavioral Medicine*, 7(2), 143–159. https://doi.org/10.1207/S15327558IJBM0702_4

Reverri, E. J., Randolph, J. M., Kappagoda, C. T., Park, E., Edirisinghe, I., & Burton-Freeman, M. (2017). Assessing beans as a source of intrinsic fiber on satiety in men and women with metabolic syndrome. *Appetite*, 118, 75–81. https://doi-org/10.1016/j.appet.2017.07.013

Ryan, R. M., & Deci, E. L. (2019). Supporting autonomy, competence, and relatedness: The coaching process from a self-determination theory perspective. In S. English, J. M. Sabatine, & P. Brownell (Eds.), *Professional coaching: Principles and practice* (pp. 231–245). Springer Publishing Company.

Schulte, E. M., Smeal, J. K., Lewis, J., & Gearhardt, A. N. (2018). Development of the Highly Processed Food Withdrawal Scale. *Appetite*, 131, 148–154. https://doi.org/10.1016/j. appet.2018.09.013

Shively, C. A., Register, T. C., & Clarkson, T. B. (2009). Social stress, visceral obesity, and coronary artery atherosclerosis: Product of a primate adaptation. *American Journal of Primatology*, 71(9), 742–751. https://doi.org/10.1002/ajp.20706

Taube-Schiff, M., Van Exan, J., Tanaka, R., Wnuk, S., Hawa, R., & Sockalingam, S. (2015). Attachment style and emotional eating in bariatric surgery candidates: The mediating role of difficulties in emotion regulation. *Eating Behaviors*, 18, 36–40. https://doi. org/10.1016/j.eatbeh.2015.03.011

Tomasello, M. (2016). *A natural history of human morality.* Harvard University Press. https:// doi.org/10.4159/9780674915855

Tronieri, J. S. (2021). Cognitive and behavioral treatments for obesity. In A. Wenzel (Ed.), *Handbook of cognitive behavioral therapy: Applications* (pp. 453–476). American Psychological Association. https://doi-org/10.1037/0000219-014

Tsai, A. G., & Wadden, T. A. (2006). The evolution of very-low-calorie diets: An update and meta-analysis. *Obesity*, 14(8), 1283–1293. https://doi.org/10.1038/oby.2006.146

Vink, R. G., Roumans, N. J., Arkenbosch, L. A., Mariman, E. C., & van Baak, M. A. (2016). The effect of rate of weight loss on long-term weight regain in adults with overweight and obesity. *Obesity (Silver Spring, Md.)*, 24(2), 321–327. https://doi.org/10.1002/oby.21346

Winchester, K. (2023) *Weight Watchers new complete cookbook 2023: 1200 day quick, easy & delicious recipes for weight loss. Eat well everyday improve your lifestyle.* Independently Published.

Wing, R. R., Lang, W., Wadden, T. A., Safford, M., Knowler, W. C., Bertoni, A. G., Hill, J. O., Brancati, F. L., Peters, A., Wagenknecht, L., & the Look AHEAD Research Group. (2011). Benefits of modest weight loss in improving cardiovascular risk factors in overweight and obese individuals with Type 2 diabetes. *Diabetes Care*, 34(7), 1481–1486. https://doi.org/10.2337/dc10-2415

Wong, K. (2017) How to find a therapist. *The Cut.* December 1, 2017.

Wrangham, R. (2017). Control of fire in the Paleolithic: Evaluating the cooking hypothesis. *Current Anthropology*, 58 (S16), S303–S313. https://10.1086/692113

Patients' Weight Management Journeys and the Therapeutic Relationship

part II

Kill the Messenger

7

Helping Patients Deal with 'Bad Numbers'
(i.e., weight, BMI, calories, blood glucose,
cholesterol, blood pressure)

One of the first uncertainties that arises in psychotherapy for weight management is ascertaining whether a patient needs to lose weight and what it means to be overweight. How much weight is too much weight? This question is challenging to answer because it arises for both cosmetic and medical reasons. In terms of physical attractiveness patients worry about what is too thin or too fat to look physically attractive. On this dimension there are many cross-cultural and individual differences as to what is found to be physically attractive in terms of body weight (Rosinger & Puts, 2018). Patients may have low self-esteem for not living up to certain ideal body standards though different cultures and different individuals possess different conceptions of what constitutes an ideal body type (Robinson & Christiansen, 2015).

Some dieting, especially among younger individuals, is motivated by a desire to look more physically attractive and to be found more sexually desirable to a target audience. Patients may desire thin romantic partners and believe that they need to be thin to attract such partners. Such dieting motivations could be driven in part by internalized weight stigma as patients may reject themselves as well potential romantic partners for failing to live up to a cultural idealization of thinness that may be an unattainable goal for many individuals.

To the extent ideal body types are unrealistic the treatment goal may be alleviation of internalized weight stigma instilled by explicit and implicit 'fat shaming' concurrent with the cultivation of body acceptance and body positivity (O'Hara, Ahmed, & Elashie, 2021; Pearl, Bach, & Wadden, 2022). The treatment may attempt to cultivate intuitive eating and the alleviation of orthorexia nervosa (Rodgers, White, & Berry, 2021) so patients can eat without undue shame and guilt about their eating habits. This approach may be appropriate when it is concluded that weight loss is contraindicated, and patients are healthy at their current size.

Stan came for treatment in his late twenties because he was a virgin who never had a girlfriend though he was a successful lawyer and had many platonic female friends. Stan had always considered himself overweight and was teased as a child for having 'man boobs'. Shame over his physical appearance made him self-conscious around romantic interests who he automatically assumed would not think his physique sufficiently manly. Those assumptions were questioned in psychotherapy as it was suggested that some women might be attracted to his big and bearish body.

Questioning those assumptions precipitated a confrontation rupture to the therapeutic relationship. Stan complained that I was being falsely reassuring because everyone knew that women were not attracted to 'fat' men. I validated that all things being equal that many women might prefer a partner who is slimmer given the cultural prevalence of weight stigma

DOI: 10.4324/9781003402336-11

but that women evaluated potential romantic partners for their personality attributes as well as physical looks. I noted that some women might be attracted to big and bearish men even if that wasn't a normative preference in the culture-at-large.

The rupture was repaired as Stan conceded that I had a point once I noted the kernel of truth in his viewpoint while still suggesting a more nuanced and less either/or perspective on cisgendered heterosexual women's romantic preferences. Stan remained skeptical, nevertheless. Repairing ruptures to the therapeutic relationship can be facilitated by validating what appears valid in the patient's underlying assumptions though those assumptions may still constitute self-defeating overgeneralizations despite possessing a substantial kernel of truth. Further clarification and qualification of the therapist's viewpoint can be helpful if the therapist's viewpoint is experienced by the patient as a gross overgeneralization that invalidates the patient's experience of feeling rejected by women due to his weight.

Despite his skepticism, the idea that some desirable women could be attracted to him began to sink in. Stan found a big woman whom he found attractive and who found him attractive. As they initiated a sexual relationship, Stan's body acceptance increased dramatically without having to lose any weight. They eventually married. Body image satisfaction, regardless of weight, is associated with having a satisfying sex and love life (Kvalem, Træen, Markovic, & von Soest, 2019).

In contrast to Stan, Margaret was a recently divorced middle-aged woman who gained weight while married. Ready to resume dating as a single cisgender heterosexual woman she wanted to look good for her age and wanted to date men who looked physically fit. Margaret wanted help with dieting and exercise as she was not interested in dating men that she perceived as overweight. Margaret had ended the marriage in part because she had married her husband for emotional security but had never felt any sexual chemistry with him. She reported that her husband was not her physical type. Margaret was determined to 'get in shape' through diet and exercise to finally win the type to whom she was most physically attracted.

I noted that men varied in the body type to whom they were most attracted and that some men were attracted to women they perceived as voluptuous. Margaret responded with barely contained sarcasm saying 'That might be true but I must like what I see in the mirror so I can feel confident when I resume dating. I don't like what I see when I look in the mirror, so you must help me lose weight until I like what I see'. My comment precipitated a confrontation rupture. I conceded her point and said I would help her with weight loss rather than try to help her accept her body as it was. Margaret lost weight rapidly on a raw foods diet but when she started looking too thin, she reintroduced cooked foods into her diet to gain weight.

Sometimes repairing the rupture to the therapeutic relationship means acknowledging that one's intervention was off and insensitive to where the patient is at even if it is well-intended and has proven effective with other patients with similar problems. Sometimes patients function in effect as the therapist's supervisor and coach the therapist on how to best repair the rupture. Margaret didn't want me to question or reframe her weight loss goals but to take them at face value.

The Problem of 'Bad' Numbers

When there is goal consensus to work on weight loss goals, it is quickly discovered that achieving such goals is quite challenging. Losing weight and keeping it off is challenging because of genetic predispositions towards overeating in obesogenic environments

(Farooqi, 2018), reliance on emotional eating for emotion regulation given a history of trauma and insecure attachment (Ansari, Shakiba, Mousavi, Mohammadkhani, Aminoroaya, & Poor, 2018; Taube-Schiff, Van Exan, Tanaka, Wnuk, Hawa, & Sockalingam, 2015), and the addictive properties of calorie-dense processed foods (Schulte, Smeal, Lewis, & Gearhardt, 2018).

Food addiction, like any other addiction, can be considered a disease of denial (Kearney, 1996). Addictions are impulse control disorders (Rosenberg & Curtiss Feder, 2014). Denial of addictive behavior is therefore a defiant assertion to others as well as oneself that one can control the addictive behavior when personal history suggests otherwise. Denial is often accompanied by rationalizations that try to offer plausible explanations of why behavior that appears out of control to external observers really isn't as out of control as it seems to be. Denial is often buttressed by dissociation, a defense mechanism by which individuals simply tune out the addictive behavior by not thinking about it as though it's a nonissue. Mindless eating has been associated with overeating (Long, Vartanian, Herman, & Polivy, 2020).

What are often difficult for food addicted individuals to deny, rationalize, and dissociate are 'bad' numbers. 'Bad' numbers are numbers that suggest that patients' weight might constitute a serious health risk and that if they don't lose weight and keep it off, they might suffer a life-threatening metabolic illness. Mortality salience, a heightened fear of dying, constitutes a threat to one's autonomous existence. Yet high autonomous self-determination attenuates the need for a defensive response, like worldview defense, to existential threats (Vail, Conti, Goad, & Horner, 2020). Ultimately everyone dies and that's an autonomy threatening event that nobody has any control over. Yet if one engages in health promoting rather than health compromising behavior one might be able to avoid premature disability and demise.

Food addicted patients may become torn between denying, rationalizing, and dissociating their out-of-control eating behavior as a defensive assertion of their threatened autonomy and acknowledging their food addiction and their need for recovery to live a healthier lifestyle. Consequently, patients are of two minds about facing 'bad' numbers. High weight patients believe that they 'should' face 'bad' numbers as biomarkers of their health status, but they don't want to because 'bad' numbers will be upsetting. Those high in autonomous self-determination are more likely to accept their mortality and do what they can to live a healthful lifestyle. In contrast those whose autonomy is threatened by mortality reminders are more likely to respond defensively by rationalizing their health compromising behaviors.

Patients in denial may avoid weighing themselves, avoid calculating their BMIs, avoid counting calories, and avoid the yearly physicals that might detect the biomarkers of various metabolic syndromes. Once exposed to 'bad' numbers, patients may rationalize such 'bad' numbers and stop thinking about it (i.e., I've added muscle weight rather than fat, weight isn't related to calories but which foods you eat, I can control my blood pressure, cholesterol, and blood sugar with medication, so I need not lose weight). Being reminded of 'bad' numbers may generate considerable reactance because those reminders challenge the denial, rationalization, and dissociation that keeps awareness of the autonomy threatening 'bad' numbers at bay.

Helping patients come to terms with autonomy threatening 'bad' numbers is challenging for a variety of reasons: 1) It is difficult to have an open-minded discussion of 'bad' numbers when contemplating such numbers threatens patients' automatic tendencies to deny, rationalize, and dissociate such numbers. 2) Patients tend to think of numbers reflective of their underlying health status in dichotomous all good or all bad ways rather than as useful information that exists on a continuum. 3) Such numbers are open to multiple interpretations and psychotherapists are neither nutritionists nor physicians whose job it is to obtain and interpret such health markers. 4) Psychotherapists generally don't weigh patients, track patients' daily caloric intake, take their blood pressure, or take their blood samples to assess their cholesterol and blood glucose levels. Therapists wouldn't know what those numbers are without patients sharing such numbers. 5) Patients have difficulty thinking about 'bad' numbers without blaming themselves for those numbers. 6) Patients might not want to make the difficult lifestyle changes they would need to make to attain 'good' numbers if 'bad' numbers are a product of a food addiction from which patients would need to recover. 7) Ruptures to the therapeutic relationship are likely when discussion of 'bad' numbers threatens patients' autonomy and produces considerable reactance.

Despite patients' aversion to facing bad numbers, patients often bring their emotional reactions to 'bad' numbers to their psychotherapists as their all-purpose sounding boards. Therapists therefore must try to help patients resolve their ambivalence about facing 'bad' numbers and figuring out what to do about it.

Blaming Oneself for 'Bad' Numbers

Psychodynamic psychotherapists have long recognized that the analysis of psychological defenses like denial, rationalization, and dissociation often provoke further defensiveness (Freud, 1923). Patients defend their defenses. Such defenses serve a useful psychological function in attenuating the shame patients feel after failures of impulse control. Analysis of those defenses therefore can threaten and destabilize patients' psychological equilibrium (Cramer, 2006). A therapist that attempts to address patients' defensiveness may therefore constitute an autonomy threat resulting in a rupture to the therapeutic relationship. The therapist is experienced as undermining rather than supporting patients' fragile sense of autonomy. Patients may then either lash out in anger against or withdraw in fear from the autonomy threatening psychotherapist.

Food addicted patients may oscillate between denying, rationalizing, and dissociating 'bad' numbers and blaming oneself for 'bad' numbers. From an early age weight can be a shame sensitive issue because of internalized weight stigma (Lucibello, Nesbitt, Solomon-Krakus, & Sabiston, 2021) as is loss of self-control such as urinary or fecal incontinence (Devendorf, Bradley, Barks, Klanchar, Orozco, & Cowan, 2021). Experiences of 'fat shaming', both explicit and implicit beginning in early childhood establishes that 'thin' is the desirable body type (Schulte, Bach, Berkowitz, Latner, & Pearl, 2021). It is challenging to discuss 'bad' numbers as a health issue without simultaneously activating patients' internalized weight stigma.

Poor body image is a source of self-blame because the underlying assumption is that anyone can readily possess a more ideal body type if they eat less and exercise more. From the perspective of food addiction this self-blame is irrational. 1) It's not one's fault if one possesses an endomorphic body type prone to weight gain in obesogenic environments. 2) It's not one's fault if trauma and insecure attachment led to emotional eating as an emotion regulation strategy. 3) Getting 'hooked' on high processed carbohydrate/high fat/low fiber foods is not one's fault if one has been fed such 'comfort' foods since early childhood.

Cognitive reappraisal of these irrational beliefs is challenging because even though the more 'rational' perspective alleviates patients' self-blame it also diminishes patients' sense of autonomy. To alter the beliefs that justify self-blame requires accepting beliefs in which one has much less control over one's eating behavior than one would like to believe one has. One can't change one's genetic predisposition and one has limited ability to extricate oneself from an obesogenic environment. One has limited ability to avoid the stresses of love, work, and family life. Childhood trauma and insecure attachment may have created a dependence on emotional eating that is not easily overcome. One may need to treat one's favorite foods as addictive substances to be avoided entirely or eaten only in carefully moderated ways. Perhaps it's better to believe that through a heroic effort of autonomous self-determination and willpower that one can force oneself to eat less and exercise more even in high stress/ high temptation environments. Beating up on oneself for failures of self-control seems to supply the necessary motivation to do better next time, overlooking the fact that self-flagellation is an ineffective motivator of health promoting behavior.

Psychological defenses are deployed like denial, rationalization, and dissociation to alleviate the shame and self-blame that derives from compulsive overeating (Moore, Sabino, Koob, & Cottone, 2019). Shame motivates hiding behavior (Shen, 2018). The universal facial expression for shame is to avoid eye contact by looking down and away from what is anticipated to be the disapproving gaze of judgmental others (Tracy, Robins, & Schriber, 2009). Psychological defenses against shame are ways of avoiding the judgmental gaze of others as well as one's own harsh inner critic. That inner critic would like to believe that if one were sufficiently autonomous one could eat whatever one likes without suffering negative consequences and if not, at least possess the willpower to eat less and exercise more.

'Bad Numbers', Confrontation, and the Therapeutic Relationship

Psychotherapists as parental surrogates/authority figures might be perceived as believing that patients who receive 'bad' numbers have only themselves to blame for their misfortune. After all, if patients have been in denial of their weight management problems and have avoided assuming responsibility for those problems, wouldn't therapists be right to blame their overweight patients for their deteriorating health situation as much as such patients blame themselves? Patients may be reluctant to raise the issue of 'bad' numbers because they fear their psychotherapists' judgment as well as their own self-blame. Patients might assume that psychotherapists who draw patients' attention to such an avoided topic are trying to expose patients' hidden shame just to make them feel badly about their weight management problems. It might not seem like their therapists are trying to help them acknowledge and reflect on their health compromising behavior so they can try to alter it for the better. Patients might be skeptical that therapists are trying to facilitate acceptance of 'responsibility without blame' (Pickard, 2017).

Patients may raise the issue of 'bad' numbers on their own initiative because they are disturbed by those numbers when they weigh themselves, calculate their daily caloric intake on a smartphone application, or are informed by their physicians about their high blood pressure, high cholesterol, and high blood glucose. As therapists help patients process those numbers it may seem like therapists are 'forcing' patients to think about something they would rather not think about and face 'bad' news they would rather not face even though patients raised the issue themselves. Patients may raise 'bad' numbers hoping to obtain reassurance that there is nothing to worry about rather than to learn to accept 'bad' news with self-compassion rather than moralistic judgment and figure out a plan of action that will help them achieve better numbers in the future.

Confrontation is a therapeutic technique that serves to help patients face painful realities that have been denied, rationalized, or dissociated (Buie & Adler, 1972). Confrontation, though, is a controversial therapeutic technique because it can be experienced as a personal attack and a moralistic judgment by an authoritarian therapist who is applying coercive pressure to make patients submit to therapists' worldview and the recommendations that derive from that worldview (Friedman-Daugherty, 1998).

Confrontations not infrequently result in ruptures to the therapeutic relationship (Moeseneder, Ribeiro, Muran, & Caspar, 2019). Addicted patients may lash out in anger (i.e., a confrontation rupture) or withdraw in fear (i.e., withdrawal rupture) by confrontations that are experienced as autonomy threatening and thereby produce considerable reactance (Karno & Longabaugh, 2005). Though confrontations may result in rupture, use of confrontation to resolve ruptures has been associated with better psychotherapy outcome (Moeseneder, Ribeiro, Muran, & Caspar, 2019).

This is not to say that confrontation should be avoided in order to avoid ruptures to the therapeutic relationship. Sometimes patients appreciate confrontations when they are close to being ready to face a painful reality and need therapists who will help them find the courage to 'face the music'. It is reassuring to patients that therapists are not as frightened and avoidant of facing painful realities as their patients are. Some patients don't want a therapist who will be falsely reassuring because patients are assumed to be too fragile to handle the truth and therapists are frightened of either offending or losing patients. Confrontation may empower patients to face rather than avoid painful realities and then do something constructive about it.

Therapists might not know in advance how patients will respond to confrontations so confrontations may seem like high-risk interventions. It seems like it must be 'bad' therapy if patients feel emotionally damaged by confrontation and lash out in anger or quit treatment. Nevertheless, avoidance of confrontation could result in withdrawal ruptures because the avoidance of painful realities keeps the treatment at a superficial level that does not address core issues. Patients may then prematurely terminate treatments that aren't going anywhere. Patient and therapist become a conflict avoidant couple whose relationship remains superficial and such couples can drift apart (Holman & Jarvis, 2003).

As weight-related metabolic syndromes are progressive illnesses time may be of the essence in addressing such weight-related health issues before the cumulative and perhaps irreversible effects of such syndromes add up. So, on the one hand, confronting weight-related health issues patients don't seem quite ready to face could potentially damage the therapeutic relationship. On the other hand, avoidance of weight-related health issues means that patients continue to engage in health compromising behavior as their metabolic syndromes progress when weight loss along with medication might be able to arrest the progression of such illnesses.

From a psychodynamic perspective, inner conflicts may get worked through by externalizing such conflicts and enacting them in the therapeutic relationship (i.e., transference) where those relational conflicts can be interpreted (Guilfoyle, 2009). That is a key principle of transference-focused psychotherapy (Levy, Yeomans, & Spina, 2022), an evidence-based treatment approach. Therapists become the representative of patients' inner critics (i.e., superegos) providing an opportunity for patients to work through their struggles with their own inner critics in the therapeutic relationship (Gray, 1987). Therapists may need to nondefensively tolerate being perceived as the representative of patients' harsh inner critic as part of the therapeutic process as patients work through their fears of facing painful realities.

Confrontation ruptures may help patients work through their conflicts with authority figures who seem to be undermining their autonomy as perhaps their parents once did. Power struggles with the therapist may ensue as the patient defiantly asserts their sense of personal choice, control, and autonomy by asserting their right to diet or not diet in their own individual way for better or worse. Learning to stand up for oneself rather than begrudgingly submit to the dictates of an unreasonably demanding authority figure is generally good for one's personal growth and development. It can be therapeutic as patients discover the courage to speak their minds openly and assert a difference of opinion with their therapists.

Unassertive patients can learn to be assertive rather than aggressive or passive by learning to assert themselves with therapists perceived as moralistic and unreasonably demanding authority figures as their parents once were or still are. Constructive dyadic communication during conflict discussions requires an ability to disagree without becoming disagreeable in contrast to the more volatile demand-withdraw communication pattern that exacerbates conflict (Domingue & Mollen, 2009).

Therapists need not avoid conflict discussions with patients to always be empathizing with and validating patients' viewpoints. Conflict discussions are inevitable aspects of close relationships (Roels, Rehman, Goodnight, & Janssen, 2022). Conflict discussions with therapists can serve as laboratories in which patients acquire the communication skills to have constructive and autonomy-enhancing conflict discussions with significant others. Treatments in which conflict discussions are avoided may be lost therapeutic opportunities.

Eric, a single 40-year-old man, initiated video-therapy because he regularly went to strip clubs for lap dances. He worried that he might suffer from a sex addiction that might make it difficult for him to have a monogamous long-term relationship. It emerged that Eric used casual sex for stress management, and he felt that paying for sex was an expensive habit that he wished to break. We began discussing the need to cultivate more constructive ways of managing stress.

I noticed that Eric seemed to be a very high weight person from what could be seen on the computer screen. I inquired whether emotional eating, like paying for casual sex, might be for Eric a maladaptive form of stress management. I appreciated that in raising a topic that Eric had not raised I could be perceived as engaging in fat shaming that might give offense. Eric denied that he was overweight and stated that he looked like he was heavier than he really was on video. He did concede that he might be more successful with women if he lost some weight as he felt that the slim women on dating apps to whom he was attracted didn't want to date 'fat' men. I let it drop as I sensed that this was a shame sensitive issue for Eric that he wasn't particularly motivated to address. My intention was only to put out a trial balloon to let Eric know that I was open to working on that issue if weight management was problematic for him. It did occur to me that he might have preferred to pay for sex rather than date to avoid being rejected for his weight by the slim women to whom he was most attracted.

A week after raising the issue of his weight, Eric missed his next regularly scheduled session without calling in advance to cancel. I sent him a text to find out what was up. Privately, I worried that perhaps he was prematurely terminating because I raised weight as a potentially problematic issue. Eric reached out to me a few days later. He had suffered an unanticipated medical emergency. He had to be hospitalized to have part of his foot amputated. Eric had been suffering undiagnosed diabetes and had developed serious vascular problems that interfered with the blood circulation in his foot. At that point he began consulting with a nutritionist and started to diet.

In retrospect Eric was glad that I had confronted him on his denied weight problem though he had resented it at the time and responded defensively. The rupture to the therapeutic relationship was repaired only after it became apparent in retrospect that he had been in denial regarding his health compromising eating behavior. Eric was grateful that his diabetes was diagnosed and treated before his physical condition further deteriorated.

Don't Make Me Think About my Body Mass Index

Body Mass Index (BMI) is the criteria that health care professionals had traditionally used to assess whether someone is underweight, overweight, or normal weight for their height. The Body Mass Index provides an estimate of how much weight is too much weight. The BMI provides a weight range for one's height that determines whether one's weight is within a range that is underweight (below 18.5), normal (18.5 to 24.9), overweight (25.0 to 29.9), obese (30.0 to 39.9), or morbidly obesity (over 40) (https://www.cdc.gov/healthyweight/assessing/bmi/adult_bmi/english_bmi_calculator/bmi_calculator.html). BMI might not be an exact science because it doesn't factor in variables like muscle mass, bone density, or age (Humphreys, 2010) as well as ethnic/racial variability in body builds. The question is whether it provides a useful ballpark estimate no matter how imprecise.

The risk of suffering a metabolic syndrome with increased mortality is highest for those with the highest BMIs, the morbidly obese (Kawada, et al., 2011; Zajacova & Burgard, 2012). Advocates of 'Health at Every Size' suggest that one can be a healthy person (i.e., lack the biomarkers of a metabolic syndrome like high cholesterol or blood glucose) despite being officially overweight according to one's BMI (Frederick, Tomiyama, Bold, & Saguy, 2020). It helps if one is lucky enough to lack the genetic predisposition towards various weight-related diseases, lives a reasonably active lifestyle, and avoids smoking or overconsumption of alcohol. Consequently, it is difficult to know with certitude who can be healthy at any size and who can't be. There is always some risk that the adverse effects of high weight might catch up with individuals with advancing age even though their biomarkers look good for the time being despite the high weight.

It can be unclear how much individuals should be concerned about their weight as they age if their BMIs are high, but their biomarkers look good. Should they worry about losing weight for health reasons if they have yet to show any of the biomarkers of an incipient metabolic syndrome (i.e., high cholesterol, high blood pressure, plaque build-up in a heart artery scan, prediabetic blood glucose levels). Should individuals without biomarkers of medical risk just live their lives without worry until a yearly physical suggests increased health risk or an actual problem? That approach may be normative in contemporary American culture given the 'obesity epidemic' (Moss, 2014).

The alternative attitude, increasingly promoted in a health-conscious media, is that achieving and maintaining a normal BMI is simply good risk management and preventative medicine at any age. [For example, see the benefits of dietary goal setting for gestational weight gain for pregnant women with normal BMIs (Olson, Strawderman, & Graham, 2019)]. Patients are often of two minds when it comes to preventative medicine. Individuals with low risk tolerance will be more likely to diet and exercise as preventative medicine so they never have to worry about receiving 'bad' numbers. Individuals with higher risk tolerance are more likely to assume they are healthy at their current size if their biomarkers look good and will adjust accordingly if at some point in the future, they receive 'bad' numbers. Most likely psychotherapy cannot easily change patients' risk tolerance through a rational cost/benefit analysis if risk tolerance and propensities towards risky behavior reflect genetic predispositions (Li, Zhang, Cai, Wang, Luo, Ma, Li, & Xiao, 2020).

Dissociating Weight Concerns

Patients concerned about their weight can avoid thinking about their weight (i.e., dissociate weight concerns) by avoiding looking at themselves in the mirror, only wearing loose fitting clothes, and never weighing themselves. It may briefly bother them when they notice that they have gained weight but then distract themselves by getting lost in other activities, like work, that take their mind off their weight. They might believe that they need to lose weight but dissociate that concern by deciding to wait for the right time to diet; preferably sometime in the future when their stress level is reduced, and they have more time to exercise.

Physicians, nutritionists, and dieticians may routinely track their patients' weight and BMI when treating disordered eating (Attia & Walsh, 2009). Traditionally, psychotherapists do not weigh patients and calculate their BMIs. Consequently, therapists might just wait until patients spontaneously share such numbers or therapists would have to be willing to inquire about what is likely a shame sensitive issue if patients are not reporting such numbers of their own volition.

The underlying problem is high weight patients' disturbed relationship with numbers. In general patients love numbers, like weight and BMI, when numbers make them look good and hate numbers when numbers make them look bad. 'Good' numbers, like weight loss or a normal BMI, are a source of pride and accomplishment to be shared and celebrated. 'Bad' numbers in contrast become a source of shameful feelings of failure and defeat to be hidden from view. Patients will become more open in discussing bad numbers when they can look at those numbers without judgment but with self-compassion when they are bad and assume their therapists can do similarly. Once patients can look at such numbers dispassionately, they can better contemplate what to do about it.

Behavioral approaches to weight loss do require patients to regularly deal with what might be 'bad' numbers in terms of weight, BMI, calories consumed, and calories burned (Gomez-Rubalcava, Stabbert, & Phelan, 2018). Dieters who routinely monitor their weight and daily caloric intake are more likely to maintain lost weight than dieters who don't (Gold, Carr, Thomas, Burrus, O'Leary, Wing, & Bond, 2020). Patients will be more likely to conscientiously self-monitor if they can do so without dread of obtaining 'bad' numbers. Avoidance of self-monitoring to avoid confrontation with 'bad' numbers is self-defeating in terms of treatment approaches that require self-monitoring. Empathic confrontation of self-defeating behavior can be a component of both schema therapy and transference-focused psychotherapy (Behary & Dieckmann, 2011; Levy, Yeomans, & Spina, 2022). Patients may require considerable moral support in dealing with the emotional fallout of being faced with 'bad' numbers.

Don't Make Me Think About Calories

Patients generally appreciate what foods are most calorie dense, like ice cream or pizza, and which are least like fruits, vegetables, and lean sources of protein such as fish or skinless chicken breast. Sometimes high weight patients do eat those low-calorie foods daily so believe that their diet is healthful. High weight patients may generally understand that dieting involves eating less and exercising more while increasing the ratio of low-calorie (i.e., 'good healthy foods') to calorie-dense foods (i.e., 'bad fattening foods') in their diet. For these reasons many patients with elevated BMIs believe they already know the basic principles of how to diet more successfully. They then berate themselves for lacking the motivation and self-discipline to do it. Some high weight patients may even say they are addicted to certain foods, like chocolate chip cookies, but mean it more figuratively than literally.

The least restrictive approach to losing weight would be to simply try to alter the ratio of high calorie to low calorie foods in one's diet and to generally limit portion size so that one doesn't seem to be overeating anything. The least restrictive approach to losing weight may prove insufficient if the total calorie count remains high, the ratio of high calorie to low calorie foods is still too highly tilted towards the higher calorie foods, the portion sizes of the lower calorie foods might be too small to be a filling replacement for the higher calorie foods, and the reduced portion sizes of the higher calorie foods that are most addictive still prime increased craving for those foods. In the end, the least restrictive diet fails because it requires too much willpower to avoid incremental portion creep of the higher calorie foods in the diet. Willpower is not a reliable control mechanism in high stress/high temptation environments. Compliance motivation wanes over time because of the chronic strain on willpower's limited capacity in stressful circumstances.

Counting calories may become a necessity, the road not traveled, for patients who repeatedly try and fail with less restrictive approaches but who do not want to give up on dieting and weight loss entirely. Patients who fail with less restrictive diets may give up on dieting or become 'anti-diet' (Jovanovski & Jaeger, 2022) because failure is so demoralizing. The same can happen with patients who try and fail repeatedly with overly restrictive diets as well. Possibly one reason that diets frequently fail is that weight cycling might sometimes derive from oscillating between diets that are too permissive and diets that are too strict. Individuals prone to dichotomous thinking may be vulnerable to all or none approaches to dieting without taking the time to discover a middle ground approach that might be more sustainable. Addressing dichotomous thinking in general as well as addressing dichotomous thinking as expressed in the transference are cardinal features of transference-focused psychotherapy (Levy, Yeomans, & Spina, 2022).

Without counting calories high weight patients would generally not know what their daily calorie count is, what their daily calorie budget would need to be to achieve their weight loss goals, how much calories they would need to eliminate from their daily diets, and where they would need to make painful cuts in their daily consumption. Many high weight patients don't want to know these numbers so they dread being confronted with a 'bad' number, a number that would make it painfully clear the full extent that they eat well beyond their daily calorie allowance and the need for making painful cutbacks in their daily consumption. Consequently, they are flying blind when they attempt to diet without counting calories. Most individuals underestimate their daily calorie count (Lichtman et al., 1992) so becoming aware of the true number might be a shock to the system they would rather not endure.

Patients may complain that counting calories is too tedious, so they don't want to do it even if they concede that it might provide useful information. They overlook that counting calories can be quite simple, easy, and convenient now that free calorie counting applications can be downloaded to one's smartphone. Nevertheless, patients may not want to discover how easy it is to count calories because they don't want to know in caloric terms exactly how much they eat beyond their daily calorie budget and see how much they would have to cut back to achieve their weight loss goals. At that point painful choices would need to be made as to what to reduce or cut out of one's diet entirely. It would also become readily apparent that one's favorite calorie-dense foods account for the lion's share of one's daily caloric intake despite having increased one's consumption of fruits, vegetables, and lean sources of protein.

The question then arises as to what degree it is the therapist's task to enable patients to think about calories despite their disinclination to do so. Autonomy support means being an encouraging and sympathetic traveling companion on high weight patients' weight manage-ment journeys. It's appreciating that patients will frequently want to give the least restrictive approaches a fair chance at succeeding before giving more restrictive approaches like counting calories a try. At the point that patients are becoming frustrated and demoralized by their repeated failures with less restrictive approaches, therapists might suggest the more restrictive alternatives such as counting calories as an antidote.

Patients will either be ready to hear and adopt a more restrictive approach or they won't. Autonomy support means not forcing the issue and respecting patients' independent decision making. From the perspective of reflective functioning and facilitating constructive conflict discussions, psychotherapists have done their job if they have raised an alternative perspec-tive at a point when patients' are frustrated by the limitations of their own perspectives, enabled patients to give the alternative perspective some consideration, explored patients' thoughts and feelings about the alternative perspective, and then respect patients' decisions about how to move forward on their weight management journeys. Respectful dialogue means patients feel free to consider and reject alternative perspectives and that therapists are attuned to potential ruptures to the therapeutic relationship if patients feel coercive pressure to adopt therapists' alternative perspectives.

It has been observed that attempts at caloric restriction often fail and can result in dele-terious rebound effects (Dulloo, 2007). That point of view may be an overgeneralization that isn't true for everybody as some individuals do succeed in long-term weight loss mainten-ance (Gold, Carr, Thomas, Burrus, O'Leary, Wing, & Bond, 2020). It doesn't consider that many attempts at dieting are overly ambitious, lack a sufficient emotional support struc-ture, do not consider the priming effect of the more addictive foods, and do not incorporate strategies for managing withdrawal symptoms. It doesn't factor in that in recovery from any addiction that relapse is common in search of a more sustainable approach. Dealing with relapse would be part of recovery from food addiction (Epstein, 2015). It would not necessarily be a reason to give up on dieting (i.e., recovery) if weight cycling is reflective of the tendency to relapse in trying to recover from addictive behavior.

Felicia aspired to lose 20 pounds and wanted to lose those 20 pounds before a big party that was planned for her 40th wedding anniversary. She wanted to look as thin as she had looked on the day she was married. Felicia had already tried and failed with less restrictive approaches, so we were discussing the possibility of counting calories which Felicia had been reluctant to do. Felicia said that she didn't need to count calories because she made healthful food choices. As an example, she said that Thai food was her favorite food and that when she went out to a Thai restaurant, she would choose Pad Thai noodles with shrimp rather than beef as she knew that shrimp was lower calorie than beef. I inquired if she wanted me to check the calorie count of Pad Thai noodles with shrimp on my calorie counter app. Felicia said: 'Sure!' confident that it would come in at a low number.

I didn't know exactly how many calories were in a restaurant serving of Pad Thai noodles with shrimp but suspected it was high because of the noodles and the sauce if not the shrimp. I rapidly checked the calorie count on my smartphone. I discovered it was 1000 calories per restaurant serving and I understood that a low-calorie diet for someone like Felicia would probably be around 1500 calories per day to achieve her weight loss goals. Felicia looked shocked and crestfallen when I told her the bad news. Yet after that intervention Felicia downloaded the app on her smartphone as she didn't want to drastically underestimate her daily caloric intake if she wanted to lose 20 pounds by the time of her big anniversary party.

Don't Make Me Think about Cholesterol, Blood Pressure, and Blood Glucose

The most upsetting numbers that patients concerned about their weight would rather not face are the numbers that suggest a heightened risk if not the actual presence of a metabolic syndrome like arteriosclerosis or diabetes. Patients who worry that they weigh too much may avoid yearly checkups because they don't want to know if their blood pressure, cholesterol, and blood glucose levels are elevated. They don't want to know the extent of plaque buildup in the arteries around their hearts. They don't want to know if there is retinal damage from either high blood pressure or high blood sugar.

Arteriosclerosis and Type 2 diabetes are progressive diseases that progress relatively slowly (Rybarczyk & Shamaskin-Garroway, 2019). That means that with yearly checkups such diseases can be detected in their early stages and their further development arrested with the proper treatment. First time diagnosis of such diseases at an advanced stage of development only happens when there is an avoidance of early detection through yearly checkups.

'Good' numbers affirm that for the time being patients are healthy at their current size and perhaps, if they are lucky, that they lack the genetic predispositions for the diseases associated with higher BMIs. Such high weight individuals may not want to be pressured into what they see as unnecessary dieting as preventative medicine for an illness they might never acquire or at least not acquire for decades if they are young.

Receiving 'bad' numbers in a yearly physical is often a tipping point for patients who have been ambivalent about dieting. 'Bad' biomarkers convince them that it is finally time to get serious about dieting. They want to receive a 'good' number when they return for their yearly physical. For these high weight patients, a 'bad' number can be a wake-up call if they hope to avoid early disability and demise due to acquiring a weight-related metabolic syndrome. Increased mortality salience is associated with increased intention to seek a medical specialist as well as increased monitoring of markers of poor health (Menzies, Sharpe, & Dar-Nimrod, 2021).

Sylvia was a single 50-year-old woman whose BMI was in the obese range. She often discussed wanting to lose weight to improve her love life though Sylvia often attracted slim boyfriends who were attracted to her vivacious personality. Sylvia had not made much progress on dieting despite her constant self-flagellation for that lack of progress. We worked on decreasing her self-flagellation and increasing her self-acceptance and body positivity without much success. Sylvia was not interested in any dieting advice as she believed she already knew all she needed to know about how to diet but wasn't yet ready to apply it. The treatment appeared to be at an impasse in which Sylvia assumed I was as frustrated with her as she was with herself.

One night Sylvia started having what felt like a panic attack, but she decided to go to the emergency room just to play it safe in case it was something more serious. It turned out that her blood pressure was dangerously high, and she needed to be placed on medication for high blood pressure. That incident terrified her. Sylvia decided to get serious about dieting and found a nutritionist with whom to work. Sylvia began to lose weight motivated by the dread of early disability and demise.

Weight loss is associated with improved biomarkers such as lower blood pressure, lower cholesterol, and lower blood sugar levels (Welsh, Cezard, Gill, Wallia, Douglas, Sheikh, Wild, Tuomilehto, McKnight, Murray, Bhopal, Lean, & Sattar, 2016). Thus, weight loss can be a useful adjunct to whatever medications physicians might prescribe for high weight patients' metabolic syndromes. Nevertheless, it remains controversial whether possessing an intentional weight loss agenda facilitates or impedes achieving improvements in the biomarkers of healthy metabolic functioning. That may be in part because one-size-fits-all approaches do not apply. Some individuals benefit from behavioral weight loss interventions that have clear weight loss goals whereas others appear to benefit from a more intuitive approach that fosters weight acceptance.

References

Ansari, N., Shakiba, S., Mousavi, M. E., Mohammadkhani, P., Aminoroaya, S., & Poor, N. S. (2018). Role of emotional dysregulation and childhood trauma in emotional eating behavior. *Journal of Practice in Clinical Psychology*, 6(1), 21–28. https://doi.org/10.29252/nirp.jpcp.6.1.21

Attia, E., & Walsh, B. T. (2009). Behavioral management for anorexia nervosa. *The New England Journal of Medicine*, 360(5), 500–506. https://doi.org/10.1056/NEJMct0805569

Behary, W. T., & Dieckmann, E. (2011). Schema therapy for narcissism: The art of empathic confrontation, limit-setting, and leverage. In W. K. Campbell & J. D. Miller (Eds.), *The handbook of narcissism and narcissistic personality disorder: Theoretical approaches, empirical findings, and treatments* (pp. 445–456). John Wiley & Sons, Inc.

Buie, D. H., & Adler, G. (1972). The uses of confrontation with borderline patients. *International Journal of Psychoanalytic Psychotherapy*, 1(3), 90–108.

Cramer, P. (2006). *Protecting the self: Defense mechanisms in action.* Guilford Press.

Devendorf, A. R., Bradley, S. E., Barks, L., Klanchar, A., Orozco, T., & Cowan, L. (2021). Stigma among veterans with urinary and fecal incontinence. *Stigma and Health*, 6(3), 335–343. https://doi-org/10.1037/sah0000260

Domingue, R., & Mollen, D. (2009). Attachment and conflict communication in adult romantic relationships. *Journal of Social and Personal Relationships*, 26(5), 678–696. https://doi.org/10.1177/0265407509347932

Dulloo A. G. (2007). Suppressed thermogenesis as a cause for resistance to slimming and obesity rebound: Adaptation or illusion? *International Journal of Obesity* (2007 Feb.), 31(2), 201–203. https://doi.org/10.1038/sj.ijo.0803537

Epstein, E. B. (2015). The experience of recovery from food addiction. *Dissertation Abstracts International: Section B: The Sciences and Engineering*, 76(5-B(E)).

Farooqi, I. S. (2018). Genetics of obesity. In T. A. Wadden & G. A. Bray (Eds.), *Handbook of obesity treatment* (pp. 64–74). The Guilford Press.

Frederick, D. A., Tomiyama, A. J., Bold, J. G., & Saguy, A. C. (2020). Can she be healthy at her weight? Effects of news media frames on antifat attitudes, dieting intentions, and perceived health risks of obesity. *Stigma and Health*, 5(3), 247–257. https://doi.org/10.1037/sah0000195

Freud, S. (1923). *The ego and the id. Standard Edition.* S. E., 19, 1–66.

Friedman-Daugherty, L. R. (1998). What do borderline's say they want from their therapists? *Dissertation Abstracts International: Section B: The Sciences and Engineering*, 59(4-B), 1849.

Gold, J. M., Carr, L. J., Thomas, J. G., Burrus, J., O'Leary, K. C., Wing, R., & Bond, D. S. (2020). Conscientiousness in weight loss maintainers and regainers. *Health Psychology*, 39(5), 421–429. https://doi-org/10.1037/hea0000846

Gomez-Rubalcava, S., Stabbert, K., & Phelan, S. (2018). Behavioral treatment of obesity. In T. Wadden & G. A. Bray (Eds.), *Handbook of obesity treatment* (pp. 336–348). The Guilford Press.

Gray, P. (1987). On the technique of analysis of the superego: An introduction. *The Psychoanalytic Quarterly*, 56(1), 130–154.

Guilfoyle, M. (2009). Theorizing relational possibilities in narrative therapy. *Journal of Systemic Therapies*, 28(2), 19–33. https://doi.org/10.1521/jsyt.2009.28.2.19

Holman, T. B., & Jarvis, M. O. (2003). Hostile, volatile, avoiding, and validating couple-conflict types: An investigation of Gottman's couple-conflict types. *Personal Relationships*, 10(2), 267–282. https://doi.org/10.1111/1475-6811.00049

Humphreys, S. (2010). The unethical use of BMI in contemporary general practice. *British Journal of General Practice*, 60(578), 696–697. DOI: https://doi.org/10.3399/bjgp10X515548

Jovanovski, N., & Jaeger, T. (2022). Demystifying 'diet culture': Exploring the meaning of diet culture in online 'anti-diet' feminist, fat activist, and health professional communities. *Women's Studies International Forum*, 90, 1–10.

Karno, M. P., & Longabaugh, R. (2005). An examination of how therapist directiveness interacts with patient anger and reactance to predict alcohol use. *Journal of Studies on Alcohol*, 66(6), 825–832. https://doi.org/10.15288/jsa.2005.66.825

Kawada, T., Otsuka, T., Inagaki, H., Wakayama, Y., Li, Q., Li, Y. J., & Katsumata, M. (2011). Optimal cut-off levels of body mass index and waist circumference in relation to each component of metabolic syndrome (MetS) and the number of MetS component. *Diabetes & Metabolic Syndrome*, 5(1), 25–28. https://doi.org/10.1016/j.dsx.2010.05.012

Kearney, R. J. (1996). *Within the wall of denial: Conquering addictive behaviors*. W. W. Norton & Co.

Kvalem, I. L., Træen, B., Markovic, A., & von Soest, T. (2019). Body image development and sexual satisfaction: A prospective study from adolescence to adulthood. *Journal of Sex Research*, 56(6), 791–801. https://doi.org/10.1080/00224499.2018.1518400

Levy, K. N., Yeomans, F. E., & Spina, D. S. (2022). Transference-focused psychotherapy. In S. K. Huprich (Ed.), *Personality disorders and pathology: Integrating clinical assessment and practice in the DSM-5 and ICD-11 era* (pp. 211–235). American Psychological Association. https://doi-org.adelphi.idm.oclc.org/10.1037/0000310-010

Li, H., Zhang, C., Cai, X., Wang, L., Luo, F., Ma, Y., Li, M., & Xiao, X. (2020). Genome-wide association study of creativity reveals genetic overlap with psychiatric disorders, risk tolerance, and risky behaviors. *Schizophrenia Bulletin*, 46(5), 1317–1326. https://doi-org/10.1093/schbul/sbaa025

Lichtman, S. W., Pisarska, K., Berman, E. R., Pestone, M., Dowling, H., Offenbacher, E., Weisel, H., Heshka, S., Matthews, D. E., & Heymsfield, S. B. (1992). Discrepancy between self-reported and actual caloric intake and exercise in obese subjects. *The New England Journal of Medicine*, 327(27), 1893–1898. https://doi.org/10.1056/NEJM199212313272701

Long, E. V., Vartanian, L. R., Herman, C. P., & Polivy, J. (2020). What does it mean to overeat? *Eating Behaviors*, 37, 101390. https://doi.org/10.1016/j.eatbeh.2020.101390

Lucibello, K. M., Nesbitt, A. E., Solomon-Krakus, S., & Sabiston, C. M. (2021). Internalized weight stigma and the relationship between weight perception and negative body-related self-conscious emotions. *Body Image*, 37, 84–88.

Menzies, R. E., Sharpe, L., & Dar-Nimrod, I. (2021). The effect of mortality salience on bodily scanning behaviors in anxiety-related disorders. *Journal of Abnormal Psychology*, 130(2), 141–151. https://doi.org/10.1037/abn0000577

Moeseneder, L., Ribeiro, E., Muran, J. C., & Caspar, F. (2019). Impact of confrontations by therapists on impairment and utilization of the therapeutic alliance. *Psychotherapy Research: Journal of the Society for Psychotherapy Research*, 29(3), 293–305. https://doi.org/10.1080/10503307.2018.1502897

Moore, C. F., Sabino, V., Koob, G. F., & Cottone, P. (2019). Dissecting compulsive eating behavior into three elements. In P. Cottone, V. Sabino, C. F. Moore, & G. F. Koob (Eds.), *Compulsive eating behavior and food addiction: Emerging pathological constructs* (pp. 41–81). Elsevier Academic Press. https://doi-org.10.1016/B978-0-12-816207-1.00003-2

Moss, M. (2014). *Salt sugar fat: How the food giants hooked us*. New York: Random House.

O'Hara, L., Ahmed, H., & Elashie, S. (2021). Evaluating the impact of a brief Health at Every Size®-informed health promotion activity on body positivity and internalized weight-based oppression. *Body Image*, 37, 225–237. https://doi.org/10.1016/j.bodyim.2021.02.006

Olson, C. M., Strawderman, M. S., & Graham, M. L. (2019). Use of an online diet goal-setting tool: Relationships with gestational weight gain. *Journal of Nutrition Education and Behavior*, 51(4), 391–399. https://doi.org/10.1016/j.jneb.2019.01.024

Pearl, R. L., Bach, C., & Wadden, T. A. (2022). Development of a cognitive-behavioral intervention for internalized weight stigma. *Journal of Contemporary Psychotherapy: On the Cutting Edge of Modern Developments in Psychotherapy*. https://doi-org.libproxy.adelphi.edu/10.1007/s10879-022-09543-w

Pickard, H. (2017). Responsibility without blame for addiction. *Neuroethics*, 10(1), 169–180. https://doi-org.adelphi.idm.oclc.org/10.1007/s12152-016-9295-2

Robinson, E., & Christiansen, P. (2015). Visual exposure to obesity: Experimental effects on attraction toward overweight men and mate choice in females. *International Journal of Obesity* (2015, Sep.), 39(9), 1390–1394. https://doi.org/10.1038/ijo.2015.87 1

Rodgers, R. F., White, M., & Berry, R. (2021). Orthorexia nervosa, intuitive eating, and eating competence in female and male college students. *Eating and Weight Disorders: EWD*, 26(8), 2625–2632. https://doi.org/10.1007/s40519-020-01054-8

Roels, R., Rehman, U. S., Goodnight, J. A., & Janssen, E. (2022). Couple communication behaviors during sexual and nonsexual discussions and their association with relationship satisfaction. *Archives of Sexual Behavior*. https://doi-org/10.1007/s10508-021-02204-4

Rosenberg, K. P., & Curtiss Feder, L. (Eds.). (2014). An introduction to behavioral addictions. In K. P. Rosenberg & L. Curtiss Feder (Eds.), *Behavioral addictions: Criteria, evidence, and treatment* (pp. 1–17). Elsevier Academic Press.

Rosinger, A. Y., & Puts, D. A. (2018). It's complicated: Why raters' BMI poorly explained attractiveness ratings. *Obesity*, 26(3), 461–462. https://doi-org/10.1002/oby.22125

Rybarczyk, B., & Shamaskin-Garroway, A. M. (2019). Aging and age-related disability. In D. S. Dunn (Ed.), *Understanding the experience of disability: Perspectives from social and rehabilitation psychology* (pp. 204–219). Oxford University Press.

Schulte, E. M., Bach, C., Berkowitz, R. I., Latner, J. D., & Pearl, R. L. (2021). Adverse childhood experiences and weight stigma: Co-occurrence and associations with psychological well-being. *Stigma and Health*, 6(4), 408–418. https://doi-org.adelphi.idm.oclc.org/10.1037/sah0000341

Schulte, E. M., Smeal, J. K., Lewis, J., & Gearhardt, A. N. (2018). Development of the Highly Processed Food Withdrawal Scale. *Appetite*, 131, 148–154. https://doi.org/10.1016/j.appet.2018.09.013

Shen L. (2018). The evolution of shame and guilt. *PloS ONE*, 13(7), e0199448. https://doi.org/10.1371/journal.pone.0199448

Taube-Schiff, M., Van Exan, J., Tanaka, R., Wnuk, S., Hawa, R., & Sockalingam, S. (2015). Attachment style and emotional eating in bariatric surgery candidates: The mediating role of difficulties in emotion regulation. *Eating Behaviors*, 18, 36–40. https://doi.org/10.1016/j.eatbeh.2015.03.011

Tracy, J. L., Robins, R. W., & Schriber, R. A. (2009). Development of a FACS-verified set of basic and self-conscious emotion expressions. *Emotion (Washington, D.C.)*, 9(4), 554–559. https://doi.org/10.1037/a0015766

Vail, K. E. III, Conti, J. P., Goad, A. N., & Horner, D. E. (2020). Existential threat fuels worldview defense, but not after priming autonomy orientation. *Basic and Applied Social Psychology*, 42(3), 150–166. https://doi.org/10.1080/01973533.2020.1726747

Welsh, P., Cezard, G., Gill, J. M., Wallia, S., Douglas, A., Sheikh, A., Wild, S. H., Tuomilehto, J., McKnight, J., Murray, G., Bhopal, R., Lean, M. E., & Sattar, N. (2016). Associations between weight change and biomarkers of cardiometabolic risk in South Asians: Secondary analyses of the PODOSA trial. *International Journal of Obesity* (2016 Jun.), 40(6), 1005–1011. https://doi.org/10.1038/ijo.2016.35

Zajacova, A., & Burgard, S. A. (2012). Shape of the BMI-mortality association by cause of death, using generalized additive models: NHIS 1986–2006. *Journal of Aging and Health*, 24(2), 191–211. https://doi.org/10.1177/0898264311406268

Recommending or Demanding? Helping Patients Choose an Approach to Weight Management

8

Once there is goal consensus for losing weight patients must decide what their weight loss goals will be and which approach they will choose to lose weight. Psychotherapists as all-purpose sounding boards will be consulted on this consequential decision. Patients will need to decide whether to try an approach to weight loss such as an 'anti-diet approach' (Lister, Rosen, & Wright, 1985). without dietary prescriptions or an approach like cognitive-behavioral treatment (Tronieri, 2021) that would prescribe caloric restriction. Do they try an approach like mindful eating (Yu, Song, Zhang, & Wei, 2020) that cultivates improved self-regulation of eating behavior or an approach like cue avoidance (Bennett, 1986) that is not reliant on improving self-control in high temptation environments but on avoiding such environments so one's self-control is not put to the test? Do they try to lose weight quickly through a very low-calorie diet (Tsai & Wadden, (2006) or more slowly? If they believe that they suffer a food addiction, to what degree do they abstain from trigger foods or try to learn to eat such foods in moderation (Eddie, Bergman, Hoffman, & Kelly, 2022)? And finally, do they choose a diet with a particular macronutrient composition, be it low fat or low carbohydrate (Gardner et al., 2018)?

How psychotherapists respond to patients' deliberations on these questions will influence the therapeutic relationship. Do therapists adopt a stance of neutrality without taking sides when patients want their therapists' advice? Do therapists recommend a particular approach to weight loss? Ruptures to the therapeutic relationship can occur when patients would like advice and guidance, but therapists decline to offer an opinion or make a recommendation. Ruptures to the therapeutic relationship can also occur when therapists make recommendations, but patients experience those recommendations as imperious demands to which they are expected to submit by know-it-all therapists. How free do patients feel to manage their weights in their own way with supportive therapists following their lead? To what extent can patients rely on their therapists for guidance when they feel they are lost on their weight management journeys and are looking to their therapists to provide them with a roadmap to help them achieve their goals?

Traveling Companion or Guide?

A traveling companion is someone who provides companionship on one's journey. They see the same sights so share the same experiences. With a traveling companion one is not alone on one's journey. It might be a difficult journey with many obstacles to overcome. The traveling companion provides emotional support that one has the stamina to make

DOI: 10.4324/9781003402336-12

the journey and reassurance that one will make it to the destination. In contrast, a guide leads the way. They've been this way many times before, so they know exactly where they're going and how to get there. If one follows the guide's lead reaching one's destination is a sure thing. Just tell the guide where you want to go, and they'll get you there in the quickest and safest way possible.

Psychodynamic and humanistic therapists are more like traveling companions whereas cognitive-behavioral therapists are more like guides. The fundamental rule of psychoanalysis is free association (Thompson, 2004). The patient is instructed to honestly say everything that comes to mind without self-censorship. The assumption is that patients' problems, like overeating, are symptoms of deeper unconscious conflicts of which patients might be unaware. Those unconscious conflicts can be the result of childhood traumas, dysfunctional family dynamics, and/or developmental arrest. The journey is into the deepest reaches of patients' psyches. The destination of the journey is to help patients face painful truths honestly and facing those painful truths honestly will set them free from their psychological symptoms. The psychoanalyst doesn't provide guidance or advice but only empathy and insight.

From the psychoanalytic point of view autonomy support is to remain neutral regarding patients' inner conflicts when patients are of two minds about something and can't decide what to do (Wallwork, 2012). Psychodynamic treatment is considered a supportive/ expressive approach (Luborsky, 1984). Since Freud, psychodynamic therapists have been cautioned about the pitfalls of giving advice, be it solicited or unsolicited (Prass, Ewell, Hill, & Kivlighan, 2021). It has been thought best for psychotherapy outcome to let patients to decide for themselves what to do with the empathy and insight that psychodynamic psychotherapy provides. Some approaches to emotional eating, like the anti-diet approach (Lister, Rosen, & Wright, 1985), would just explore patients' underlying reasons for emotional eating in the hopes that insight into those reasons will be therapeutic without telling patients how to diet. There is concern that telling patients how to think or what to do could be infantilizing if not authoritarian and undermine patients' capacities to think for themselves with minds of their own.

Patients may be happy with an exclusively supportive expressive approach when they want a traveling companion who will help them better understand their most private thoughts and feelings about their weight and eating behavior. Such a companion will let them discover their own approach to weight management. Patients might be frustrated by such an approach when they want a guide who will coach them on how to manage their weight more successfully, be it by teaching mindful eating or by helping them develop a meal plan that remains within a daily calorie budget. Ruptures to the therapeutic relationship occur when patients want their nondirective therapists to become more directive, but nondirective therapists decline to change their approach as a matter of principle.

Humanistic therapists are also more traveling companions than guides. In fact, Carl Rogers's (1951) client or person-centered therapy is a nondirective treatment approach. The goal of humanistic psychotherapies, like person-centered psychotherapy, is to help patients actualize their true selves (Schlegel & Hicks, 2009). The support and empathy patients receive from the therapeutic relationship provides the safety, security, and encouragement to discover who they are and who they want to be. The goals and direction of the treatment comes from patients as they figure out who they are and how to live up to their fullest potentials. Their authentic values will lead the way and therapists will follow patients' leads.

From the humanistic perspective autonomy support is respecting patients' unique individuality and affirming its authentic self-expression. When it comes to weight management, it would be for patients to decide which weight management strategy is reflective of their core values. If patients are of two minds, it is for therapists to respect that inner struggle as they try to figure who they are and who they wish to be and become. Humanistic therapists don't tell their patients who they are but help them discover who they are and learn to accept who they are. Patients must ascertain for themselves to what degree their motivations for managing their weight in a particular way derive from intrinsic motivations (i.e., authentic self-expression) versus extrinsic motivations (i.e., conformist social pressure like weight stigma).

Motivational interviewing derives from the humanistic tradition as an approach to helping patients when they are of two minds about who they are and who they hope to be and become (Butryn, Schumacher, & Forman, 2018). Motivational interviewing empathizes with the perspectives of both states of mind. Autonomy support means supporting patients' process of self-discovery and autonomous decision making when they are confused about who they are and who they hope to become.

Patients looking for a therapist who will help them discover who they are and help them become the person they were meant to be will be happy with this approach. In fact, the first empirical measure of the therapeutic relationship, the Barrett-Lennard *Relationship Inventory* (Barrett-Lennard, 2015), was based on Rogers's approach and was comprised of three subscales: 1) Unconditional positive regard, 2) Empathy, and 3) Therapist Congruence. Nevertheless, patients can be frustrated by such a nondirective approach if they wish to work with a therapist who has more definite opinions about what is or isn't healthful when it comes to weight, eating habits, and lifestyle choices and can provide a clear roadmap for healthful living to which patients can subscribe.

The frustrations that patients may have with the nondirective approaches to psychotherapy are not problematic with more cognitive-behavioral approaches to treatment. There is acceptance that obesity is a medical problem because of its association with various metabolic syndromes (Tronieri, 2021). Cognitive behavioral approaches to weight loss attempt to change cognitions through techniques such as cognitive reappraisal and change behavior through techniques such as behavior chain analysis and cue avoidance (Tronieri, 2021).

Cognitive behavior therapists would be more guides than traveling companions on patients' weight management journeys. The destination is weight loss, and the itinerary is clearly spelled out in advance. The patient is provided with a clear roadmap of how to arrive at the destination on the quickest route possible as cognitive behavioral treatment approaches are often short-term. Patients who want a guide on their weight loss journeys will be happy with this approach. Autonomy support is helping patients achieve their weight loss goals by coaching them on how to best achieve those goals.

Ruptures to the therapeutic relationship are likely when patients respond with reactance to being told what to do when they want to find their own way and try out their own approaches to weight management with their therapists' support. Weight loss specialists could be perceived as authoritarian if they appear to be trying to get patients to conform to a one-size-fits-all approach to weight management. Patients may not want to have to count calories, avoid high temptation situations, eat mindfully when they would rather 'wolf' down their food without savoring every bite, or eat more fruits, vegetables, and whole grains because all that fiber gives them gas and that kind of diet is perceived as boring.

Approaches to health that center on social justice are becoming more common in clinical practice (Mitchell & Raque, 2022). Much emotional suffering as well as health problems derive from being a victim of social prejudice be it for one's gender, sexual orientation, race, ethnicity, or religion. Weight stigma is the social prejudice against high weight individuals (Pearl, Bach, & Wadden, 2022). The antidote may be appreciating that one can be healthy at any size, intuitive eating, and body positivity to overcome fat phobia. This would also be a directive approach for which the therapist would be a guide who provides a clear roadmap to the destination – acceptance of one's body as it is. Patients who are tired of diets and dieting and want to feel better about being the high weight individuals they currently are, have been, and expect to be in the future might find such an approach a welcome relief from the relentless pressure to lose weight and then feel badly about themselves if they don't.

Ruptures to the therapeutic relationship are likely if patients remain privately skeptical of such an approach. Patients might worry that sexual attraction has some basis in evolutionary biology so they are skeptical that they can be attractive at any size. They might not want to overcome their own preference for thin romantic partners. What if one can't be healthy at any size as one possesses a family history of heart disease and diabetes that high weigh might exacerbate? What if one is healthy at one's current weight for now but the ill effects of high weight might catch up with one in the future with advancing age?

There is no therapeutic approach that is immune to patients' skepticism and reactance. Repair of therapeutic ruptures may mean addressing that skepticism even if left unsaid. Integrative therapists can try to minimize some of these pitfalls by adjusting their approach to patients' apparent needs and desires for what they want in a therapist. Integrative therapists may cultivate the flexibility to sometimes respond as traveling companions and other times as guides, sometimes look at weight management from a social justice perspective and other times from an evolutionary viewpoint, sometimes from a self-actualization model and other times from a medical model. Looking at things from multiple perspectives can be good for fostering a reflective attitude and practice (Price & Deveci, 2022).

Patients can be of two minds about whether they want a traveling companion or a guide. Consequently, even integrative therapists will have to address ruptures to the therapeutic relationship. Patients may sometimes act like 'help rejecting complainers' (Kowalski & Erickson, 1997) who will want the therapist to be more of a guide whenever the therapist is trying to be a good traveling companion and will want the therapist to be more of a traveling companion whenever the therapist is trying to be a good guide. In such no-win situations ruptures are inevitable. From the perspective of reflective functioning, negotiating the clash of perspectives in conflict discussions between therapists and their patients can improve communication skills and enhance reflective functioning. Increasing reflective functioning may be a common factor in all successful psychotherapies (Fonagy, Campbell, & Luyten, 2023; Goodman, 2013).

Donald was a 25-year-old single heterosexual cisgendered man who came for treatment suffering from depression mostly triggered by a history of failed relationships with women. Secondarily he realized that he engaged in emotional eating and wanted help losing weight. Donald explicitly stated that he wanted a therapist who would coach him about how to lose weight and didn't want a therapist who just sat and listened. We seemed to have consensus on the methods and goals of the treatment. Donald was very appreciative of the dieting advice that I gave him. Yet as the treatment proceeded it became apparent that he wasn't implementing any of my dieting recommendations. Donald started beating up on himself for knowing what he should do but not doing it and assumed that I was as critical of him for not following my advice as he was of himself. We seemed to be at an impasse due to a withdrawal rupture as the patient became demoralized about the effectiveness of the treatment.

I inquired if perhaps Donald was of two minds about losing weight and wondered why he might not be as motivated as he would like to be to lose weight at this point in his life despite feeling that he should. Donald developed the insight that he was much less depressed being single than in his last relationship with a woman who cheated on him and left him for another man. Why lose weight just to end up back in a depressing relationship with a woman who might betray his trust? Wasn't it better to just remain single, eat what he liked, and not worry about having to attract a woman that might be more faithful to him than his previous girlfriend? We established that he might not be that motivated to lose weight until he was convinced that he could have more trustworthy and fulfilling relationships with women than in years past. At this point he was still cynical about that possibility. We concluded that Donald felt that he 'should' work with a directive therapist who would coach him on weight loss strategies but that deep down he just wanted a traveling companion who would support his current depression management strategy – stay single and eat what he liked.

To Permit or to Prohibit?

In general, the greater the demands of the weight management approach the greater the reactance. The greater the dietary restrictions the greater the threat to one's sense of freedom to eat what, when, and how much one wants. The most restrictive approaches may advocate very low or low daily calorie budgets, require abstention from or only the smallest portions of 'forbidden' foods, require time-consuming lifestyle changes in terms of an exercise and/or meditation routine, require avoidance of high temptation environments, and require time-consuming therapeutic activities like weekly psychotherapy, nutritional counseling, and self-help support groups. Such lifestyle changes may mean less time for work, less time for friends and family, eating out less frequently, less snacking while engaged in mindless entertainment like watching television, and having to eat on weekends, holidays, and vacations not that differently than the way one eats during the work week.

Such an approach might seem like overkill. Patients may not subscribe to such an approach unless they are convinced it's an absolute necessity and that the substantial costs of such an approach are worth the benefits. A skeptical patient might believe that such an approach is excessive, that it might not work, that even if it works in the short-term it might not be sustainable in the long-term, and even if it works and is sustainable it just wouldn't be a reasonably gratifying way to live one's life.

Some patients could feel that even if high weight makes them less attractive and less healthy, they don't care enough about their looks or health to subject themselves to such an onerous lifelong ordeal. Such a severely restricted lifestyle might not seem like a life worth living (i.e., live free or die). The freedom to enjoy eating what they like is worth being perceived as less attractive by normative standards and possibly having to suffer a metabolic syndrome later in life that could be managed through medication. Though most people want to be attractive by normative standards and healthy, it's not necessarily everyone's highest priority in life and the less so the more onerous it becomes to achieve those two goals.

It's also quite possible that for some initially skeptical individuals that once they adopt such substantial lifestyle changes and become acclimated to those changes that they come to prefer that way of living to their previous lifestyles. The more restrictive weight management strategy may not be unduly onerous in the long-term when cravings subside for foods not eaten at all or only in moderation, after achieving a higher level of physical fitness that is not too difficult to maintain with a certain exercise routine, when significant others are supportive of this alternative lifestyle, and when they've developed sufficient assertiveness to manage those who subject them to divergent weight management stigma.

The more restrictive the approach therapists appear to be recommending the more likely patients will experience therapists' recommendations as unreasonable demands. This may be due in part to the problem of 'delayed reward discounting' (Amlung, Gray, & MacKillop, 2016). Patients balk at having to suffer for sure in the short-term for an uncertain long-term benefit that might not be as rewarding as the immediate pleasures that would have to be sacrificed. Patients may feel that they 'should' make such sacrifices and feel guilt-ridden that they don't but when push comes to shove, they don't want to. Ruptures arise as patients assume their therapists are as critical of them as they are of themselves for not doing what they 'should' do to achieve their weight loss goals.

The more permissive the approach to weight management the less the reactance to it. Consequently, patients are more likely to give less restrictive approaches a try if it seems that a less restrictive approach could result in reasonable weight loss and sustainable weight loss maintenance. That is the appeal of many commercial diets – a quick, easy, and painless approach to sustainable weight loss and a flat stomach.

Approaches such as intuitive and mindful eating may not be perceived as demanding in terms of dietary restrictions but could still be perceived as psychologically demanding. It takes psychological effort to eat mindfully rather than mindlessly. Patients may not want to put in the effort to eat mindfully when stressed and hungry or out for a good time. Overcoming 'fat phobia' and developing 'body positivity' are hard work given the tenacity of internalized weight stigma. Learning to look at one's body without moralistic judgment and learning to replace harsh self-blame with self-compassion and self-affirmation is not easy when self-blame is automatic and unrelentingly reinforced by daily reminders of culturally prevalent weight stigma. Perfectionistic self-criticism can be a treatment resistant personality trait that contributes to depression (Blatt, 1995).

Patients might fear that their therapists will perceive them as vain, superficial, narcissistic, excessively appearance-oriented, and prejudiced individuals if they still aspire to conform to normative standards of beauty and be with romantic partners who also conform to those standards. Such patients might fear being subject to divergent weight management stigma if beliefs in the benefits of dietary restrictions are perceived by their therapists as evidence of psychological rigidity, perfectionism, and obsessive-compulsive disorder that would need to be overcome.

Some therapists, usually more psychodynamic or humanistic, choose to be more the traveling companion than the guide because they assume that giving advice is inherently authoritarian. Nevertheless, some patients can experience a non-directive approach as an authoritarian demand to figure everything out on their own without professional guidance. They don't believe it is unreasonable for a therapist to provide weight management advice and they don't want to be made to feel deficient or immature if they can't find their own way without guidance. Some patients will avoid or terminate treatments with therapists who won't 'teach coping skills' in favor of working with therapists who will.

All treatments have 'demand characteristics' (Whitehouse, Orne, & Dinges, 2002) that can potentially feel oppressive to patients and generate reactance. The task then is not to search for a treatment approach that lacks demand characteristics but to appreciate the demand characteristics of the various treatment approaches that therapists provide. Patients may respond with reactance to those demand characteristics when those demand characteristics are autonomy threatening.

Colin, a 30-year-old single man, had lost weight eating a diet of fruits, vegetables, and lean meats that did not include any grains because of the carbohydrate content. Colin felt deprived and was looking for a way to maintain his weight loss where he wouldn't feel quite so deprived. Colin read about the benefits of whole grain for weight management so decided to add whole grain foods to his diet. He bought a grain mill and started making his own freshly milled whole grain flour. Colin learned how to make whole grain breads and whole grain pastas with freshly milled whole grain flour. His friends and dates were quite impressed.

Soon enough, though, eating his own homemade whole grain breads and pastas became his favorite foods in his daily diet. Next thing he knew he was gaining weight and started feeling that his eating was starting to get out of control. Colin began to appreciate that even whole grain foods were somewhat addictive for him if not for others. It would be difficult for him to eat whole grain foods daily without overeating it. He decided that whole grain foods would have to be a special treat on weekends.

The therapist mirrored Colin's excitement when he discovered how to make his own freshly milled whole grain flour. The therapist also supported Colin's decision when he reluctantly decided that he could not eat whole grain foods daily without regaining the weight he had lost. To lessen reactance therapists may support a process of dietary self-discovery through trial and error whether it takes patients in a more restrictive or a more permissive direction.

Self-Control or Emotional Support?

Patients not only need to choose a weight management approach that is on a continuum from more permissive to more restrictive. Patients also need to choose a treatment approach that is relatively more reliant on improved self-control and self-regulation or one that is relatively more reliant on an external support system. These two approaches are not mutually exclusive but there does tend to be some tension between the two approaches. Individuals who hope to eat their favorite calorie-dense foods in moderation daily and who also plan to keep living in high temptation environments will need to cultivate high levels of self-control in the face of constant temptations to overeat. They will need to manage craving when small portions of addictive foods arouse craving daily, and they will need to manage constant temptation to overeat if continuing to live in environments in which calorie-dense foods are readily available.

Individuals who plan to mostly abstain from addictive foods and avoid high temptation environments in which the more addictive foods are readily available will need a support system to make that approach work. Will family members agree to keep the more addictive foods out of the house? Will friends serve low calorie meals and meet up at restaurants that serve low-calorie options? Will friends and families ensure that weekends, holidays, and vacations aren't entirely high calorie feasts without lower calorie options? Will significant others approve of a more restrictive approach to weight management, or try to undermine it by encouraging the adoption of a more flexible approach that weakens one's resolve to adhere to a more restrictive program of recovery?

Managing withdrawal symptoms may require a sufficient level of therapeutic support. Does one have a supportive psychotherapist, a supportive nutritionist, a self-help support group, or a sponsor? The guiding assumption is that self-control will fail in high temptation/high stress environments so such environments must be avoided as much as possible. Considerable emotional support is required to create and live in a small subculture that supports rather than undermines a non-normative lifestyle choice that might be perceived as overly rigid and excessively self-denying by significant others.

From the perspective of reactance, approaches that emphasize increasing the capacity for self-control in high temptation/high stress situations will be preferred over situations that require avoiding high temptation/high stress environments and relying on an external support structure to maintain one's recovery. To eat what one likes and whenever one likes but to be able to exercise moderation no matter how stressed or tempted seems like a proud assertion of autonomous self-determination. That's the way most thin people can eat (i.e., individuals who do not suffer food addiction) and it would be nice to be able to eat like 'normal' people. To maintain self-control in high temptation environments like restaurants or family holiday feasts without fear of relapsing asserts a high level of autonomous self-discipline.

It can seem like a shameful defeat to acknowledge the lack of that kind of self-control and the inability to acquire that kind of self-control through an effort of will. It may be humbling to have to acknowledge a lifelong dependence on an external support structure to consistently eat in a more low-calorie way to compensate for a self-control deficit that appears to be beyond fixing. Considerable reactance is therefore to be expected to any approach that requires avoiding high temptation environments as much as possible, even on vacations, while relying on an extensive external support system to compensate for self-control deficits.

Though increasing patients' capacities for self-control seems as though it would support patients' autonomous self-determination, it can also be experienced as an infringement on one's freedom of choice in high temptation and/or high stress environments. Patients may resent the expectation to exercise self-control when tempted by a favorite calorie-dense but addictive food or when emotional eating seems a well-deserved reward for having to deal responsibly with stressful life circumstances. Reactance arises whenever freedom of choice seems limited by external demands.

Patients may want to defend the freedom to eat 'mindlessly' without having to think about it. Eating thoughtfully, slowly, and/or with self-restraint can be experienced as an oppressive demand when eating freely is being able to eat without having to think about one's food choices or without having to savor every bite when feeling ravenous. Reactance may be defending the right to eat without having to think about it and without self-restraint when that right is threatened. From the perspective of food addiction significant others become 'enablers' (Vernig, 2011) when they encourage others to eat freely for pleasure without restrictions or aforethought. From the perspective of autonomy support such enablers could be perceived as benign subversives who support defying oppressive strictures so to live more freely and pleasurably.

Being mindless has been considered a dissociative frame of mind (Schooler, Reichle, & Halpern, 2004) and dissociation has been associated with eating disorders (Meneguzzo, Garolla, Bonello, & Todisco, 2022). Mindlessness can be a pleasurable state of mind achieved through emotional eating because it provides a welcome relief from stressful realities (Kristeller, Wnuk, & Du, 2018). Reactance arises when people are denied the escapist pleasures that help them deny unpleasant existential realities (Solomon, Greenberg, & Pyszczynski, 2005).

Patients are often of two minds about self-control. After losses of self-control patients feel ashamed and become self-critical so are motivated to work on improving their self-control. Yet at the point patients are in high temptation and/or high stress environments they want the freedom to eat what they want without constraints. It seems like a right of autonomous self-determination to eat what one wants in the present moment and there is resentment of anything that infringes on that right of free choice. What appears like loss of control in retrospect, may feel in the present moment like a defiant assertion of the right to make one's own autonomous choices and then live with the consequences. It is only when negative consequences arrive that there might be regret for prior choices that seem like poor choices in retrospect.

This is one reason to avoid high temptation and/or high stress environments because a side of oneself will angrily erupt that defiantly asserts one's freedom of choice to eat what one wants, whenever one wants, and how much one wants without either external or internal constraints. In the end it might be easier to avoid situations that trigger a defiant side of oneself than learn to restrain that side of oneself once it's been activated by temptation and stress. It may be difficult, though, to entirely avoid high temptation/high stress situations that activate a defiant side of oneself. There may still be a need to the degree possible to learn how to be aware of and down-regulate that defiant side of oneself once activated.

Joseph had learning disabilities growing up and was always advised to make a structure for himself to do his best. Joseph resented having to subject himself to that structure as it felt oppressive. He wanted to be like 'normal' people who he assumed didn't need a structured routine. Though he was a thin teenager, he gradually put on weight over the years. In his 40s he wanted to lose weight by eating less and exercising more without having to put himself on a diet. That approach didn't work as he continued to gain weight, so he consulted with a nutritionist who suggested adopting a weekly meal plan.

Joseph resented the suggestion as he didn't want to have to eat in a structured pre-planned way. He wanted to be able to eat freely the way 'normal' people eat. I noted that structured routines are not just for people with learning disabilities. Many people who are trying to do their best, like professional athletes, embrace a structured routine. Joseph acknowledged that he had never thought of structured routines in that way but as an oppressive imposition to which he begrudgingly submitted that 'normal' people didn't require. His reactance to his nutritionist's recommendation for a weekly meal plan significantly lessened once he appreciated that 'normal' people might subject themselves to a demanding routine to live up to their full potential.

Defiant Self-Destructiveness

Therapists of all approaches are proponents of supporting patients' autonomy. Nevertheless, patients who suffer addictions can be defiantly self-destructive. To assert their agency and freedom of choice they defiantly engage in the addictive behavior almost daring anybody to try to stop them. Engaging in the addictive behavior with wild abandon is an assertion of their freedom of choice that they will zealously defend. Such patients are almost inviting therapists to engage them in a power struggle over their addictive behavior just so they can triumph over an authoritarian therapist who is trying to control their behavior.

Addictions have been associated with oppositional defiant disorder (Kiefer & Frischknecht, 2021). The lack of empathy that individuals with oppositional defiant disorder have for the impact of their behavior on others makes such individuals difficult to treat. They don't want to have to reflect on others' points of view or how they impact others' mental states. Thus, treatment may focus on increasing their capacity for mentalization of others' mental states as well as their own (Fonagy & Luyten, 2018).

Evan was a wealthy single businessman who never had children. His BMI was still in the morbidly obese range though he had suffered a serious heart attack several years back. He came for treatment because his relationships with women always became contentious around what his partners saw as his poor self-care and ended with considerable mutual animosity. Evan believed he didn't need to lose weight or change his diet because he believed he could control his heart disease by taking medication to lower his cholesterol. He was only willing to date slim women with model good looks because he felt it would be a fair exchange to provide a slim future partner with an affluent lifestyle in exchange for her physical beauty. Yet he complained that few slim women with model good looks were willing to date him because he was fat.

The few girlfriends he had didn't see the exchange the way he saw it. They all tried to get him to diet and exercise to no avail. This routinely led to escalating power struggles around his weight that ultimately ended the relationship. Evan was hurt and angry that these slim physically attractive women treated him as a 'fixer-upper' and would not accept him as he was.

I was met with open expressions of contempt if I noted his unwillingness to date higher weight women or to lose weight to better manage his heart disease as problems we might work on together. Evan became argumentative if I pressed on any of these issues or noted his dismissive attitude towards my interventions. I suggested that maybe we could work on learning how to have a difference of opinion without getting into an argument. He wasn't interested. Evan just wanted to use the sessions to vent his grievances with women to a sympathetic audience as he searched for a thin attractive woman who didn't have a prejudice against 'fat' men.

With high reactance patients like Evan, therapists might have to tolerate the lack of goal consensus and considerable push back to their interventions for long periods of time. Therapists don't have to support patient goals that therapists think are unrealistic or self-defeating. I didn't think Evan would be able to have a successful romantic relationship despite poor communication skills, poor self-care skills, low empathy for others' viewpoints, prejudicial attitudes towards higher weight women, and resentment of average weight women who found his poor self-care problematic. Nevertheless, if such patients do not terminate treatment because of the lack of goal consensus, therapists can remain stubbornly persevering in trying to have a constructive dialogue with such patients in the hopes of eventually being able to achieve a negotiated solution to the treatment impasse.

References

Amlung, M., Gray, J. C., & MacKillop, J. (2016). Delay discounting and addictive behavior: Review of the literature and identification of emerging priorities. In C. E. Kopetz & C. W. Lejuez (Eds.), *Addictions: A social psychological perspective* (pp. 15–46). Routledge/ Taylor & Francis Group.

Barrett-Lennard, G. T. (2015). *The Relationship Inventory: A complete resource and guide.* Wiley-Blackwell

Bennett, G. A. (1986). Cognitive rehearsal in the treatment of obesity: A comparison against cue avoidance and social pressure. *Addictive Behaviors*, 11(3), 225–237. https://doi.org/10.1016/0306-4603(86)90051-1

Blatt S. J. (1995). The destructiveness of perfectionism. Implications for the treatment of depression. *The American Psychologist*, 50(12), 1003–1020. https://doi.org/10.1037//0003-066x.50.12.1003

Butryn, M. L., Schumacher, L. M., & Forman, E. M. (2018). Alternative behavioral weight loss approaches: Acceptance and commitment therapy and motivational interviewing. In T. A. Wadden & G. A. Bray (Eds.), *Handbook of obesity treatment* (pp. 508–521). The Guilford Press.

Eddie, D., Bergman, B. G., Hoffman, L. A., & Kelly, J. F. (2022). Abstinence versus moderation recovery pathways following resolution of a substance use problem: Prevalence, predictors, and relationship to psychosocial well-being in a U.S. national sample. *Alcoholism: Clinical and Experimental Research*, 46(2), 312–325. https://doi-org/10.1111/acer.14765

Fonagy, P., Campbell, C., & Luyten, P. (2023). Alliance rupture and repair in mentalization-based therapy. In C. F. Eubanks, L. W. Samstag, & J. C. Muran (Eds.), *Rupture and repair in psychotherapy: A critical process for change* (pp. 253–276). American Psychological Association. https://doi.org/10.1037/0000306-011

Fonagy, P., & Luyten, P. (2018). Conduct problems in youth and the RDoC approach: A developmental, evolutionary-based view. *Clinical Psychology Review*, 64, 57–76. https://doi.org/10.1016/j.cpr.2017.08.010

Gardner, C. D., Trepanowski, J. F., Del Gobbo, L. C., Hauser, M. E., Rigdon, J., Ioannidis, J. P. A., Desai, M., & King, A. C. (2018). Effect of low-Fat vs low-carbohydrate diet on 12-month weight loss in overweight adults and the association with genotype pattern or insulin secretion: The DIETFITS Randomized Clinical Trial. *JAMA*, 319(7), 667–679. https://doi.org/10.1001/jama.2018.0245

Goodman, G. (2013). Is mentalization a common process factor in transference-focused psychotherapy and dialectical behavior therapy sessions? *Journal of Psychotherapy Integration*, 23(2), 179–192. https://doi-org.adelphi.idm.oclc.org/10.1037/a0032354

Kiefer, F., & Frischknecht, U. (2021). Addressing the associated conditions of drug and alcohol abuse. In A. R. Felthous & H. Saß (Eds.), *The Wiley international handbook on psychopathic disorders and the law: Diagnosis and treatment* (pp. 957–975). Wiley Blackwell. https://doi-org/10.1002/9781119159322.ch39

Kowalski, R. M., & Erickson, J. R. (1997). Complaining: What's all the fuss about? In R. M. Kowalski (Ed.), *Aversive interpersonal behaviors* (pp. 91–110). Plenum Press. https://doi.org/10.1007/978-1-4757-9354-3_5

Kristeller, J., Wnuk, S., & Du, C. (2018). Mindfulness-based therapies in severe obesity. In S. Cassin, R. Hawa, & S. Sockalingam (Eds.), *Psychological care in severe obesity: A practical and integrated approach* (pp. 175–198). Cambridge University Press. https://doi.org/10.1017/9781108241687.011

Lister, M., Rosen, K., & Wright, A. (1985). An anti-diet approach to weight loss in a group setting. *Transactional Analysis Journal*, 15(1), 69–72. https://doi-org/10.1177/036215378501500112

Luborsky, L. (1984). *Principles of psychoanalytic psychotherapy: A manual for supportive/expressive treatment*. New York, NY: Basic Books.

Meneguzzo, P., Garolla, A., Bonello, E., & Todisco, P. (2022). Alexithymia, dissociation and emotional regulation in eating disorders: Evidence of improvement through specialized inpatient treatment. *Clinical Psychology & Psychotherapy*, 29(2), 718–724. https://doi.org/10.1002/cpp.2665

Mitchell, A. M., & Raque, T. L. (2022). Addressing health in psychotherapy: Future directions from a community wellness lens. *Psychotherapy*, 59(2), 296–301. https://doi-org/10.1037/pst0000444

Pearl, R. L., Bach, C., & Wadden, T. A. (2022). Development of a cognitive-behavioral intervention for internalized weight stigma. *Journal of Contemporary Psychotherapy: On the Cutting Edge of Modern Developments in Psychotherapy*. https://doi-org.libproxy.adelphi.edu/10.1007/s10879-022-09543-w

Prass, M., Ewell, A., Hill, C. E., & Kivlighan, D. M., Jr. (2021). Solicited and unsolicited therapist advice in psychodynamic psychotherapy: Is it advised? *Counselling Psychology Quarterly*, 34(2), 253–274. https://doi-org/10.1080/09515070.2020.1723492

Price, H., & Deveci, Y. (2022). 'One size does not fit all': Understanding the situated nature of reflective practices. *Journal of Social Work Practice*, 36(2), 227–240. https://doi-org/10.1080/02650533.2022.2058920

Rogers, C. R. (1951). *Client-centered therapy*. Houghton Mifflin.

Schlegel, R. J., Hicks, J. A., Arndt, J., & King, L. A. (2009). Thine own self: True self-concept accessibility and meaning in life. *Journal of Personality and Social Psychology*, 96(2), 473–490. https://doi.org/10.1037/a0014060

Schooler, J. W., Reichle, E. D., & Halpern, D. V. (2004). Zoning out while reading: Evidence for dissociations between experience and metaconsciousness. In D. T. Levin (Ed.), *Thinking and seeing: Visual metacognition in adults and children* (pp. 203–226). MIT Press.

Solomon, S., Greenberg, J., & Pyszczynski, T. (Jan. 20–Jan. 22, 2005). Teach these souls to fly: Existential reactance and the flight to freedom [Conference session abstract]. *6th Society of Personality and Social Psychology Annual Meeting*, New Orleans, Louisiana. https://doi.org/10.1037/e633942013-125

Thompson, M. G. (2004). *The ethic of honesty: The fundamental rule of psychoanalysis*. Editions Rodopi.

Tronieri, J. S. (2021). Cognitive and behavioral treatments for obesity. In A. Wenzel (Ed.), *Handbook of cognitive behavioral therapy: Applications* (pp. 453–476). American Psychological Association. https://doi-org/10.1037/0000219-014

Tsai, A. G., & Wadden, T. A. (2006). The evolution of very-low-calorie diets: An update and meta-analysis. *Obesity*, 14(8), 1283–1293. https://doi.org/10.1038/oby.2006.146

Vernig, P. M. (2011). Family roles in homes with alcohol-dependent parents: An evidence-based review. *Substance Use & Misuse*, 46(4), 535–542. https://doi.org/10.3109/10826084.2010.501676

Wallwork, E. (2012). Ethics in psychoanalysis. In G. O. Gabbard, B. E. Litowitz, & P. Williams (Eds.), *Textbook of psychoanalysis* (pp. 349–366). American Psychiatric Publishing, Inc.

Whitehouse, W. G., Orne, E. C., & Dinges, D. F. (2002). Demand characteristics: Toward an understanding of their meaning and application in clinical practice. *Prevention & Treatment*, 5(1), 34. https://doi.org/10.1037/1522-3736.5.1.534i

Yu, J., Song, P., Zhang, Y., & Wei, Z. (2020). Effects of mindfulness-based intervention on the treatment of problematic eating behaviors: A systematic review. *Journal of Alternative and Complementary Medicine*, 26(8), 666–679. https://doi.org/10.1089/acm.2019.0163

Coaching or Policing? Helping Patients Self-Monitor

9

All approaches to weight management require some form of self-monitoring for the approach to work. In behavioral weight loss treatment patients would need to monitor calories consumed and monitor calories burned to insure a daily calorie deficit (Gomez-Rubalcava, Stabbert, & Phelan, 2018). In a Twelve-step approach to food addiction that is reliant on high levels of social support to maintain abstinence, there would still be a need to monitor when one is in danger of relapse and then assume responsibility for going to a meeting or calling one's sponsor (Rodríguez-Martín & Gallego-Arjiz, 2018). Mindful eating requires heightened self-monitoring of tendencies towards judgmental thinking or bodily experiences in the moment like the taste, smell, and stomach feel of the food one is eating (Shaw & Cassidy, 2021).

The guiding assumption in all approaches is that some form of increased self-monitoring will be useful in managing one's eating behavior. Increased self-monitoring means that eating behavior will be more regulated by higher level executive functioning and less so by automatic unconscious processes. Once patients choose a weight management strategy, they will need to begin implementing it and that will require monitoring their eating behavior much more than they usually do for their chosen approach to work.

Conscious self-monitoring is part of what Kahneman (2011) calls 'System 2' (i.e., thinking slow) which is a deliberate and logical mode of thought. Thinking slow is an effortful process so can be painstaking. This contrasts with 'System 1' (i.e., thinking fast) which is intuitive and emotional. System 1 is an effortless automatic process that can be pleasurable. Even intuitive eating requires 'thinking slow' because it requires one to be thoughtful about whether one is experiencing genuine physiological hunger or a desire to eat something just to alleviate stress when one isn't experiencing physiological hunger (Tylka, 2006).

Neuroscientists assume that brain resources are subjected to the principle of the conservation of energy (Brem, Fried, Horvath, Robertson, & Pascual-Leone, 2014). There is a human tendency towards expending as little energy as possible to accomplish a task. For most people eating their favorite foods is an effortless and pleasurable activity that can be implemented mindlessly. Weight management, whatever the approach, requires conscious effort and aforethought. Consequently, consistently implementing any weight management strategy is challenging due to the ubiquitous human tendency to revert to System 1 modes of functioning because it's easier and conserves energy.

Judging oneself lazy for reverting to System 1 modes of functioning is being self-punitive and lacking self-compassion for the inevitable difficulty of overriding what is an automatic human tendency. Suffering hunger, craving, fatigue, and other forms of stress only makes the effortful conscious override of System 1 even more challenging (Baumeister, Tice, &

DOI: 10.4324/9781003402336-13

Vohs, 2018). Thus, strengthening System 2 functioning relative to System 1 functioning is likely to be a slow, effortful, and sometimes painful process. With sufficient practice intentional self-monitoring can get easier, faster, and more automatic as in learning to play a musical instrument. Yet one would still have difficulty performing at one's best when suffering hunger, craving, fatigue, and other forms of stress that deplete the energy available for conscious self-monitoring and self-control.

Given the ubiquitous tendency to revert to effortless System 1 functioning, the question is to what extent should psychotherapists monitor the consistency of patients' self-monitoring (i.e., the consistency of implementating a weight management strategy). Should therapists monitor patients' failures of self-monitoring and then buttress patients' self-monitoring after detecting such failures? How might patients feel about their therapists' monitoring their self-monitoring, pointing out their lapses of self-monitoring, and offering midcourse corrections?

Patients may be of two minds about their psychotherapists monitoring their implementation of a weight management strategy. On the one hand, patients may want their therapists' support as a monitor who keeps them honest and on track with the difficult task at hand. They may wish their therapists to function as weight management coaches who provide encouragement and advice about how to improve their implementation. On the other hand, patients may want to prove that they can implement the weight management strategy on their own without their psychotherapists' oversite or input. They don't want their therapists policing their eating behavior or calling them out on their implementation failures. They will prefer to rely on their own capacity for self-correction if they require one.

Ruptures to the therapeutic relationship are likely when patients are trying to implement a weight management strategy in a more self-sufficient way, but therapists want to monitor patients' progress and coach them on ways that they could improve their implementation. Ruptures to the therapeutic relationship are also likely when patients seek their therapists' assistance in monitoring their progress and coaching them on their implementation, but therapists refrain from adopting such a directive therapeutic role. Sometimes therapists are damned if they do and damned if they don't. Patients complain when their therapists monitor their implementation because they feel policed, and the same patients may then complain when their therapists don't monitor their implementation because they feel left to their own devices.

I Can Do it Myself

Not all patients will use their therapists as sounding boards for their weight management concerns. Many patients will try to manage their body weights in self-sufficient ways without seeking consultation with a professional. Innumerable books, newspaper and magazine articles, television segments, and commercials suggest ways that individuals can better manage their weights through diet, exercise, and various psychological techniques that individuals can try out on their own. For example, patients can pay for Noom, an online behavioral weight loss service, that offers behavioral advice patients can use on their own timetable in their own way.

High weight patients who are in psychotherapy for other issues may not raise their weight management struggles or their experiments with different ways of managing those struggles.

There may be a variety of reasons patients may keep these struggles to themselves: 1) It's not sufficiently pressing in comparison to other issues with which patients are grappling. 2) It's a shame-sensitive issue patients don't want exposed in fear of their therapists' judgment. 3) Patients want to resolve this issue in a self-sufficient way so don't want to raise the issue because they fear their therapists might tell them what to do. The latter two reasons imply a latent trust issue in the therapeutic relationship. Patients don't trust that their therapists will address patients' weight management concerns in ways that are nonjudgmental and will respect their autonomy. Therefore, they don't raise the issue at all.

Some patients will mention their weight management strategies in passing. For example, they might briefly mention a new weight management strategy they are attempting. Such patients appear to believe that it's important to keep their therapists abreast of what they are up to on this front. The intention of such brief updates may be to implicitly seek their therapists' approval under the assumption that their therapists will say something if their approach seems problematic. Otherwise, it's a good idea with which to proceed. The update is not being raised as a topic for in-depth discussion. The assumption is that if their plan is a good idea that their therapists will not ask exploratory questions or provide feedback.

The weight management strategy could be announcing an intention to eat less and exercise more as though saying it out loud to their therapists will somehow commit them to following through on that intention. They might want reassurance that simply asserting such a vague intention will be sufficient to lose weight despite their worry that it won't be. Or it might be announcing some sort of very low-calorie approach, like only eating 500 calories a day while taking gonadotropin hormone, that they might worry the therapist will think is 'crackpot'. They raise the issue to obtain reassurance that the therapist doesn't think it's a 'crazy' idea. Such patients might get upset if they don't obtain the reassurance that they seek to proceed with an approach they worry might be excessively restrictive.

In these situations, patients are not seeking an in-depth discussion but are raising the issue to alleviate some self-doubt about the wisdom of their approach. They may want reassurance that their approach is not too permissive to lose weight or too strict to be sustainable. They may be trying to push away a nagging concern that in the end their weight management strategy will fail because it is misguided with which to begin. An approving comment or a lack of comment by their therapists can provide the necessary reassurance that their approaches are not essentially misguided. Such patients might feel threatened by more in-depth discussion because the need for such discussion suggests that their therapists might have some concern that the strategy might turn out to be misguided once subjected to greater scrutiny. Consequently, patients may prefer to briefly raise their intention and then let it drop without further discussion.

It is a complex clinical judgment whether to systematically address such passing comments about patients' new weight management strategies or to let such comments pass given the likelihood patients will respond defensively to a more thoughtful discussion about the issue. Autonomy support could be letting patients discover on their own through trial and error what works for them. Perhaps patients must learn for themselves which approaches are too permissive or too restrictive without their therapists seeming to prejudge the issue in advance. If such is the case, it might be best to let such comments pass and perhaps revisit the issue months later when the jury is in as to how patients' new weight management approaches have fared.

What is important to appreciate is that once patients inform their therapists, even if only in passing comments, about a new weight management approach they are implicitly letting their therapists know that they wish to begin taking their therapists along with them on their weight management journeys, at least as a traveling companion if not a guide. Patients may not want to be alone on this journey though they want to make this journey in the most autonomous and self-sufficient way possible. At this point all they may want out of their therapists is a witness to their journey who is sympathetic to their struggle. They may want someone who is a source of reassurance rather than of doubt as to whether they are going down the right path.

Ruptures to the therapeutic relationship may occur when patients press for explicit validation of their new strategy and experience a more neutral position as though it were a vote of no confidence. Gabriel was an overweight 25-year-old single male who was a successful software engineer. He sought psychotherapy because he was depressed about his love life. Gabriel felt that the thinner women he desired would not date him because of his weight but he claimed he had no interest in dieting. He was resigned to being forever overweight and single. He would just live for his career. Thus, weight management issues were put off the table as a topic for discussion.

One day Gabriel came in for a session excitedly declaring that he was starting an 800 calorie a day liquid diet that would be medically supervised. He expected me to be excited for him and say with enthusiasm something like 'That's great!' I was taken aback by his announcement because I didn't know he was even considering a diet and I was skeptical of such very low-calorie diets without careful consideration in advance of what might be more sustainable in the long-term once the weight loss goal is achieved. Responding to the look on my face Gabriel pressed: 'Don't you think this is great?'

I clarified that I would support whatever his weight loss goals were. I acknowledged my skepticism about the very low-calorie approach without aforethought about what comes after. Gabriel responded to my stated reasons for skepticism with a counterargument of why his very low-calorie approach would be effective when other approaches he had tried had failed. That disclosure also took me aback because I didn't even know that he was trying other approaches as he had led me to believe that he didn't care about losing weight. I had mistakenly assumed that he had not been actively trying and failing with other approaches to dieting.

I saw that we were starting to fall into a debate about the pros and cons of very low-calorie dieting. I decided that autonomy support would not be to try to win this debate through logical argument but rather to support his new weight management strategy and let him discover through trial and error if this approach would work despite my skepticism. This appeared to satisfy Gabriel as my support of his independent decision making was more important to him than my support of his final decision. At this point in his weight management journey, he only wanted me as a supportive traveling companion rather than as a guide who might provide oversite of and input into his weight management strategy.

Patients who want to monitor their implementation of a weight management strategy on their own or with the help of other weight management specialists, like nutritionists, have their reasons. Autonomy support would mean respecting that exclusion. Such a nondirective role will be comfortable for therapists who are generally nondirective in their approach to therapy but potentially frustrating for therapists who prefer to coach their patients when it comes to behavior change.

With the passage of time therapists will see whether the approaches that patients are implementing without their therapists' oversite and input are achieving patients' weight management goals. Therapists will observe if patients are losing weight or gaining weight. As it turned out with Gabriel, he was not able to sustain the very low-calorie diet and at that point solicited my input as to what might be a more sustainable approach for him.

To some extent in everyday life, everybody monitors everybody else's weight. Individuals implicitly make assessments of how much people weigh and if there are changes in their weight. In a culture that idealizes thin, high weight individuals are generally complimented for weight loss and told how good they look. Weight stigma is often expressed more covertly as explicit fat shaming is often considered rude though many judgmental people feel entitled to do it anyhow. Weight stigma has been associated with greater difficulty with weight loss maintenance among those whose weight is 10% below their highest weight (Puhl, Quinn, Weisz, & Suh, 2017).

These everyday social dynamics can be recreated in psychotherapy. Patients would expect their psychotherapists to validate and affirm their weight loss successes while overlooking their weight loss failures without comment unless patients raise the topic of their own initiative.

Patients who proudly announce their new weight management strategies with excited anticipation of good results may be reluctant to revisit the issue if results are not forthcoming. The complex clinical judgment is then whether to raise the issue of the failure of the patients' weight management strategies when they don't bring it up of their own accord, a kind of dissociation of a shame-sensitive issue.

Dissociation is a defense mechanism in which one simply doesn't think about something distressing as though it doesn't exist or isn't real. Dissociated material is commonly experienced as too threatening, too conflict-laden, or too anxiety-provoking to be allowed into awareness and fully acknowledged by the subject (Perry, 1990). Dissociation creates a pretense or illusion of normality as though everything is just fine when in fact it isn't (Boevink & Corstens, 2012). Dissociation doesn't necessarily require denying the painful reality or rationalizing it if that reality is never mentioned or discussed (Perry, 1990). Dissociation can be maintained by avoiding anything that would remind oneself of the distressing reality. High weight might be dissociated by not looking at oneself in the mirror or never weighing oneself. In psychotherapy patients can simply not raise a dissociated issue, prioritize other issues for discussion, and hope their psychotherapists follow their lead in avoiding certain shame-sensitive topics.

Therapists would still be observing the fact that patients have not lost weight despite their declared intention to do so or to gain weight despite a stated effort to maintain their weight at its current level. When dissociation is operative, the expectation is that therapists will keep such observations to themselves so a pretense can be maintained that patients' weight management strategies are working when in fact they aren't. It's not unlike a situation in which someone is dying of a terminal illness, but everyone pretends the terminally ill person isn't because it's too upsetting to acknowledge the impending loss. Do therapists respect that dissociation and patiently wait until patients raise of their own accord their difficulties with their weight management strategies and now seek their therapists' input? Or do therapists call patients' attention to a dissociated issue to help them address something of which they have been avoidant?

The psychodynamic literature is of two minds about this topic. On the one hand, addressing topics of which patients are avoidant and exploring uncomfortable feelings are defining techniques of psychodynamic psychotherapy [See the Comparative Psychotherapy Process Scale (Hilsenroth, Blagys, Ackerman, Bonge, & Blais, 2005)]. On the other hand, some psychodynamic writers recommend waiting until patients are ready to address such issues of their own accord when the dissociated material is of a traumatic and/or highly shame-sensitive nature (Bromberg, 1998). It can be retraumatizing to feel 'forced' to deal with a traumatic issue before one is emotionally ready to do so (McGee, 2009).

Patients can feel ashamed that they weren't able to succeed implementing their weight management strategy in a more self-sufficient way. It feels like a shameful dependency to need their therapists' help with implementing their weight management strategy because their own self-monitoring is unreliable. It can feel like a shameful weakness to require their therapists' oversite and input to stay on track with a weight management strategy as well as keep themselves honest in their self-assessment. They may need therapists who can provide midcourse corrections when an approach is proving too permissive to lose weight or too strict to be sustainable.

Therapists who fail to provide such necessary input could be implicitly making patients feel that they 'should' be able to successfully implement such strategies without their therapists' guidance and there is something 'wrong' with them if they can't. The stance of nondirective therapists can be implicitly shaming if it makes patients feel that there is something immature or overly dependent about requiring their therapists' explicit direction and guidance to stay on track.

For patients to welcome their psychotherapists help with implementation and self-monitoring they would have to overcome their shame about becoming dependent on their therapists for that kind of oversite and input. Until that time therapists would be providing unsolicited and unwanted oversite and input that would be experienced as infringing on patients' autonomy. Therapists can let patients know that they are willing to provide oversite and input but if patients decline the offer therapists can't force the issue without becoming an autonomy threat. Therapists would need to patiently wait until patients conclude that they can't implement their weight management strategy without more oversite and input from their therapists and that there is no shame in being dependent on their therapists for that kind of assistance.

The Problem of Cheating

Some patients welcome and solicit their therapists' help in implementing a weight management strategy. They want a weight management coach who will guide them through the process – offering encouragement, directions, tips for improvement, and midcourse corrections as it becomes apparent what is too permissive or too restrictive. Such patients may provide regular progress reports hoping to obtain validation of and affirmation for their successful weight management efforts. They seek their therapists' input on weight management challenges such as how avoid or manage being in high temptation/high stress environments, finding stress management strategies other than emotional eating, how to find the right daily calorie allowance, how to find the right macronutrient mix of foods, how to figure out what are one's trigger foods, to what extent to abstain from or moderate the consumption of those trigger foods, how to find the time for exercise, discovering the extent to which the diet can be modified on weekends, holidays, or vacations, etc.. Much of these deliberations involve 'tweaking' an approach that patients have started implementing as they discover what works and what doesn't.

'Cheating' is the term that is colloquially used when deviating from a chosen dietary approach (Peel, Parry, Douglas, & Lawton, 2005). Cheating can be intentionally stopping the calorie count knowing that one plans to go well above the daily calorie allowance, consuming trigger foods from which one had committed to abstain, overeating such trigger foods one had committed to eating in moderation, skipping regularly scheduled exercise routines because one wasn't in the mood, mindlessly wolfing down a meal when feeling ravenously hungry, eating for emotional reasons rather than for physiological hunger, giving oneself more 'cheat' days than had been decided upon, and avoidance of regularly weighing oneself when there has likely been incremental weight gain.

Such lapses from consistent adherence to a weight management strategy are called 'cheating' because patients feel guilty about failing to honor a commitment, they made to themselves as well as to others to adhere to a diet, an exercise routine, or a more thoughtful approach to eating. They feel badly about themselves because their self-monitoring and self-control was insufficient to adhere to the weight management strategy. They might hide 'cheating' from their therapists' because they fear their therapists' judgment. They then feel badly about hiding things from their therapists because they appreciate that the effectiveness of psychotherapy rests upon patients being open and honest with their therapists.

Patients highly value their therapists' approval, validation, and affirmation when their weight management approaches are succeeding so they dread their therapists' disapproval, disappointment, frustration, blame, and criticism when they fail. Their therapists begin to seem less like helpful coaches and more like police officers who are keeping them under surveillance waiting to punish them after catching them breaking the rules and then covering it up. Ruptures to the therapeutic relationship will need to be repaired when therapists are experienced as policing patients' eating behavior so that patients' no longer feel comfortable being open about their struggles implementing and complying with a particular weight management strategy.

From a psychotherapeutic viewpoint noncompliance with an approach is not a moral offense to be exposed and punished but rather a problem to be analyzed and solved. The problem to be solved is to ascertain to what extent there is room for improvement in patients' implementation of a certain approach or to what extent is the approach too permissive or too restrictive to be sustainable so needs to be changed? For example, patients might go into high temptation/high stress environments hungry mistakenly believing they will be able to exercise self-restraint despite their hunger and stress level. It might not occur to them that self-control in such an environment is more likely to fail when hungry than when not hungry. A potential solution may be to have something to eat before going into a high temptation environment so one is not as hungry.

Patients would then have to try out that potential solution to see if that solution might work for them. Some patients might discover that no matter how much they fill up in advance on low calorie foods that they overeat the high calorie foods anyhow once they enter the high temptation environment. Creative problem solving could be trying out a therapeutic approach like distress tolerance that can increase patients' capacities to better endure distress when distressful situations are unavoidable (Garceau, 2017) Distress tolerance has been used in behavioral weight loss treatment (Butryn, Schumacher, & Forman, 2018). Nevertheless, it might be discovered that there are limits as to how much distress one can tolerate without relapsing in a high temptation/high stress environment.

Maybe after trying and failing with a wide variety of approaches designed to facilitate exercising self-restraint in high temptation/high stress environments it might be concluded that one will never learn to exercise self-restraint in such environments and those environments are best avoided. Yet it might not be feasible to forever avoid such environments. Periodically, entering such high temptation/high stress environments and overeating in such environments may have to be accepted as part of life. Positive interpretation (Woldemariam, 2020) can help patients accept periodic relapse without self-flagellation. Cognitive reframing can undercut catastrophizing when therapists clarify that one's weight management strategy is not doomed forever if one periodically overeats.

Patients may need to learn that it's acceptable to try and fail in the implementation of one's weight management strategy as one tries to discover a sustainable approach that isn't too permissive or too restrictive. Perfect compliance is neither realistic nor necessary to achieve a good-enough result. To benefit from a trial-and-error approach patients would need to feel free to speak about their failed weight management experiments openly and honestly without fear of their therapists' judgment. The Serenity Prayer (Reich, 2015) suggests that self-acceptance may come down to discovering through trial and error a way to change what can be changed, accept what can't be changed, and acquire the wisdom to know the difference. That is unlikely to happen if therapists who are trying to guide patients on their weight management journeys are experienced as policing rather than constructively monitoring patients' eating behavior.

Patients and their therapists must be able to ascertain if a weight management approach is ineffective, if it has yet to be adequately implemented, or if it can be effective with certain adjustments. Answering such questions require honest and open-minded discussions after giving an approach a fair trial run. Nevertheless, the freedom to have such honest and open-minded discussions cannot be taken for granted. Trust in the therapist may have to be earned through the test of time before patients feel that they can speak freely about such shame-sensitive issues.

Wendy was a 21-year-old college student who wished to lose weight by eating in a healthier way. She wanted to shift her diet from eating mostly processed junk foods to eating mostly whole, natural, and raw foods that she believed were healthier. I was supportive of her weight loss strategy. Yet after several months, she expressed frustration with herself that she hadn't lost any weight and was wondering why. I asked if she wanted my help with figuring out why by going through her daily diet. I noticed a look of hesitance in her face, the look of someone worried about being caught in an impropriety so she didn't feel entirely comfortable saying yes to my offer.

I inquired about the anxious look and Wendy confessed that she frequently went out drinking with her girlfriends where she drank too much alcohol and ate too much junk food. She didn't want to talk about it because she assumed I would disapprove not only about her eating habits but about her drinking habits as well. I clarified that it was not for me to decide if she should diet or drink less but that it seemed unlikely to me that she would learn how to control her eating habits while intoxicated with only bar food available to eat. Wendy didn't argue with that assertion.

Wendy dropped the topic of diet and drinking for several months choosing to focus on academic issues instead. One day she came in proudly announcing that she wouldn't go out drinking with her girlfriends more than once a week and thought that would make me happy. I said it did make me happy to see her pride in taking charge of her life, but I wondered why she had dropped discussion of the issue. Wendy said she had been angry at me for making her feel like she shouldn't go out drinking so much when college is the time to be carefree and have fun. She assumed I would disapprove if she continued to do so. Yet she came to realize that she was angry at herself because she felt she was beginning to fall into an unhealthy lifestyle that was starting to get out of control but hadn't been ready to admit it to herself.

The Problem of Plateauing

The advocates of Health at any Size claim that dieting is hazardous to one's health because weight cycling may mean that patients lose a significant amount of weight only to gain it back and then some (Burgard, 2009). Advocates of behavioral weight loss intervention claim that their approach yields an average weight loss of around 10% only half of which is regained in long-term follow-up (Gomez-Rubalcava, Stabbert, & Phelan, 2018). Another common pattern is that of plateauing. Patients lose weight and do not regain it. Yet they plateau well above their weight loss goals.

A problem arises when patients aspire to achieve a normal BMI and they plateau somewhere in the overweight or obese range. They have lost a substantial percentage of their body weight from their highest weight. That by itself is often a remarkable achievement and maintaining the lost weight without reverting to their highest weight could be considered an even more remarkable achievement. Yet patients may not see it that way. It seems like if they got this far, they should be able to go all the way. The issue with such patients is a matter of perspective; is the cup is half empty or half full?

The legitimate question in such situations is whether there is an adjustment that can be made to the weight management strategy that would make achieving and sustaining a normal BMI attainable. Is it possible to tolerate a lower daily calorie allowance? Would a more demanding exercise routine burn sufficient calories? Would more dietary fat, protein, fiber, whole foods, or raw foods in one's diet make the difference? Could total abstinence from trigger foods make the difference? Would intermittent fasting help? Is it worth it to try a new weight loss drug despite the possible side effects like gastrointestinal distress?

Such patients are hoping their therapists can suggest a 'tweak' to their weight management strategy that will help them descend from the plateau where their weight appears to have settled so they can achieve and sustain a normal BMI. Such patients are highly motivated to engage in collaborative problem solving so welcome therapists' oversite and input into their weight management strategies. What they might not want to hear is that their weight loss achievement is good enough and is in fact a remarkable achievement. They don't want to consider the possibility that it may beyond them to lose further weight and keep it off. They don't want to hear that they may need to work on overcoming their residual fat phobia because they are never going to eliminate all their stomach fat. These are all words of defeat to such patients, and they don't want their therapists to give up on helping them go all the way with further words of encouragement and advice.

Self-acceptance for high weight individuals may require learning to accept having to live as someone with an endomorphic disposition who must adapt to an obesogenic environment that can only be partially controlled. Ruptures to the therapeutic relationship are likely when therapists are experienced as being unsupportive of the dream of achieving a normal BMI because therapists don't believe that dream is realistic. Therapists do not actually know what is realistically possible for patients but must learn along with their patients what is possible through trial and error over time. Therapists may have a rough estimate of what the prognosis is but only time will tell if therapists' prognostications are correct. Thus, there must be some tolerance of uncertainty when embarking on a weight management journey with high weight patients because only time will tell the degree to which patients' long-term weight management goals are more wishful than realistic.

Ivan decided to lose weight after a prediabetic diagnosis. His initial BMI was in the morbidly obese range, and he was able to get down to slightly below the cutoff for an obese BMI. This was an impressive achievement as he had lost 33% of his body weight and had maintained that weight for five years. His blood sugar had returned to the normal range. Nevertheless, he was frustrated with himself for not being able to lose the additional 30 pounds he would need to lose to make it to a normal BMI.

Ivan wanted me to help him go all the way and would bring in his daily diet diary to try to figure out where to make cuts. We tried to tweak his daily diet, but his daily diet seemed reasonable, so I didn't understand exactly why he wasn't continuing to lose weight. I started to probe how he was eating on weekends, holidays, and vacations because I suspected that he might not be following his diet when he wasn't working. Ivan seemed evasive when I inquired so I asked why. Ivan confessed that during weekends, holidays, and vacations he wanted to eat like a normal person who would eat what he wanted, when he wanted, and as much as he wanted and assumed I would disapprove. Ivan felt that eating like a normal person on the weekend was his well-deserved reward for conscientiously following a strict diet during the work week.

I clarified that although I didn't think he could achieve a normal BMI managing his weight in that manner that it was his goal rather than mine to achieve a normal BMI. I was only trying to support his effort to achieve a normal BMI because he seemed to want my help with that. Given that he appeared to be healthy at his current size it was not a problem for me if he just maintained his current weight for the foreseeable future. I noted that it might be disappointing to him that he couldn't eat like a normal person on weekends, holidays, and vacations and still lose further weight. I clarified that the choice was his whether to adhere to his diet on weekends, holidays, and vacation. I said I would support whichever choice he made. Ivan became less self-critical of his failure to achieve a normal BMI and more appreciative of his enduring capacity to avoid regaining the hundred pounds he had lost.

References

Baumeister, R. F., Tice, D. M., & Vohs, K. D. (2018). The strength model of self-regulation: Conclusions from the second decade of willpower research. *Perspectives on Psychological Science*, 13(2), 141–145. https://doi.org/10.1177/1745691617716946

Boevink, W., & Corstens, D. (2012). My body remembers; I refused: Childhood trauma, dissociation, and psychosis. In J. Geekie, P. Randal, D. Lampshire, & J. Read (Eds.), *Experiencing psychosis: Personal and professional perspectives* (pp. 119–126). Routledge/ Taylor & Francis Group.

Brem, A. K., Fried, P. J., Horvath, J. C., Robertson, E. M., & Pascual-Leone, A. (2014). Is neuroenhancement by noninvasive brain stimulation a net zero-sum proposition? *NeuroImage*, 85 Pt 3(0 3), 1058–1068. https://doi.org/10.1016/j.neuroimage.2013.07.038

Bromberg, P. M. (1998). *Standing in the spaces: Essays on clinical process, trauma, and dissociation.* Analytic Press.

Burgard, D. (2009). What is "Health At Every Size"? In E. Rothblum & S. Solovay (Eds.), *The fat studies reader* (pp. 41–53). New York: NYU Press.

Butryn, M. L., Schumacher, L. M., & Forman, E. M. (2018). Alternative behavioral weight loss approaches: Acceptance and commitment therapy and motivational interviewing. In T. A. Wadden & G. A. Bray (Eds.), *Handbook of obesity treatment* (pp. 508–521). The Guilford Press.

Garceau, M. K. (2017). Comparing domain-general and domain-specific measures of distress tolerance in adherence to diet. *Dissertation Abstracts International: Section B: The Sciences and Engineering*, 77(8-B(E)).

Gomez-Rubalcava, S., Stabbert, K., & Phelan, S. (2018). Behavioral treatment of obesity. In T. Wadden & G. A. Bray (Eds.), *Handbook of obesity treatment* (pp. 336–348). The Guilford Press.

Hilsenroth, M. J., Blagys, M. D., Ackerman, S. J., Bonge, D. R., & Blais, M. A. (2005). Measuring psychodynamic-interpersonal and cognitive-behavioral techniques: Development of the Comparative Psychotherapy Process Scale. *Psychotherapy: Theory, Research, Practice, Training*, 42(3), 340–356. https://doi.org/10.1037/0033-3204.42.3.340

Kahneman, D. (2011). *Thinking, fast and slow*. Farrar, Straus and Giroux.

McGee, J. (Nov. 2009). Avoiding retraumatization in treatment when working with complex trauma and addictions [Conference session abstract]. *26th Annual Conference of the International Society for the Study of Trauma and Dissociation*, Washington, D. C. https://doi.org/10.1037/e608902012-102

Peel, E., Parry, O., Douglas, M., & Lawton, J. (2005). Taking the biscuit? A discursive approach to managing diet in Type 2 diabetes. *Journal of Health Psychology*, 10(6), 779–791. https://doi.org/10.1177/1359105305057313

Perry, C. (1990) *Defense Mechanism Rating Scale Fifth Edition*.

Puhl, R. M., Quinn, D. M., Weisz, B. M., & Suh, Y. J. (2017). The role of stigma in weight loss maintenance among U.S. adults. *Annals of Behavioral Medicine: A Publication of the Society of Behavioral Medicine*, 51(5), 754–763. https://doi.org/10.1007/s12160-017-9898-9

Reich, J. W. (2015). *Mastering your self, mastering your world: Living by the serenity prayer*. Psyche Books/John Hunt Publishing Ltd.

Rodríguez-Martín, B. C., & Gallego-Arjiz, B. (2018). Overeaters Anonymous: A mutual-help fellowship for food addiction recovery. *Frontiers in Psychology*, 9, 1491. https://doi.org/10.3389/fpsyg.2018.01491

Shaw, R., & Cassidy, T. (2021). Self-compassion, mindful eating, eating attitudes and wellbeing among emerging adults. *The Journal of Psychology: Interdisciplinary and Applied*. https://doi-org/10.1080/00223980.2021.1992334

Tylka, T. L. (2006). Development and psychometric evaluation of a measure of intuitive eating. *Journal of Counseling Psychology*, 53(2), 226–240. https://doi.org/10.1037/0022-0167.53.2.226

Woldemariam, S. A. (2020). Positive interpretation as a tool in psychotherapy. In E. Messias, H. Peseschkian, & C. Cagande (Eds.), *Positive psychiatry, psychotherapy and psychology: Clinical applications* (pp. 417–421). Springer Nature Switzerland AG. https://doi-org/10.1007/978-3-030-33264-8_34

Accepting or Judging? Weight Cycling and Relapse Recovery

10

The research literature suggests that individuals frequently lose weight and regain the weight that they lost, so-called 'yo-yo dieting' (Hutchinson, 2011). There has been some degree of pessimism in the weight loss literature on the feasibility of long-term weight loss as relapse has been more the rule than the exception (Elfhag & Rössner, 2010). Repeated relapse gives rise to weight cycling as individuals oscillate between losing significant weight and then regaining that weight (Elfhag & Rössner, 2010). Consequently, greater clinical attention has been paid to the challenges of long-term weight loss maintenance by incorporating relapse prevention techniques in cognitive behavior therapy for weight loss (Dalle Grave, Sartirana, & Calugi, 2020). Extended care focusing on weight loss maintenance does help limit weight regain (Perri & Ariel-Donges, 2018).

Dieting often begins with high levels of motivation and compliance and losing weight is highly rewarding. Weight loss maintenance doesn't appear to be as rewarding so that motivation and compliance declines leading to weight regain (Perri & Ariel-Donges, 2018). Individuals trying to lose weight may become disappointed and demoralized if they do not achieve unrealistic weight loss goals and then regain the lost weight because of lack of motivation to stick with the diet (Cooper & Fairburn, 2001).

Compensatory health beliefs (Knäuper et al., 2004) may rationalize deviations from an effective diet. Individuals who have lost weight may believe that they deserve to reward themselves with more calorie-dense food to celebrate their achievement. They may believe they could afford to be more flexible with their diet because they could always reinstitute stricter controls if they start to regain lost weight. Perhaps weight loss was achieved with an approach that was too restrictive to be sustainable in the long-term, like very low-calorie diets, though it was sufficiently sustainable in the short-term to achieve significant and rapid weight loss.

Weight cycling has been associated with food addiction (Parylak, Koob, & Zorrilla, 2011). From the perspective of recovery from addiction, periodic relapse on the road to a more stable recovery is to be expected. Vulnerability to relapse may be considered a lifelong vulnerability because addiction can be considered a disease that is never cured but only managed. An addicted individual is never recovered but is always in a lifelong process of recovery that might require attending regular meetings and trying to live one's life according to 12-step precepts (Rodríguez-Martín & Gallego-Arjiz, 2018). From the 12-step perspective, relapse recovery is more about obtaining the necessary social support rather than trying to repair the self-control deficit. That may require learning to accept that the self-control deficit might be beyond repair so one should avoid as much as possible situations in which self-control failure is likely.

DOI: 10.4324/9781003402336-14

From the food addiction perspective, psychotherapists may serve as traveling companions as well as guides in a lifelong process of recovery on patients' weight management journeys. Psychotherapists may be called upon to help with both relapse prevention and relapse recovery (i.e., trying to recover after substantial weight regain). Helping patients recover from relapse will be common though preventing future relapse would be the more optimal outcome. Patients can be ambivalent about relapse prevention to the degree that the demands of weight loss maintenance seem too onerous to be endured for a lifetime. Patients can also be ambivalent about relapse recovery as they might be tired of repeatedly trying and failing to diet successfully. They don't see why the next attempt will be any more sustainable than the last attempt.

Autonomy support is supporting patients' independent decision making (Kors, Paternotte, Martin, Verhoeven, Schoonmade, Peerdeman, & Kusurkar, 2020). It is for patients to decide whether to remain on a diet that has worked but seems to be becoming progressively intolerable. It also means respecting patients' independent decision making regarding reinstitution of an effective but ultimately intolerable diet prior to relapse and hope that one can better tolerate it the next time around with some tweaking. Patients can be ambivalent about whether they want to commit to getting ever better at tolerating the intolerable or to just accept the limits of what they can learn to tolerate without falling back into old patterns of behavior that lead to weight regain.

Relapse Prevention

Relapse prevention strategies are routinely incorporated into contemporary cognitive behavioral approaches to weight loss (Tronieri, 2021). Relapse prevention centers on identifying high risk situations in which relapse is likely. Those situations can be avoided if possible or problem solving can be used to identify coping strategies for dealing with such situations without relapsing (Perri, Nezu, McKelvey, Shermer, Renjilian, & Viegener, 2001).

Lapses can be differentiated from relapses as compliance with any weight management approach is likely to be less than perfect. In addition, weight regain of up to 50% of weight lost is common and should not necessarily be considered treatment failure (Dalle Grave, Sartirana, & Calugi, 2020). Thus, relapse could be defined as something that approximates total weight regain of the lost weight. To prevent catastrophizing lapses (i.e., less than perfect adherence) or partial weight regain, cognitive reappraisal could be used to help patients put such lapses and partial weight regain in perspective. The hope is to prevent patients from giving up in frustration and demoralization and consequently regaining all the lost weight. Patients can be reminded that perfect adherence is neither realistic nor necessary. In addition, maintaining 50% of the original weight loss is still a significant achievement that has measurable psychological and health benefits (Elfhag & Rössner, 2010).

Relapse prevention requires motivating consistent adherence to the standard cognitive behavioral weight loss strategies despite patients' frustration and demoralization with the process. Those strategies include meal planning, self-monitoring, regular exercise, problem solving obstacles, establishing realistic goals, and cue avoidance (Tronieri, 2021). The coping strategies used to lose weight are largely the same strategies required for weight loss maintenance. The challenge of weight loss maintenance is motivating patients to continue to adhere to the strategies that initially resulted in effective weight loss.

Patients' unrealistic expectations about how much weight they will lose or how easy it will be to lose the weight and keep it off may have to be corrected. On average, it appears that losing 10% of body weight and regaining back 50% is average with behavioral weight loss treatment (Gomez-Rubalcava, Stabbert, & Phelan, 2018). Doing better than that would be doing better than average whereas doing worse than that might be a greater cause of concern about the efficacy of the approach.

Disappointment is less when individuals have more realistic goals. Motivation for weight loss maintenance might decline when weight loss was motivated by an expectation of quick, easy, and substantial weight loss that could be effortlessly maintained. Achieving a normal BMI and a flat stomach might only be a realistic goal for those whose BMIs are only slightly overweight if maintaining a long-term 5% weight reduction from their highest weight is what is achievable on average. Individuals with higher BMIs would have to reconcile themselves to, and learn to take pride in, weight loss that still leaves one with an elevated BMI. That may require working on their fat phobia as achieving a fat free body would not be a realistic goal.

Motivation enhancement (Smith, Hay, & Raman, 2015) becomes an essential element of relapse prevention when patients become demoralized by having to deal with dashed expectations, periodic lapses, and weight regain be it slight or substantial. Acceptance and commitment approaches have been used to address patients' declining motivation to adhere to a weight management strategy. That approach tries to enhance self-control skills that revolve around a willingness to choose behaviors that may be perceived as uncomfortable in the moment, for the sake of a more valuable future objective (Forman & Butryn, 2016). The idea is that if one keeps in mind one's core values and the long-term goals that derive from those core values that one can better tolerate the immediate distress one must endure to achieve those long-term goals. As such it is a manner of trying to overcome the problem of 'delayed reward discounting' (Amlung, Gray, & MacKillop, 2016).

Teaching distress tolerance, a core component of Dialectical Behavior Therapy, has been used in the treatment of addiction (Richards, Daughters, Bornovalova, Brown, & Lejuez, 2011). To the extent recovery from food addiction requires suffering withdrawal symptoms, distress tolerance can be helpful with relapse prevention. Distress tolerance helps individuals better endure distress by better understanding that emotional distress doesn't last forever. Appreciating that emotional distress is temporary and will eventually pass if one rides it out, helps one endure it without doing something self-defeating to make oneself feel better like emotional eating. Recovery is facilitated when food addicted individuals can tolerate their withdrawal symptoms without lapsing or relapsing on their diet until the withdrawal symptoms pass and cravings subside.

Mindfulness has been used to facilitate relapse prevention in behavioral weight loss treatment (Sperry, Knox, Edwards, Friedman, Rodriguez, Kaly, Albers, & Shaffer-Hudkins, 2014). Mindfulness training could help patients regard lapses, partial weight regains, or complete weight regain without judgment but with self-compassion. Such events could therefore better be appreciated as problems to be solved rather than as moral offenses to be punished. Mindfulness can also facilitate distress tolerance by looking at withdrawal symptoms and temptations to 'cheat' without judgment for feeling what one feels. Instead, such suffering can be responded to with self-compassion and self-acceptance as enduring the suffering of unfulfilled human desires is an inescapable part of life.

Motivational interviewing could be utilized to address ambivalence about relapse prevention and long-term treatment follow through for various addictive behaviors (Ruger, Weinstein, Hammond, Kearney, & Emmons, 2008). Ambivalence about relapse prevention, relapse recovery, and weight loss maintenance can be acknowledged. Therapists can respond without judgment but with empathy for all the reasons for not sticking with a diet as well as the reasons for sticking with the diet. Maybe the privations of dieting aren't worth the benefits, maybe a less restrictive and less demanding approach could be equally effective, or maybe one should become anti-diet and give Health at any Size a try? Autonomy support would be supporting patients' independent decision making when patients remain skeptical of the value of a treatment approach after giving it a fair trial. After all, even if cognitive behavioral treatment for weight loss is the approach with the best empirical support that doesn't mean it works for everybody.

Fifty percent average weight regain suggests that the average person finds the original protocol for cognitive behavioral weight loss treatment too demanding or too restrictive to be sustainable at the level of adherence that resulted in the initial weight loss. Yet the average individual can maintain 50% of the original weight loss long-term. Possibly patients settle on a higher daily calorie count, incorporate 'cheat days' during which they overeat trigger foods, indulge in 'lazy' days without exercise, do not eat as mindfully as they could have, periodically put themselves in high temptation environments where they know their self-control will fail because they don't want to exclude themselves, etc. Patients may settle on hybrid approaches which combine cognitive behavioral weight loss strategies with eating mindlessly like a 'normal' person.

Frank had substantial plaque buildup in his widow maker artery. His cardiologist put him on a low dose of a statin to lower his cholesterol and recommended losing weight on a low-fat diet. Initially, alarmed by the thought of dropping dead of a heart attack he lost weight and the combination of medication, weight loss, and a low-fat diet dramatically reduced his blood cholesterol levels. Frank was proud of his accomplishment and his fear of dropping dead of a heart attack subsided. Frank began to feel that his good numbers gave him wiggle room on his diet and he started to consume a higher calorie/higher fat diet. He started to gain weight but that did not alarm him because he assumed the medication would ensure good blood cholesterol levels at his next yearly check-up. Yet his cholesterol levels increased significantly at his next check-up and his cardiologist suggested that increasing the dosage of his medication could be of help.

Frank came to therapy extremely upset with himself for having let himself become complacent and not sticking with a diet that had helped to generate such good numbers. I used cognitive reappraisal to reduce his catastrophizing as his cardiologist didn't seem unduly alarmed as his most recent stress test was still good. I encouraged self-acceptance by suggesting that he had conducted an experiment to see how flexible with the diet he could be and still get good numbers and now he knew the answer. I noted that he appeared to have two options from which to choose: Maintain the current diet but increase the dosage of medication as his doctor recommended or resume the original diet to see if he could get his numbers back down on the lower dose as he seemed inclined to do. Autonomy support was highlighting that this was ultimately his choice to make. Frank decided to recommit to his original dietary approach. His cardiologist recommended repeating the blood test in three months to assess if his numbers went back down without having to increase the dosage of his medication.

Relapse Recovery

Complete relapse (i.e., total weight regain) is not uncommon (Hutchinson, 2011). Consequently, psychotherapists will be called upon to work with patients who have successfully dieted but have regained all the lost weight and on occasion gain more weight than they lost. Such patients may be frustrated, demoralized, and down on themselves for their failure to keep off the lost weight. They had put in considerable time and self-sacrifice to lose weight and now it seems all for naught. Such patients may believe that sustainable weight loss is beyond them and do not feel good about that possibility. They believe it makes them less attractive and less healthy despite attempts to convince themselves otherwise. Understanding weight stigma doesn't take away the memory of all the compliments they received about how good they looked after losing weight. It's difficult to feel healthy when one is taking medication for diabetes or heart disease and had gotten better blood test results at lower weights.

Approaches like acceptance and commitment therapy, distress tolerance, mindfulness, and motivational interviewing that are used to enhance motivation for relapse prevention can also be used to motivate relapse recovery, recommitment to a weight loss and weight loss maintenance regimen after total weight regain. From the perspective of addiction psychology, the road to recovery may entail temporary or prolonged relapses of varying levels of severity. Individuals might need to 'hit bottom' before they achieve a sustainable recovery (Young, 2011). Hitting bottom becomes the tipping point at which the costs of the addiction undeniably outweigh the benefits of the addictive behavior. That alteration in the cost-benefit equation provides the impetus to engage in relapse recovery.

Some people have a 'high bottom' (Young, 2011). They function well despite the addiction but as that high functioning becomes endangered by the addictive behavior there is motivation to seek help. Others have a 'low bottom' (Young, 2011). Their lives must fall apart before they acknowledge the need for help. For food addiction, a high bottom might be finding oneself single again and trying to lose weight to help with dating or it might be wanting to lose weight because one is prediabetic, has high cholesterol, or has high blood pressure but is not diabetic and does not yet have significant arterial plaque buildup. A low bottom might be having no marital sex life because high weight precludes vaginal intercourse, having significant orthopedic and ambulation issues because of high weight, having had a serious heart attack, or suffering complications of Type 2 diabetes.

Relapse recovery doesn't necessarily have to wait until hitting bottom becomes the tipping point that motivates patients to recommit to a weight management strategy that had been previously effective. Patients can be helped to appreciate that weight cycling is not uncommon when individuals suffer food addiction (Parylak, Koob, & Zorrilla, 2011). Just because food addicted individuals regain lost weight doesn't mean the next time around that they won't be able to keep it off. Perhaps the weight management approach can be tweaked so it will be more sustainable the next time around. Maybe one is at a different place in one's life, more mature or a better life situation, that will make it easier to consistently adhere to the weight management strategy than previously.

Patients may hit bottom while under their therapists' care despite their therapists' best efforts to motivate their patients to recommit to a weight loss strategy before the negative consequences of their high weight catches up with them. It becomes more difficult to deny or rationalize the negative consequences of addictive behavior when therapists have been predicting those negative consequences well in advance of their occurrence and patients did not take heed of their therapists' forewarnings. For some food addicted individuals weight cycling might not be overcome until they finally become convinced that problems in their love lives or their health, that are weight related, will never be resolved to their satisfaction without not only losing the weight but keeping it off in the long-term. That painful and humbling realization might provide the necessary impetus for sustainable weight loss maintenance.

Moralization and the Therapeutic Relationship

Weight moralization is the belief that weight is controllable across the weight spectrum (Täuber, Flint, & Gausel, 2020). Believing that weight is controllable is associated with increased defensive avoidance among high BMI individuals but with decreased defensive avoidance among individuals with low BMIs (Täuber, Flint, & Gausel, 2020). Such results appear reflective of the self-serving bias whereas positive results are attributed to oneself while negative results are attributed to forces outside of one's control. The self-serving bias serves to maintain a positive view of oneself in response to self-threat (Campbell & Sedikides, 1999). The self-serving bias appears to influence individuals' nutrition beliefs throughout the lifespan though individuals do report better intentions to adhere to a healthy diet as they grow older and gain weight (Renner, Knoll, & Schwarzer, 2000).

The clinical dilemma is this: Relapse is a self-threat as it is perceived as a failure of self-control of something that 'should' be controllable. The self-serving bias can alleviate that self-threat by attributing that failure to factors beyond one's control like genetic predisposition, an obesogenic environment, or weight stigma that makes one feel that one needs to lose weight to be attractive and healthy when in fact one doesn't. To the extent high weight is attributed to external factors beyond one's control there would be no point to trying to lose weight once again if it will only be regained. That's a wasted effort and an exercise in futility. Thus, motivation enhancement may require the remoralization of weight. Perhaps one will never acquire adequate self-control in high temptation/high stress environments but at least one can choose to avoid those high-risk situations as much as possible and seek out high levels of social support for living an alternative lifestyle.

Relapse prevention and relapse recovery is about remoralization of weight. It's helping patients feel that if they recommit to a weight loss and weight loss maintenance strategy it might be possible to regain control of their weight in some sustainable way. Yet remoralization of weight results in greater defensive avoidance among high BMI individuals because it increases their self-blame for their previous failure at weight loss maintenance. Ruptures to the therapeutic relationship will occur whenever patients believe that their therapists are making them feel badly about themselves. The challenge is helping patients assume 'responsibility without blame' (Pickard, 2017) for relapse recovery.

Remoralizing weight may make patients feel badly about themselves because it makes them feel that they 'should' continue to try to better manage their weight when they don't want to because they're not good at it. Thus, power struggles between patients and therapists can arise to the extent therapists try to remoralize the weight loss effort and patients resist that remoralization of weight. Of course, patients can also feel that their therapists now perceive them as lost causes if therapists give up the remoralization effort while still believing that patients' high weight will only continue to compound their relationship and health problems.

The evidence that weight cycling is hazardous to one's health is questionable (Elfhag & Rössner, 2010). Perhaps high weight puts undue pressure on individuals' metabolic functioning. Temporary weight loss may at least, for a time, take the pressure off those biological systems and result in at least temporary improvements in measures of cholesterol, blood pressure, and blood glucose. Some weight management specialists suggest that weight cycling might be a preferable alternative to steady weight gain over time (Elfhag & Rössner, 2010). Remoralization may be helping patients appreciate that although weight loss maintenance is optimal, weight cycling might still be healthier than continuing to gain weight or remaining at one's highest weight forever.

Growing up, Stanley was criticized by his father and teased by other boys for being 'chubby' leading to a high level of internalized weight stigma. As a young adult he was able to achieve his weight loss goals by using Weight Watchers and jogging three miles a day. Nevertheless, Stanley still saw himself as 'chubby' because he didn't have a 'six-pack' though complimented by others for his weight loss. Stanley married a woman who thought he was handsome and sexy.

Stanley and his wife had three children together and Stanley tried to share childcare responsibilities. Because of not having enough time to exercise and eating the same 'junk food' that the children ate, Stanley's weight was higher than it had ever been in his life. Stanley was disgusted by his 'dad bod' though his wife reassured him that he was still as handsome and sexy as ever. Stanley came for therapy because he constantly bickered with his wife about how to discipline the children among other things. As a dual career couple, they were both stressed out and dumped their spillover stress on each other. The issue of his weight came up as a side issue as Stanley would make off-hand comments berating himself for being 'disgustingly fat' and failing to diet and exercise when he knew better because of his prior success with Weight Watchers and daily jogging.

I suggested that Stanley was of two minds about dieting and exercise. I noted that on the one hand he felt that he should diet and exercise as it would make him feel better about himself, and in the past he had done it successfully for many years. I then noted that on the other hand emotional eating and taking it easy on his free time seemed like a psychological necessity raising three rambunctious children, having a demanding full-time job, frequently bickering with his wife, and having to live with his own excessively harsh inner critic. It might be difficult returning to Weight Watchers and resume daily jogging in such trying circumstances.

I was trying to reframe the issue from a moral issue to a practical issue of which Stanley was of two minds – if he was up to dieting at this point in his life that was OK and if he wasn't up to dieting at this point that was OK also. Both choices had their pros and cons. I was trying to support his autonomy by making it clear that this was his choice to make. This line of interpretation alleviated his self-criticism for not dieting when he felt that he should.

One day Stanley came in with a look of self-satisfaction telling me that he had returned to Weight Watchers and jogging three days a week and had already lost six pounds. After a marital argument, his wife to reconcile would make him his favorite oatmeal chocolate chip cookies. To practice cue avoidance, Stanley told her that although he greatly appreciated her effort to make him happy, he'd rather not have such tempting high-calorie foods around the house. It was already sufficiently challenging to avoid eating the children's junk food. Stanley became re-moralized to diet and exercise as he began to feel that it wasn't impossibly overwhelming if he chose to multitask more than he already was by adding the burdensome demands of dieting and exercise to his other burdensome responsibilities. As therapy alleviated some of the burden of managing his harsh inner critic, Stanley felt strong enough to assume the additional burden of dieting and exercise.

References

Amlung, M., Gray, J. C., & MacKillop, J. (2016). Delay discounting and addictive behavior: Review of the literature and identification of emerging priorities. In C. E. Kopetz & C. W. Lejuez (Eds.), *Addictions: A social psychological perspective* (pp. 15–46). Routledge/Taylor & Francis Group.

Campbell, W. K., & Sedikides, C. (1999). Self-threat magnifies the self-serving bias: A meta-analytic integration. *Review of General Psychology*, 3(1), 23–43. https://doi.org/10.1037/1089-2680.3.1.23

Cooper, Z., & Fairburn, C. G. (2001). A new cognitive behavioural approach to the treatment of obesity. *Behaviour Research and Therapy*, 39(5), 499–511. https://doi-org.adelphi.idm.oclc.org/10.1016/S0005-7967(00)00065-6

Dalle Grave, R., Sartirana, M., & Calugi, S. (2020). Personalized cognitive-behavioural therapy for obesity (CBT-OB): Theory, strategies and procedures. *BioPsychoSocial Medicine*, 14, 5. https://doi.org/10.1186/s13030-020-00177-9

Elfhag, K., & Rössner, S. (2010). Weight loss maintenance and weight cycling. In P. G. Kopelman, I. D. Caterson, & W. H. Dietz (Eds.), *Clinical obesity in adults and children* (pp. 351–365). Wiley Blackwell.

Forman, E. M., & Butryn, M. L. (2016). *Effective weight loss: An acceptance-based behavioral approach: Clinician guide.* Oxford University Press.

Gomez-Rubalcava, S., Stabbert, K., & Phelan, S. (2018). Behavioral treatment of obesity. In T. Wadden & G. A. Bray (Eds.), *Handbook of obesity treatment* (pp. 336–348). The Guilford Press.

Hutchinson E. (2011). Systems neuroscience: The stress of dieting. *Nature Reviews Neuroscience*, 12(2), 65. https://doi.org/10.1038/nrn2985

Knäuper, B., Rabiau, M., Cohen, O. & Patriciu, N. (2004) Compensatory health beliefs: Scale development and psychometric properties. *Psychology & Health*, 19(5), 607–624, https://doi.org/10.1080/0887044042000196737

Kors, J. M., Paternotte, E., Martin, L., Verhoeven, C. J., Schoonmade, L., Peerdeman, S. M., & Kusurkar, R. A. (2020). Factors influencing autonomy supportive consultation: A realist review. *Patient Education and Counseling*, 103(10), 2069–2077. https://doi.org/10.1016/j.pec.2020.04.019

Parylak, S. L., Koob, G. F., & Zorrilla, E. P. (2011). The dark side of food addiction. *Physiology & Behavior*, 104(1), 149–156. https://doi.org/10.1016/j.physbeh.2011.04.063

Perri, M. G., & Ariel-Donges, A. H. (2018). Maintenance of weight lost in behavioral treatment of obesity. In T. A. Wadden & G. A. Bray (Eds.), *Handbook of obesity treatment* (pp. 393–410). The Guilford Press.

Perri, M. G., Nezu, A. M., McKelvey, W. F., Shermer, R. L., Renjilian, D. A., & Viegener, B. J. (2001). Relapse prevention training and problem-solving therapy in the long-term management of obesity. *Journal of Consulting and Clinical Psychology*, 69(4), 722–726. https://doi.org/10.1037/0022-006X.69.4.722

Pickard, H. (2017). Responsibility without blame for addiction. *Neuroethics*, 10(1), 169–180. https://doi-org.adelphi.idm.oclc.org/10.1007/s12152-016-9295-2

Renner, B., Knoll, N., & Schwarzer, R. (2000). Age and body make a difference in optimistic health beliefs and nutrition behaviors. *International Journal of Behavioral Medicine*, 7(2), 143–159. https://doi.org/10.1207/S15327558IJBM0702_4

Richards, J. M., Daughters, S. B., Bornovalova, M. A., Brown, R. A., & Lejuez, C. W. (2011). Substance use disorders. In M. J. Zvolensky, A. Bernstein, & A. A. Vujanovic (Eds.), *Distress tolerance: Theory, research, and clinical applications* (pp. 171–197). The Guilford Press.

Rodríguez-Martín, B. C., & Gallego-Arjiz, B. (2018). Overeaters Anonymous: A mutual-help fellowship for food addiction recovery. *Frontiers in Psychology*, 9, 1491. https://doi.org/10.3389/fpsyg.2018.01491

Ruger, J. P., Weinstein, M. C., Hammond, S. K., Kearney, M. H., & Emmons, K. M. (2008). Cost-effectiveness of motivational interviewing for smoking cessation and relapse prevention among low-income pregnant women: A randomized controlled trial. *Value in Health: The Journal of the International Society for Pharmacoeconomics and Outcomes Research*, 11(2), 191–198. https://doi.org/10.1111/j.1524-4733.2007.00240.x

Smith, E., Hay, P., & Raman, J. (2015). Cognitive remediation therapy for obesity. In K. Tchanturia (Ed.), *Cognitive remediation therapy (CRT) for eating and weight disorders* (pp. 176–191). Routledge/Taylor & Francis Group.

Sperry, S., Knox, B., Edwards, D., Friedman, A., Rodriguez, M., Kaly, P., Albers, M., & Shaffer-Hudkins, E. (2014). Cultivating Healthy Eating, Exercise, and Relaxation (CHEER): A case study of a family-centered and mindfulness-based cognitive-behavioral intervention for obese adolescents at risk for diabetes and cardiovascular disease. *Clinical Case Studies*, 13(3), 218–230. https://doi-org/10.1016/j.applanim.2022.105765

Täuber, S., Flint, S. W., & Gausel, N. (2020). Exploring responses to body weight criticism: Defensive avoidance when weight is seen as controllable. *Frontiers in Psychology*, 11, 598109. https://doi-org/10.3389/fpsyg.2020.598109

Tronieri, J. S. (2021). Cognitive and behavioral treatments for obesity. In A. Wenzel (Ed.), *Handbook of cognitive behavioral therapy: Applications* (pp. 453–476). American Psychological Association. https://doi-org/10.1037/0000219-014

Young, L. B. (2011). Hitting bottom: Help seeking among Alcoholics Anonymous members. *Journal of Social Work Practice in the Addictions*, 11(4), 321–335. https://doi.org/10.1080/1533256X.2011.618067

Empowering or Pressuring? Helping Patients Deal with Prejudice

11

Kristeller, Wnuk, & Du (2018) suggest that mindless eating is rampant in American society and mindless eating has been associated with weight gain. Most people would like to be able to eat what they want, when they want, and as much as they want without giving it much thought and without weight gain. Mindless eating means allowing System 1 (i.e., thinking fast) to make the decisions about what, when, and how much to eat with minimal oversite from System 2 (i.e., thinking slow). That means eating what tastes good until feeling reasonably full without giving it a second thought. Though mindless eating is associated with weight gain, some people can eat mindlessly without weight gain and that is an enviable capacity.

Individuals with ectomorphic or mesomorphic genetic predispositions may be more likely to be able to eat mindlessly without excessive weight gain. In contrast individuals with an endomorphic genetic predisposition cannot eat mindlessly in contemporary obesogenic environments without excessive weight gain (King, 2013). That is why high weight individuals could benefit from mindfulness training to lose weight (Kristeller, Wnuk, & Du, 2018). High weight individuals then have a difficult choice to make: Continue to eat mindlessly as is the rampant trend (Kristeller, Wnuk, & Du, 2018) and learn to accept living with a high BMI or find a more thoughtful way to eat to achieve their weight management goals. The more ambitious the weight management goal the more that high weight individuals will need to cultivate System 2 oversite of mindless automatic eating behavior regulated by System 1.

Intuitive eating guided by the philosophy of Health at Any Size is the least restrictive approach to eating that still requires increased thoughtfulness (Watkins, Clifford, & Souza, 2018). There are no weight loss goals and is anti-diet as there are no dietary restrictions. Meta-analyses suggest that on average individuals' weights remain stable utilizing this approach (Linardon, Tylka, & Fuller-Tyszkiewicz, 2021). That means that this approach could be an effective weight maintenance strategy that could prevent further weight gain.

On the surface, individuals that practice intuitive eating can appear to be eating like everybody else since there would be no observable dietary restrictions. Nevertheless, such individuals are not eating mindlessly. They are eating in a way that is thoughtful about nutrition and tries to avoid emotional eating that is not based on physiological hunger (Burgard, 2009). Such individuals may eat mindfully so perhaps could be observed eating more slowly than others or declining second helpings. Intuitive eating does require cultivating a certain kind of System 2 oversite of mindless automatic eating behavior. Yet their eating habits would not necessarily make them appear visibly different than others.

To the extent intuitive and/or mindful eaters appear to eat like everybody else, others would not necessarily comment on their eating habits if they were of average weight. Yet

DOI: 10.4324/9781003402336-15

if such individuals are high weight, they could be subject to weight stigma and that might mean being criticized for not exercising sufficient dietary restraint in their eating habits (Puhl & Heuer, 2009). All high weight individuals, whether they eat mindlessly or mindfully, could be shamed for their lack of dietary self-restraint. Thus, for high weight individuals, eating in public can be fraught if eating in public makes one vulnerable to being shamed for one's eating habits.

Individuals with more ambitious weight loss goals will likely subject themselves to a more demanding approach to weight management that requires dietary restrictions. They might utilize techniques recommended by cognitive behavioral approaches (Tronieri, 2021) or 12-step approaches (Rodríguez-Martín & Gallego-Arjiz, 2018) to losing weight. They may count calories, they may abstain from certain calorie-dense foods, they may carefully control portions sizes, they may avoid certain high temptation/high stress environments, they may stick to a rigorous exercise routine, they may bring their own food to social occasions where the food served is likely to be calorie-dense, and they may still follow these rules on weekends, holidays, and vacations when others become laxer in their eating habits. Individuals who sub-scribe to such demanding weight management strategies would be observed eating differently than everybody else (i.e., mindlessly and without restrictions) unless they took pains to hide their eating habits from others to try to pass for 'normal'.

Such individuals could be criticized and shamed for their nonnormative eating habits (Romo, 2018). Those eating habits could be perceived as excessively rule-bound, rigid, and puritanical. It could be perceived as a kind of 'virtue signaling' that advertises to the world a morally superior healthful way of eating, the way everyone 'should' be eating (van de Grint, Evans, & Stavrova, 2021). As such it would be implicitly reproachful of people who don't eat as 'healthfully' by watching their portion sizes, eating whole organic foods, and avoiding processed 'junk' foods. For these reasons individuals who appear to eat in a very self-conscious rule-bound way that seems excessively restrictive may be subject to divergent weight management stigma (Romo, 2018).

Such individuals are made to feel badly about themselves for being too rule-bound, too rigid, and too puritanical in their approach to eating. If they are of high weight, the impli-cation might be that such a rule-bound approach isn't working so should be abandoned in favor of something more flexible. If they are of average weight, the implication might be that such a strict approach is unnecessary because they don't need to lose weight.

It might not occur to others that such a rule-bound approach can be adaptive for some people if it contributes to weight loss and weight loss maintenance. Engaging in divergent weight management stigma is therefore undermining what may be an effective weight man-agement strategy for some people. There wouldn't be acknowledgment that such rules pro-vide a necessary external support structure that compensates for a self-control deficit that may be beyond repair. From the point of view of addiction psychology, individuals could be viewed as enablers (Miller & Millman, 1989) when they undermine weight manage-ment strategies of which they disapprove by encouraging individuals who adhere to certain dietary restrictions to relax those restrictions.

Nora used to bring fresh baked cookies to business meetings to facilitate team building. After being diagnosed with Type 2 diabetes she still brought cookies to business meetings, but she didn't eat any. Instead, she brought a container of carrot and celery sticks that she mindfully ate by slowly savoring every little bite. Colleagues noticed that she had lost con-siderable weight and complimented her on her accomplishment. Yet the compliments were embarrassing because they were usually along the lines of 'I wish I had your self-discipline to eat as healthfully as you do' as though eating carrots and celery sticks at business meetings was a kind of virtue signaling. Nora didn't want to have to blurt out 'I'd trade places with you in a minute to go back to being able to snack on cookies without worrying about spiking my blood sugar'.

Rarely would there be recognition that individuals who suffer such self-control deficits, like those that suffer food addiction, might have to manage their diet in a way not dissimilar to someone suffering juvenile diabetes who must avoid high glycemic foods or individuals with gastric reflux who might have to avoid fried foods. The point of the diet is not 'virtue signaling' (van de Grint, Evans, & Stavrova, 2021) but managing a medical condition. Individuals who adhere to special dietary restrictions would be happy to eat mindlessly like everybody else were it not for the medical conditions that they suffer.

Divergent weight management stigma sows the seeds of doubt that adhering to dietary restrictions is perhaps not a normal or a healthful way to eat. There can be a kernel of truth to that concern if some restrictions are excessive. The daily calorie budget could be too low (i.e., a starvation diet), or the nutrient mix could be too unbalanced (i.e., too little fat or too little carbohydrates) to be healthful or sustainable. Yet questioning a person's weight management strategy, teasing a person about their weight management strategy, or making a person self-conscious about their weight management strategy is undermining what might be an effective weight management strategy that should be supported or at least respected.

Successful weight managers can seek out consistent sources of social support for their alternative lifestyle such as psychotherapists, nutritionists, and self-help support groups. Nevertheless, it is a source of chronic stress if their family, friends, colleagues, and the culture-at-large remain unsupportive or actively undermining. Learning how to manage unsupportive or actively undermining individuals may be a necessary ingredient of a successful weight management strategy. Yet it can be difficult for people to assert themselves around shame-sensitive issues like weight and eating habits as shame tends to inhibit self-assertive behavior (Breggin, 2014).

Tony decided to manage his weight by abstaining from anything that had added sugar or was grain-based such as cereal, bread, and pasta. Tony found it relatively easy to just fill up on fruits, vegetables, and lean meats when by himself. Yet whenever he was eating out with other people at work or with family and friends, he felt he needed to eat like everybody else even if that led to overeating what he discovered were his trigger foods. He was embarrassed to admit that he put himself on a special diet because he found it was easier for him to not eat his trigger foods at all then to try to eat them in moderation. It can be socially awkward for individuals like Nora and Tony to have to explain the underlying conditions that necessitate not eating what everyone else is eating were others to comment on their divergent weight management strategy.

Therapists may need to help patients assert themselves when subjected to divergent weight management stigma as well as weight stigma. The goal is to empower stigmatized patients to stand up for their themselves and their lifestyle choices however they eat and whatever their weights (Robinson & Bacon, 1996). Yet patients can feel pressured and pushed to stand up for themselves before they feel prepared to do so. Ruptures to the therapeutic relationship can occur when therapists appear to be making patients feel that they 'should' combat stigmatizing treatment, but they don't want to because that might complicate and strain their relationships with people with whom they need to get along.

Patients might fear antagonizing family, friends, and colleagues by exposing their insensitivity to patients' feelings, lifestyle choices, medical condition, and the special diets that their underlying medical conditions might entail. Patients who stand up for themselves might get belittled for believing in an imaginary medical condition like food addiction if it is not perceived as a real illness or a real addiction.

The Challenge of Confronting Stigma

There are extensive literatures on the need to fight the ill effects of stigma in general (Fabbre, Gaveras, Shabsin, Gibson, & Rank, 2020). and weight stigma in particular (Puhl, Himmelstein, & Pearl, 2020). Divergent weight management stigma has been much less researched (Romo, 2018). Therapeutic approaches have been developed that address the maladaptive ways that patients relate to other people like assertiveness training (Ballou, 1995; Gambrill, 1995) and communication skills training (Oliver & Margolin, 2009). Interpersonal effectiveness (Bhatnagar, Martin-Wagar, & Wisniewski, 2019) and learning to reflect on the impact of one's own behavior on others' mental states (Fonagy, Campbell, & Luyten, 2023) could be useful in helping patients deal with the people in their daily lives be they family, friends, or colleagues who are sources of stigmatization.

The interpersonal challenge is how to effectively encourage stigmatizing others to at least respect if not support one's approach to weight management, whatever that approach happens to be, rather than to undermine it by instilling doubt in its legitimacy. This may be challenging because individuals who engage in weight stigma tend to deny mental agency to high weight individuals relative to average weight individuals. 'De-mentalization' of high weight individuals was associated with disgust (Sim, Almaraz, & Hugenberg, 2022). Disgust with human bodies viewed as diseased is associated with dehumanization (Valtorta, Baldissarri, Andrighetto, & Volpato, 2021). It is not easy to assert oneself when perceived as a subhuman object of disgust lacking mental agency.

When it comes to weight management, the problem is that weight management critics have their own conceptions of what is a healthy weight as well as a healthy approach to eating and exercise. When weight management critics critique a family member, a friend, or a colleague for their weight and/or eating habits they believe they are engaging in constructive criticism for the person's own good. They believe their criticism will motivate health promoting behavior and discourage health compromising behavior as they see it. They assume that such criticism, be it explicit or implicit, will be an effective motivational tool (Puhl & Peterson, 2014). Such weight management critics do not see themselves as engaging in stigmatizing behavior. They view themselves as promoting healthy behavior utilizing a particular psychoeducational and motivational strategy.

It doesn't occur to weight management critics that the effects are likely to be the opposite – to make individuals feel undermined in their weight management strategy and feel badly about themselves for choosing an approach of which others disapprove. Individuals stigmatized for their weight and weight management strategies may respond with both positive and negative coping strategies (Puhl & Brownell, 2006). Negative strategies might be eating more food (i.e., emotional eating), but positive strategies might be heading off negative comments, positive self-talk, and seeking social support from others (Puhl & Brownell, 2006). Psychotherapists can therefore help patients utilize more positive and less negative coping strategies when confronted with stigmatizing treatment.

Autonomy support would be the main therapeutic intervention (Ryan & Deci, 2019). The problem with weight stigma and divergent weight management stigma is not that others have their own independent conceptions of what constitutes a healthy weight and a healthy way of eating. Everyone is entitled to a mind of their own, their own beliefs, and their own weight management strategies. There may be a need for cultural humility (Dixon, Kivlighan, Hill, & Gelso, 2022) as different individuals live in different food cultures with different beliefs about what is a healthy way to eat. What individuals are not entitled to do is to try to impose their preferred weight management strategies on others and to do so by trying to shame others into compliance. That would be undermining the autonomous self-determination of others to choose their own weight management strategy. Therapeutic provision of autonomy support is therefore an antidote to that kind of stigmatizing treatment.

Stigmatizing treatment also implies unfairly that individuals have much more conscious control over their weight and their eating behavior than they do have. It turns a psychological and/or medical challenge into a moral problem that faults individuals for choosing the wrong weight management strategy when they should know better. As previously discussed, eating behavior is largely under the control of System 1 that runs on automatic pilot. The 'natural' way to eat is to eat what tastes good until full without giving it much thought. When eating naturally results in excessive weight gain, one would have to eat more thoughtfully to prevent further weight gain. Though System 2 can override System 1 in the regulation of eating behavior it is not so easy to do. Such self-control becomes only more difficult in obesogenic environments when hungry, tired, or stressed as it depletes the energy available for volitional self-control (Baumeister, Tice, & Vohs, 2018).

Autonomy support is not only supporting patients' right to choose their own weight management strategy but is also providing that support with sensitivity to how tenuous patients' sense of autonomy is when it comes to controlling their own eating behavior. That means to try to alleviate whatever shame patients have about their fragile sense of autonomous self-determination when it comes to their eating behavior. It's appreciating the frustration and demoralization patients experience from repeatedly trying and failing to better control their eating behavior as System 1 overrides System 2 despite their best attempts to make it the other way around. Stigmatizing treatment only reinforces the shame that patients already experience regarding these repeated failures of volitional self-control.

Individuals who stigmatize others for their weight and weight management strategies suffer what social psychologists call 'the fundamental attribution error' (Coleman & Renjilian, 2014). The fundamental attribution error blames other people's personalities for their failures without empathy for the situational and contextual factors that might contribute to those failures (Ross, 1977). Stigmatizing individuals may attribute their own average weight to their mature self-control without appreciating that their average weight might be largely regulated by System 1 functioning programmed by their ectomorphic or mesomorphic genetic predispositions. In other words, they are lucky to be able to eat mindlessly without excessive weight gain. The fundamental attribution error allows stigmatizing individuals to feel morally superior to individuals who aren't so lucky. That bias relieves such individuals of the need to empathize with the plight of less fortunate individuals who have difficulty managing their weights in obesogenic environments.

Confronting stigmatizing treatment can be met with a defensive response since individuals who unwittingly stigmatize others for their weight and eating habits mistakenly believe they are offering constructive criticism and are unaware of their own fundamental attribution error. There can be resistance to awareness of unconscious bias (Hannah & Carpenter-Song, 2013). Consequently, stigmatizing individuals will feel unfairly criticized when confronted with their own unconscious biases.

Stigmatizing individuals may respond defensively to being called out on their prejudice. They may lash out in anger or withdraw from further critique of their prejudiced attitudes. No one likes to be critiqued for acting morally superior, moralistic, prejudiced, and lacking compassion when believing that they are only trying to offer constructive criticism to motivate others to engage in health promoting behavior. No one likes to feel that they are only making people feel badly about themselves when they are trying to be helpful. Thus, confronting stigma means questioning and challenging the benign self-concept of those that engage in stigmatizing behavior.

Fred was dieting by abstaining from between meal snacks and had lost some weight. Work colleagues complimented him on his weight loss though they didn't think he needed to lose weight because he was only slightly overweight according to his BMI. During work meetings bags of candy would be passed around for all to share. When the candy came around to Fred, he would just pass the candy around without taking any for himself. His boss teased Fred about taking a pass as though consuming a few pieces of candy might ruin his diet. Initially, Fred let these comments pass.

Over time as Fred's annoyance grew, he retorted sarcastically 'you love mocking my diet but if teasing me makes you happy go for it'. His boss responded 'Of course I support your diet. I was just kidding' as though Fred was a thin-skinned person who couldn't take a joke. The teasing stopped but Fred was worried his boss would hold a grudge against him. He thought his boss might be someone who liked to dish it out but couldn't take it.

Confronting stigmatizing behavior is challenging. It requires finding a way to make individuals aware of their stigmatizing behavior so they can respond more respectfully and supportively to patients' weight management strategies even if they disagree with them. It means discovering a way to increase the self-awareness of individuals who engage in stigmatizing behavior while minimizing the threat to their self-concept. It requires finding a constructive response to their defensiveness when their benign self-concept is threatened.

Interpersonal effectiveness in this circumstance means not simply getting stigmatizing individuals to suppress their stigmatizing behavior in fear of being shamed for their prejudicial attitudes. Ideally it would mean turn stigmatizing individuals into providers of the autonomy support patients' need to adhere to their weight management strategy. Hopefully, with family and friends if not in the workplace one could achieve genuine understanding and support of one's divergent approach to weight management or at least of one's right to autonomous self-determination in that regard.

Gary struggled with his weight growing up in the 1950s and '60s eating sugary cereals for breakfast, peanut butter and jelly sandwiches for lunch, burgers and fries for dinner, and ice cream for dessert. Being a child of the '60s counterculture Gary decided to switch to a diet of whole, organic, and natural foods that was largely plant-based while at college. It was difficult eating that way at home because his parents didn't think such a diet was healthy. Several years later Gary's father had a serious heart attack and quadruple bypass surgery. His father's cardiologist recommended losing weight on a low fat/low-calorie diet. At that point, Gary's father conceded that Gary's approach to eating was the heart healthier way to eat as now the whole family ate in a lower fat/lower calorie way.

Interpersonal Effectiveness in Managing Stigma

Researchers who study couple's communication in intimate long-term relationships have identified the factors that lead to communication breakdown. Gottman's (1993) 'four horsemen of the apocalypse'; criticism, defensiveness, stonewalling, and contempt predict relationship dissolution. One member of the couple has a complaint, criticism, or grievance that is expressed as a personal attack on the other's moral character. The other responds defensively which could be defensive self-justification or countercomplaint. Those defensive responses that Gottman described tend to result in escalating arguments (Honeycutt, Frost, & Krawietz, 2019). To avoid such conflicts there may be withdrawal in hurt and anger. Thus, defensive interpersonal responding can result in either criticize/defend or demand-withdraw communication patterns (Dunbar & Abra, 2021). Having collegial relationships with others, including others who possess unconscious bias, is then learning how to have respectful disagreement, how to disagree without becoming disagreeable or disconnected (Wright, 2005).

Confrontation of stigma can lead to communication breakdown because confrontation of unconscious bias can be experienced as an attack on the moral character of the stigmatizing individual (i.e., one of Gottman's four horses of the apocalypse). Consequently, stigmatizing individuals may respond to what feels like unfair character assassination with self-justification (i.e., an argument that their weight management beliefs are valid) and/or countercomplaint (i.e., an argument that the other's weight management beliefs are invalid).

Such arguments may activate dichotomous thinking in which moral virtue is attributed to one weight management belief while moral turpitude is attributed to the other. It is not simply a power struggle about the nature of reality, what is a rational or irrational belief, based on the available evidence but a power struggle about who holds the moral high ground as well. In certain contexts, the oppressed and marginalized victims of stigmatization by virtue of their oppression may lay a claim to a moral superiority and thus perpetuate an ongoing power struggle for the moral high ground (Anderson, 2001).

There is a breakdown of dialectical thinking as the conflict is framed in a polarizing way as though different beliefs couldn't each possess their significant kernel of truth or that different weight management strategies could be effective for different people (Fruzzetti, 2022). There is not a conception that the evidence that supports certain beliefs could be interpreted in other ways or that many aspects of dietary reality remain uncertain and poorly understood. The breakdown of dialectical thinking may threaten attachment security (Wang & Lopez, 2011) and reflective functioning deteriorates in the face of attachment insecurity (Tasca, 2019).

There is an inability to see and empathize with the other's point of view when feeling personally attacked. Buddhists suggest that your enemy is your teacher because it is challenging to cultivate compassion for someone who is actively trying to hurt you (Ho, Nakamura, & Swain, 2021). It is difficult to reflect on the impact of one's defensive response to personal attack on the other's mental state during an ongoing personal attack.

Stigmatizing individuals may just withdraw in hurt and anger if they fear being 'cancelled' for their politically incorrect beliefs (i.e., Gottman's stonewalling). They believe that voicing their politically incorrect beliefs is just authentic self-expression; just telling it like it is (Rosenblum, Schroeder, & Gino, 2020). Individuals might then suppress what is perceived as stigmatizing behavior to avoid further attack on their moral character without any change in their underlying attitudes and beliefs. Yet their underlying weight management prejudices could still leak out in microaggressions (Kinavey & Cool, 2019).

Assertiveness training differentiates passive and aggressive behavior from assertive behavior (Gambrill, 1995). Passive behavior is avoidant or overaccommodating behavior designed to avoid conflict. The passive person doesn't assert what they want but hopes they might get what they want if they avoid confrontation, and their accommodation is appreciated and reciprocated. Aggressive behavior is angrily demanding what one wants. It can seem like being assertive, a demand to be heard and validated, but since aggressive behavior is experienced as a personal attack it provokes a defensive response. Self-righteous indignation can express a legitimate grievance that warrants a fair hearing (West, 2020). Yet righteous rage may be an assertion of political power that can have a negative impact on political subjects (Rothbart, 2021). Making angry demands from the moral high ground may not constitute an effective strategy of communication if it only provokes a defensive response from someone who feels unfairly vilified.

Assertiveness is standing up for what one wants or how one wants to be treated but in a way that is respectful of the other person's perspective and beliefs. It consists of three sequential components: 1) A statement showing an appreciation of the other person's perspective. 2) A statement clarifying one's own perspective. 3) A request for the behavior change one would like (Gambrill, 1995). Standing up to weight stigma might sound something like this: 'I know you think if I lost weight, I'd be happier because I'd feel healthier and more attractive but I'm tired of trying to diet so I'm learning to accept myself as I am and feel that I'm good enough as I am so I'd really appreciate it if you could stop trying to motivate me to lose weight'. Standing up to divergent weight management stigma might sound something like this: 'I know you think that my approach to dieting is too rigid and probably won't work in the end and that I'd be happier if I eased up on it but more flexible approaches haven't worked for me in the past and I really want to give this approach my best shot so I'd really appreciate it if you could respect my choice though I understand why you don't agree with this approach to dieting'.

The goal of assertiveness is to achieve a mutually respectful relationship. By treating the stigmatizing individual with respect for their perspective the hope is to invite reciprocation. It is leading by example. Individuals are allowed to have their own beliefs about what is a healthy weight or an effective weight management strategy without having to debate it. The idea is that in a mutually respectful relationship one doesn't try to impose one's beliefs on others even when it's believed to be for their own good.

Weight stigma may unconsciously serve to rationalize power and privilege over high weight individuals (Kanagasingam, Norman, & Hurd, 2022). Yet to interpret that unconscious dynamic explicitly would be consciously perceived as an unwarranted attack on the stigmatizing individual's moral character. Assertiveness training is based on an appeal to the stigmatizing individual's better nature, their latent capacity to treat others with empathy for their predicament, and respect for their autonomous decision making.

Stigmatized individuals who are passive, avoidant, and/or overaccommodating may allow stigmatizing behavior to go unchallenged because their shame inhibits assertive behavior (Breggin, 2014). Yet once they own their self-righteous indignation at prejudicial treatment (West, 2020), they might lash out in righteous rage (Rothbart, 2021) at stigmatizing individuals in ways that make it less likely that they receive the respect, empathy, and autonomy support that they need and desire. Stigmatizing individuals may feel that they are being punished rather than enlightened for their prejudicial attitudes.

Stigmatized individuals who angrily confront stigma and demand its immediate cessation to proudly assert themselves may generate considerable reactance as stigmatizing individuals respond defensively to what seems like an unwarranted attack on their moral character. Anger tends to deactivate reflective functioning (Josephs & McLeod, 2014). Enraged morally indignant individuals may not appreciate their impact on their targets' mental states. Bias is not something that can be volitionally suspended in response to an angry demand if bias is an unconscious process that is rationalized and then defended when openly confronted.

Assertiveness by expressing understanding and empathy for the worldview of the stigmatizing individual tries to evoke their latent capacity to return the favor. Speaking assertively may still be met with stiff resistance if stigmatizing individuals feel an imperious need for validation of their perspective and compliance with their recommendations. They may become angry when they don't get the validation and compliance that they feel they must have. Interpersonal effectiveness may then be learning to stand one's ground without becoming aggressive/demanding/argumentative in ways that escalate conflict or avoidant/accommodating to diffuse conflict when assertiveness is met with a defensive response (Deluty, 1985).

The point of standing one's ground would not be to win a debate about the merits of one's weight management strategy but rather to stand up for one's right of autonomous self-determination in that regard. Standing one's ground might sound something like: 'I appreciate your passionate defense of your position and that you only want what you think is best for me but how I manage my weight is my choice to make and I'll have to live with the consequences of my choices so I'd rather not continue to debate this issue and would hope that you could respect that this is my call to make'. The point is to diffuse rather than escalate conflict without surrendering one's right of autonomous self-determination when showing appreciation of the other's viewpoint doesn't yield the desired reciprocation.

Individuals stigmatized for their weight or eating habits may need to find supportive subcultures of like-minded individuals where they can feel affirmed (Himmelstein, Puhl, Pearl, Pinto, & Foster, 2020) when neither angry confrontation, calm respectful self-assertiveness, or standing one's ground yields the understanding, respect, and autonomy support that they need to persevere in their weight management strategy.

Dan's mother, a pediatrician, worried that Dan was too short and too chubby while he was growing up and brought him around to various specialists trying to figure out what to do. Dan suffered from internalized height as well as internalized weight stigma worrying that he was too short and too chubby to be good at sports or to be a desirable sexual partner. Dan compensated by becoming very successful in finance and found a partner with a similar body build to his own who accepted him as he was.

Dan came for therapy because his mother continued to be overinvolved in his life in a way that he perceived as judgmental and controlling. Dan tended to placate his mother by being overaccommodating, but his wife complained as she felt that Dan deferred more to his mother than to her. Dan oscillated between begrudging accommodation to his mother and losing his temper with her. His mother would feel deeply wounded by his temper outbursts protesting that she only wanted what was best for him and she didn't want to have to 'walk on eggs' with her own son.

We worked on learning to assert himself with his mother though she did not respond well to not getting her own way. Dan often felt that I was pushing him too hard to confront his mother when life was often easier if he just ignored her or put some distance between them. Dan practiced asserting himself with me by tactfully telling me to back off when he thought

I was being too pushy with the assertiveness training. I backed off so that being assertive with me worked even if it did not yet work with his mother.

Things came to a head when his youngest son was three years old, and his mother thought his son was too short and chubby for his age so Dan should consult with medical specialists. Dan did not want 'grandma' making his son feel badly about his height and weight so decided the issue had to be confronted. Applying the principles of assertiveness training Dan was able to say to his mother something like: 'I know you only want what's best for me and my son and I respect your professional opinion as a pediatrician when it comes to most medical issues but I've always been self-conscious about my height and weight since you made such a big deal about it while I was growing up so I don't want my son having to grow up the way I did feeling self-conscious about his height and weight'. Talking to his mother this way was much better received than losing his temper and calling his mother a 'control freak'. His mother confessed that she never knew that Dan felt that way growing up, apologized for making him feel badly about himself, and reassured him that she would never want to make her grandchild feel self-conscious about his height and weight.

Becoming Ready to Assert Oneself in the Face of Stigma

Asserting oneself in the face of stigma is not easy as being stigmatized for one's weight or eating habits is shaming (Lucibello, Nesbitt, Solomon-Krakus, & Sabiston, 2021). Narcissistically vulnerable individuals defend against shame by hiding their vulnerability or lashing out in anger [see Krizan & Johar (2015) on narcissistic rage]. Psychotherapy then must help patients overcome their fear of self-assertion when they respond avoidantly to stigmatization or help with anger management if they tend to lash out in anger when feeling shamed. Avoidant and/or overaccommodating individuals may not want to threaten valued relationships with biased individuals if they were to assert themselves. Individuals that lash out in anger when feeling shamed fear that their legitimate grievances won't be heard unless fully and forcefully vented. It may seem weak to show respect towards individuals that have not shown respect towards you.

The point of assertiveness training is to empower individuals to communicate more effectively. Yet there can be reactance to assertiveness training if individuals feel pressured to assert themselves before they feel ready. Passive individuals may fear that being assertive will be perceived as aggressive. Aggressive individuals may fear that being assertive in a way that is respectful rather than dismissive of the other's viewpoint will be perceived as weak because it seems to make an accommodation or concession to the other's prejudiced way of thinking. Consequently, goal consensus may be lacking to working on asserting oneself in the face of weight stigma and divergent weight management stigma. Ruptures to the therapeutic relationship can arise when patients feel pressured by their therapists to assert themselves in the face of stigmatizing treatment prior to feeling ready to do so.

Readiness to assert oneself in the face of stigmatization is not an easy thing to achieve. Stigmatizing treatment is shaming so makes one feel less than confident. It instills low self-worth, self-doubt, and expectation of ongoing rejection for the shamed quality (Lucibello, Nesbitt, Solomon-Krakus, & Sabiston, 2021). System 1 responds automatically to such a self-threat with a fight or flight response (Mischel & DeSmet, 2000) to defend oneself against further stigmatization. Attachment security is endangered as one can't be oneself in the relationship without getting rejected for who one is (Carnelley & Hepper, 2015). That threat deactivates reflective functioning (Kuipers, van Loenhout, van der Ark, & Bekker, 2016) which includes deactivating the ability to understand and empathize with the perspective of the shaming other as well as reflect on the impact of one's defensive response on the shaming other's mental state.

These automatic responses to shaming self-threats preclude being able to respond assertively. Responding assertively requires some ability to articulate and empathize with the perspective of the shaming other, a System 2 function that is overridden when the more emotion-driven System 1 is strongly activated and operating on automatic pilot. In addition, responding assertively requires overriding one's own self-doubt and fear of further rejection to clearly articulate one's own needs, desires, and perspective. Being self-revealing in such a manner makes one vulnerable to further rejection and requires overriding the impulse to hide rather than expose one's vulnerabilities to rejecting others. It also requires a high degree of self-possession in a state of high emotional arousal. It means responding in a calm, thoughtful, and measured way when feeling hurt and angry.

When therapists role model assertive behavior they can lead by example. Role modeling might be most apparent in how therapists respond to ruptures to the therapeutic relationship. Do therapists respond to withdrawal ruptures by defensively withdrawing themselves? Do therapists respond defensively to confrontation ruptures with defensive self-justification or countercomplaint? Or do therapists articulate and empathize with patients' perspectives after ruptures to the therapeutic relationship and then try to calmly and thoughtfully clarify where they are coming from in a measured way? Can patient and therapist have a respectful difference of opinion as they work towards a meeting of minds and goal consensus regarding how to best deal with stigmatizing others?

While attempting to facilitate patients' capacities to assert themselves with stigmatizing others it is possible to work on other coping strategies as well. Therapists can help patients take stigmatizing treatment less personally to the extent it is internalized. Validation, affirmation, and autonomy support of patients' weight management strategies can counter the lack of support elsewhere. Patients can seek alternative sources of support like nutritionists, self-help groups, and readings that are more supportive of their preferred weight management strategy. Avoidance of stigmatizing others to the degree possible may prevent salt from being poured in the wound until a time when patients feel ready to stand up to such prejudicial treatment. Hiding one's weight management strategy from disapproving others is also an option until a time that one's feel prepared to 'come out of the closet' regarding one's preferred weight management strategy. Coming out of the closet could mean openly declaring to others that one is a food addict in recovery who abstains from certain foods knowing full well that stigmatizing others might think that food addiction is a bogus scientific concept and that abstaining from 'forbidden' foods is a misguided approach that will backfire.

References

Anderson, J. M. (2004). The conundrums of binary categories: Critical inquiry through the lens of postcolonial feminist humanism. *CJNR: Canadian Journal of Nursing Research*, 36(4), 11–16.

Ballou, M. (1995). Assertiveness training. In M. Ballou (Ed.), *Psychological interventions: A guide to strategies* (pp. 125–135). Praeger Publishers/Greenwood Publishing Group. https://doi.org/10.1037/0000288-007

Baumeister, R. F., Tice, D. M., & Vohs, K. D. (2018). The strength model of self-regulation: Conclusions from the second decade of willpower research. *Perspectives on Psychological Science*, 13(2), 141–145. https://doi.org/10.1177/1745691617716946

Bhatnagar, K. A. C., Martin-Wagar, C., & Wisniewski, L. (2019). DBT for eating disorders: An overview. In M. A. Swales (Ed.), *The Oxford handbook of dialectical behaviour therapy* (pp. 573–594). Oxford University Press.

Breggin, P. R. (2014). *Guilt, shame, and anxiety: Understanding and overcoming negative emotions.* Prometheus Books.

Burgard, D. (2009). What is "Health At Every Size"? In E. Rothblum & S. Solovay (Eds.), *The fat studies reader* (pp. 41–53). New York: NYU Press.

Carnelley, K. B., & Hepper, E. G. (2015). Stigma, attachment, and relationship dissolution: Commentary on meanings of intimacy. *Analyses of Social Issues and Public Policy (ASAP)*, 15(1), 401–405. https://doi.org/10.1111/asap.12088

Coleman, K. A., & Renjilian, D. (2014). *Perceiving Others: Body-Image Distortion and Dissatisfaction* [Conference session]. 122nd American Psychological Association Annual Convention, Washington, D.C. https://doi.org/10.1037/e548142014-001

Deluty, R. H. (1985). Consistency of assertive, aggressive, and submissive behavior for children. *Journal of Personality and Social Psychology*, 49(4), 1054–1065. https://doi-org/10.1037/0022-3514.49.4.1054

Dixon, K. M., Kivlighan, D. M., Hill, C. E., & Gelso, C. J. (2022). Cultural humility, working alliance, and Outcome Rating Scale in psychodynamic psychotherapy: Between-therapist, within-therapist, and within-client effects. *Journal of Counseling Psychology*, 69(3), 276–286. https://doi.org/10.1037/cou0000590

Dunbar, N. E., & Abra, G. (2021). A dyadic power theory explanation of the demand-withdraw interaction pattern. *Personal Relationships*, 28(3), 586–606. https://doi-org/10.1111/pere.12381

Fabbre, V. D., Gaveras, E., Shabsin, A. G., Gibson, J., & Rank, M. R. (2020). Confronting stigma, discrimination, and social exclusion. In M. R. Rank (Ed.), *Toward a livable life: A 21st century agenda for social work* (pp. 70–93). Oxford University Press.

Fonagy, P., Campbell, C., & Luyten, P. (2023). Alliance rupture and repair in mentalization-based therapy. In C. F. Eubanks, L. W. Samstag, & J. C. Muran (Eds.), *Rupture and repair in psychotherapy: A critical process for change* (pp. 253–276). American Psychological Association. https://doi.org/10.1037/0000306-011

Fruzzetti, A. E. (2022). Dialectical thinking. *Cognitive and Behavioral Practice*, 29(3), 567–570. https://doi-org/10.1016/j.cbpra.2022.02.011

Gambrill, E. (1995). Assertion skills training. In W. O'Donohue & L. Krasner (Eds.), *Handbook of psychological skills training: Clinical techniques and applications* (pp. 81–118). Allyn & Bacon.

Gottman, J. M. (1993). A theory of marital dissolution and stability. *Journal of Family Psychology*, 7(1), 57–75. https://doi.org/10.1037/0893-3200.7.1.57

Hannah, S. D., & Carpenter-Song, E. (2013). Patrolling your blind spots: Introspection and public catharsis in a medical school faculty development course to reduce unconscious bias in medicine. *Culture, Medicine and Psychiatry*, 37(2), 314–339. https://doi.org/10.1007/s11013-013-9320-4

Himmelstein, M. S., Puhl, R. M., Pearl, R. L., Pinto, A. M., & Foster, G. D. (2020). Coping with weight stigma among adults in a commercial weight management sample. *International Journal of Behavioral Medicine*, 27(5), 576–590. https://doi.org/10.1007/s12529-020-09895-4

Ho, S. S., Nakamura, Y., & Swain, J. E. (2021). Compassion as an intervention to attune to universal suffering of self and others in conflicts: A translational framework. *Frontiers in Psychology*, 11, 603385. https://doi.org/10.3389/fpsyg.2020.603385

Honeycutt, J. M., Frost, J. K., & Krawietz, C. E. (2019). Applying signal detection theory to conflict escalation as a consequence of victimization with physiological arousal covariates. *Journal of Aggression, Conflict and Peace Research*, 11(3), 200–212. https://doi.org/10.1108/JACPR-10-2018-0386

Josephs, L., & McLeod, B. A. (2014). A theory of mind–focused approach to anger management. *Psychoanalytic Psychology*, 31(1), 68–83. https://doi.org/10.1037/a0034175

Kanagasingam, D., Norman, M., & Hurd, L. (2022). 'It's not just to treat everybody the same': A social justice framework for caring for larger patients in healthcare practice. *Sociology of Health & Illness*, 44(6), 899–918. https://doi-org/10.1111/1467-9566.13470

Kinavey, H., & Cool, C. (2019). The broken lens: How anti-fat bias in psychotherapy is harming our clients and what to do about it. *Women & Therapy*, 42(1–2), 116–130. https://doi.org/10.1080/02703149.2018.1524070

King, B. M. (2013). The modern obesity epidemic, ancestral hunter-gatherers, and the sensory/reward control of food intake. *The American Psychologist*, 68(2), 88–96. https://doi.org/10.1037/a0030684

Kristeller, J., Wnuk, S., & Du, C. (2018). Mindfulness-based therapies in severe obesity. In S. Cassin, R. Hawa, & S. Sockalingam (Eds.), *Psychological care in severe obesity: A practical and integrated approach* (pp. 175–198). Cambridge University Press. https://doi.org/10.1017/9781108241687.011

Krizan, Z., & Johar, O. (2015). Narcissistic rage revisited. *Journal of Personality and Social Psychology*, 108(5), 784–801. https://doi.org/10.1037/pspp0000013

Kuipers G. S., van Loenhout, Z., van der Ark, L. A., & Bekker, M. H. (2016). Attachment insecurity, mentalization and their relation to symptoms in eating disorder patients. *Attachment & Human Development*, 18(3), 250–272. https://doi.org/10.1080/14616734.2015.1136660

Linardon, J., Tylka, T. L., & Fuller-Tyszkiewicz, M. (2021). Intuitive eating and its psychological correlates: A meta-analysis. *The International Journal of Eating Disorders*, 54(7), 1073–1098. https://doi.org/10.1002/eat.23509

Lucibello, K. M., Nesbitt, A. E., Solomon-Krakus, S., & Sabiston, C. M. (2021). Internalized weight stigma and the relationship between weight perception and negative body-related self-conscious emotions. *Body Image*, 37, 84–88. https://doi.org/10.1016/j.bodyim.2021.01.010

Miller, N. S., & Millman, R. B. (1989). A common cause of alcoholism. *Journal of Substance Abuse Treatment*, 6(1), 41–43. https://doi.org/10.1016/0740-5472(89)90019-6

Mischel, W., & DeSmet, A. L. (2000). Self-regulation in the service of conflict resolution. In M. Deutsch & P. T. Coleman (Eds.), *The handbook of conflict resolution: Theory and practice* (pp. 256–275). Jossey-Bass/Wiley.

Oliver, P. H., & Margolin, G. (2009). Communication/problem-solving skills training. In W. T. O'Donohue & J. E. Fisher (Eds.), *General principles and empirically supported techniques of cognitive behavior therapy* (pp. 199–206). John Wiley & Sons, Inc.

Puhl, R. M., & Brownell, K. D. (2006). Confronting and coping with weight stigma: An investigation of overweight and obese adults. *Obesity (Silver Spring, Md.)*, 14(10), 1802–1815. https://doi.org/10.1038/oby.2006.208

Puhl, R. M., & Heuer, C. A. (2009). The stigma of obesity: A review and update. *Obesity (Silver Spring, Md.)*, 17(5), 941–964. https://doi.org/10.1038/oby.2008.636

Puhl, R. M., Himmelstein, M. S., & Pearl, R. L. (2020). Weight stigma as a psychosocial contributor to obesity. *The American Psychologist*, 75(2), 274–289. https://doi.org/10.1037/amp0000538

Puhl, R. M., & Peterson, J. L. (2014). The nature, consequences, and public health implications of obesity stigma. In P. W. Corrigan (Ed.), *The stigma of disease and disability: Understanding causes and overcoming injustices* (pp. 183–203). American Psychological Association.

Robinson, B. E., & Bacon, J. G. (Sep. 1996). Take the bite out of "fat". *Clinician's Research Digest*, 14(9), 3. https://doi.org/10.1037/e327982004-006

Rodríguez-Martín, B. C., & Gallego-Arjiz, B. (2018). Overeaters Anonymous: A mutual-help fellowship for food addiction recovery. *Frontiers in Psychology*, 9, 1491. https://doi.org/10.3389/fpsyg.2018.01491

Romo, L. K. (2018). An examination of how people who have lost weight communicatively negotiate interpersonal challenges to weight management. *Health Communication*, 33(4), 469–477. https://doi.org/10.1080/10410236.2016.1278497

Rosenblum, M., Schroeder, J., & Gino, F. (2020). Tell it like it is: When politically incorrect language promotes authenticity. *Journal of Personality and Social Psychology*, 119(1), 75–103. https://doi.org/10.1037/pspi0000206

Ross, L. (1977). The intuitive psychologist and his shortcomings: Distortions in the attribution process. In L. Berkowitz, (Ed.), *Advances in experimental social psychology* (pp. 173–220). Academic Press. https://doi.org/10.1016/s0065-2601(08)60357-3

Rothbart, D. (2021). Righteous rage as political power. *Peace and Conflict: Journal of Peace Psychology*, 27(4), 681–684. https://doi.org/10.1037/pac0000544

Ryan, R. M., & Deci, E. L. (2019). Supporting autonomy, competence, and relatedness: The coaching process from a self-determination theory perspective. In S. English, J. M. Sabatine, & P. Brownell (Eds.), *Professional coaching: Principles and practice* (pp. 231–245). Springer Publishing Company.

Sim, M., Almaraz, S. M., & Hugenberg, K. (2022). Bodies and minds: Heavier weight targets are de-mentalized as lacking in mental agency. *Personality and Social Psychology Bulletin*, 48(9), 1367–1381. https://doi-org/10.1177/01461672211039981

Tasca G. A. (2019). Attachment and eating disorders: A research update. *Current Opinion in Psychology*, 25, 59–64. https://doi.org/10.1016/j.copsyc.2018.03.003

Tronieri, J. S. (2021). Cognitive and behavioral treatments for obesity. In A. Wenzel (Ed.), *Handbook of cognitive behavioral therapy: Applications* (pp. 453–476). American Psychological Association. https://doi-org/10.1037/0000219-014

van de Grint, L. T. M., Evans, A. M., & Stavrova, O. (2021). Good eats, bad intentions? Reputational costs of organic consumption. *Journal of Environmental Psychology*, 75, 101622. https://doi.org/10.1016/j.jenvp.2021.101622

Valtorta, R. R., Baldissarri, C., Andrighetto, L., & Volpato, C. (2021). Seeing others as a disease: The impact of physical (but not moral) disgust on biologization. *International Review of Social Psychology*, 34(1), 7. https://doi.org/10.5334/irsp.407

Wang, D. C., & Lopez, F. G. (2011). Attachment security as the social foundation of mindfulness-based emotional self-regulation: Dialectical thinking as a mediator [Conference session abstract]. *APA 119th Annual Convention*, Washington, D.C. https://doi.org/10.1037/e656762011-001

Watkins, P. L., Clifford, D., & Souza, B. (2018). The Health At Every Size® paradigm: Promoting body positivity for all bodies. In E. A. Daniels, M. M. Gillen, &

C. H. Markey (Eds.), *Body positive: Understanding and improving body image in science and practice* (pp. 160–187). Cambridge University Press. https://doi-org.adelphi.idm.oclc.org/10.1017/9781108297653.008

West, H. (2020). In praise of indignation. *Journal of Humanistic Psychology, 60*(4), 532–547. https://doi-org/10.1177/0022167820916378

Wright, M. R. (2005). Collegiality. *Optometry and Vision Development, 36*(1), 13–14.

Conclusion

Generalist psychotherapists are well-suited to accompany patients on their weight management journeys as patients negotiate many of life's other challenges like managing anxiety, depression, anger, and relationship problems. Weight management concerns are often intertwined with such issues. Regardless of psychotherapists' theoretical orientation, an understanding of what may be common factors in effective psychotherapy can help therapists as patients look to their therapists as companions and guides on their weight management journeys. Common factors can be finding goal consensus (Tryon, Birch, & Verkuilen, 2018), establishing a working alliance (Zilcha-Mano & Ben David-Sela, 2022), repairing ruptures to that alliance (Eubanks, 2022), autonomy support (Ryan & Deci, 2019), empathy for both frames of mind when patients are of two minds about pressing issues (Miller & Moyers, 2017), increasing attachment security (Allen, 2023), increasing self-acceptance, (Forman & Butryn, 2016), and strengthening various System 2 functions such as reflective functioning (Goodman, 2013) and dialectical thinking (Fruzzetti, 2022).

Patients' weight management journeys are likely to be characterized by weight cycling as patients' search for a sustainable approach to weight management (Elfhag & Rössner, 2010). To the extent problems with weight management are symptoms of a food addiction relapse is to be expected on the road to recovery (Gearhardt, Corbin, & Brownell, 2009). Given that the evidence-based weight management literature does not suggest that there is any one-size-fits-all approach to treatment that works for everybody, patients may need to discover through trial and error what is a sustainable approach for them.

What is or isn't too much weight might have to be decided on an individual basis as individuals vary in terms of what they consider a desirable body image, what they are willing to sacrifice to achieve a certain body size and shape, their risk tolerance for acquiring a metabolic syndrome, and/or how much they will rely on medication without weight loss to manage a metabolic syndrome that has been acquired. Therapists must be sensitive to, and respectful of, these individual differences regardless of their own beliefs regarding what is a healthy weight and a healthful approach to eating. When it comes to weight management there is a need for a 'personalized science of human improvement' (Hayes, Ciarrochi, Hofmann, Chin, & Sahdra, 2022).

Approaches to weight loss and weight loss maintenance will also vary on an individual basis on a continuum from the least restrictive to the most restrictive approaches. The least restrictive approaches like intuitive and mindful eating may be an effective form of preventing further weight gain (Linardon, Tylka, & Fuller-Tyszkiewicz, 2021; Yu, Song, Zhang, & Wei, 2020). Eating thoughtfully with an understanding of nutrition and the difference between

DOI: 10.4324/9781003402336-16

physiological hunger and emotional eating may be sufficient to prevent further weight gain. No foods are forbidden or restricted. An awareness of the nutritional values of various foods and an intention to only eat when genuinely hungry rather than just stressed may provide sufficient System 2 executive control for some individuals to put a break on mindless eating. Nevertheless, some individuals may require more restrictive approaches if they continue to gain weight utilizing the least restrictive approaches or possess more ambitious weight loss goals. What is or isn't too permissive or too restrictive for such individuals may have to be discovered on an individual basis rather than decided a priori.

When the goal is weight loss, it appears that any approach that generates an energy deficit by restricting caloric intake, restricting consumptions of the more calorie-dense foods, and increasing exercise facilitates weight loss (Marlatt & Ravussin, 2018). What remains unclear is how sustainable different approaches to weight loss are given the high rates of relapse (Hutchinson, 2011). Was the daily calorie budget too low, was their too little fat or too little carbohydrate in the diet, was the exercise regimen too demanding, were System 2 overrides like distress tolerance insufficiently strengthened, was their too little emotional support to compensate for self-control deficits, and/or was cue avoidance insufficient in the face of omnipresent environmental temptation? It may not always be possible to answer these questions in advance. These may be questions that need to be answered on an individual basis after relapse and then creative individual solutions must be discovered in the hopes of preventing future relapse.

Individual solutions to prevent relapse will be variable and may need to be discovered through trial and error. Some individuals might find it easier to abstain from a certain food than to learn to eat that food in moderation. Yet that might only be discovered after trying and failing repeatedly to eat certain calorie-dense foods in moderation. Other individuals might find it easier to just have a small taste of a calorie-dense food rather than abstain from that food entirely. Yet that might only be discovered after repeatedly trying and failing to abstain from such foods.

Some individuals might find it easier to just fill up on fruits, vegetables, and lean meats without controlling portion size or counting calories. They don't plan on eating the more calorie-dense foods and they don't want to have to stop eating until they feel reasonably full. Other individuals might find it easier to control portion size and count calories so that they can eat whatever they want as long they don't go over their daily calorie budget. Individuals might have to try out both approaches as well as other strategies to ascertain which one is preferrable for them.

Weight management raises several psychological issues with which psychotherapists may be uniquely well-suited to help patients. The basic sense of autonomous self-determination from early childhood is derived from a sense of being able to control essential bodily functions like urination and defecation (Erikson & Erikson, 1997). Appreciation of how little self-control of eating behavior and weight gain one possesses is a shame sensitive issue. It may be difficult to accept that some combination of a genetic predisposition towards an endomorphic body type (Farooqi, 2018), childhood adversity (Kazmierski, Borelli, & Rao, 2022), and trauma (Hoover, Yu, Duval, & Gearhardt, 2022), leads to emotional eating and weight gain in obesogenic environments that is not easy to control (King, 2013).

Psychological defenses like denial, rationalization, and dissociation may be activated in response to this shame sensitive issue (Kearney, 1996; Meneguzzo, Garolla, Bonello, &

Todisco, 2022). Those defenses generate considerable reactance to any therapeutic approach that threatens those defenses (Beutler, Edwards, & Someah, 2018). Consequently, any approach to weight management could be experienced as an autonomy threat to be defended against. Therapeutic expertise is therefore required to address psychological defenses against shame and the ruptures to the therapeutic relationship that arise whenever patients feel that their autonomy is threatened. Autonomy is threatened anytime patients feel pressured to manage their weights in ways that they are not yet prepared to do.

The shame that patients feel about their lack of control over their eating behavior is compounded by weight stigma (Puhl & Brownell, 2006) and divergent weight management stigma (Romo, 2018). Patients may suffer poor body image if they have been made to feel that their weight makes them unattractive and unhealthy (Watkins, Clifford, & Souza, 2018). Patients can become self-conscious about their eating habits if they have been criticized for eating too much or eating too little. It can be difficult to figure out for oneself what is the optimum weight and optimum way of eating when others are strongly opinionated about how much one should weigh to look attractive and be healthy and how one should eat to achieve those goals. Stigma is based on negative stereotypes and negative stereotypes are based on overgeneralizations (Fabbre, Gaveras, Shabsin, Gibson, & Rank, 2020). As such, stigma is disregarding and disrespectful of individual differences. Psychotherapy provides a venue in which patients' unique individuality can be discovered and affirmed, a core therapeutic process for the humanistic approaches to psychotherapy (Rogers, 1951, 1961).

Patients' weight management journeys are often difficult lessons in humility. Not everyone can be healthy at any size and some individuals who have acquired serious metabolic syndromes despite their anti-diet philosophy might find themselves dieting to lose weight (deVos, 2018). Given that relapse appears to be an inevitable aspect of the weight management journey, patients will likely experience giving a weight management strategy their best shot and then discovering that their best shot wasn't good enough. Repeated experiences of weight management failure can be enraging, depressing, humiliating, and demoralizing. Such emotions are difficult to tolerate and it's always tempting to look for someone to blame and negatively stereotype to assuage the blow to the sense of self-efficacy (Latner, Puhl, Murakami, & O'Brien, 2014).

Cultivating self-compassion after weight management failure and recommitting to the weight management effort despite demoralization is a therapeutic challenge (Genin, Vinson, Lagrange, & Le Barbenchon, 2022). Such situations are challenging for therapists as well who might worry that they are failures as therapists if their patients fail as weight managers. Therapists' self-blame might be exacerbated if their patients do blame them for weight management failures. Patients may resent therapists for their failures to provide sufficient guidance or for providing guidance of the wrong kind. Thus, psychotherapy of weight management can be a lesson in humility for therapists as well as patients.

Ruptures to the therapeutic relationship can occur at any point in patients' weight management journeys. It can occur at the beginning of such journey as patients are grappling with their lack of control of their eating behavior and defend against their shame through denial, rationalization, and dissociation. Patients can feel threatened by therapists who seem to be pressuring them to address their weight management concerns before they feel ready (Moeseneder, Ribeiro, Muran, & Caspar, 2019). Overcoming weight stigma and divergent weight management stigma can be challenging when therapists say things that seem reflective of such stigmas and appear to make patients feel badly about their weights and eating habits.

Once patients commit to a weight management strategy they can be sensitive to whether their therapists approve of their chosen strategies. They might worry that their therapists think a chosen strategy is either too permissive or too restrictive to be effective. Even when patients and therapists agree as to the preferred weight management strategy there can be a fear that therapists are monitoring patients' implementation of the strategy and will be critical if patients are implementing the strategy incorrectly. And finally, there is a fear of disappointing their therapists if they give a weight management strategy their best shot and it doesn't work and it seems like someone must be to blame for that failure.

Psychotherapy, whatever the techniques utilized, is a conversation between two people who have a relationship with each other (Norcross & Lambert, 2019). That relationship will have its conflicts and its ups and downs just like any other human relationship (Eubanks, 2022). The psychotherapeutic relationship, though, has a special function. Therapists serve as patients' all-purpose sounding boards for a wide variety of psychological problems of which weight management is but one. Weight management has its own specific technical challenges as a psychological problem (i.e., eat intuitively or count calories). Yet psychotherapy of weight management cannot be reduced to those problem-specific technical challenges alone. The relational dimensions of the psychotherapy of weight management require therapists to be reflective about how the relational dimensions of effective psychotherapy in general are at play when treating this specific clinical problem (Finsrud, Nissen-Lie, Vrabel, Høstmælingen, Wampold, & Ulvenes, 2022). Keeping an eye on those common relational factors can be helpful when psychotherapists must help patients find their way on a case-by-case basis because one-size-fits-all approaches to weight management may not apply.

References

Allen, B. (2023). *The science and clinical practice of attachment theory: A guide from infancy to adulthood.* American Psychological Association. https://doi.org/10.1037/0000333-000

Beutler, L. E., Edwards, C., & Someah, K. (2018). Adapting psychotherapy to patient reactance level: A meta-analytic review. *Journal of Clinical Psychology*, 74(11), 1952–1963. https://doi.org/10.1002/jclp.22682

deVos, K. (2018). The problem with body positivity. *The New York Times.* https://www.nytimes.com/2018/05/29/opinion/body-positivity-fat-acceptance.html

Elfhag, K., & Rössner, S. (2010). Weight loss maintenance and weight cycling. In P. G. Kopelman, I. D. Caterson, & W. H. Dietz (Eds.), *Clinical obesity in adults and children* (pp. 351–365). Wiley Blackwell.

Erikson, E. H., Erikson, J. (1997). *The life cycle completed – Revised and extended version.* New York: W. W. Norton & Company Inc.

Eubanks, C. F. (2022). Rupture repair. *Cognitive and Behavioral Practice*, 29(3). https://doi-org/10.1016/j.cbpra.2022.02.012

Fabbre, V. D., Gaveras, E., Shabsin, A. G., Gibson, J., & Rank, M. R. (2020). Confronting stigma, discrimination, and social exclusion. In M. R. Rank (Ed.), *Toward a livable life: A 21st century agenda for social work* (pp. 70–93). Oxford University Press.

Farooqi, I. S. (2018). Genetics of obesity. In T. A. Wadden & G. A. Bray (Eds.), *Handbook of obesity treatment* (pp. 64–74). The Guilford Press.

Finsrud, I., Nissen-Lie, H. A., Vrabel, K., Høstmælingen, A., Wampold, B. E., & Ulvenes, P. G. (2022). It's the therapist and the treatment: The structure of common therapeutic relationship factors. *Psychotherapy Research: Journal of the Society for Psychotherapy Research*, 32(2), 139–150. https://doi.org/10.1080/10503307.2021.1916640

Forman, E. M., & Butryn, M. L. (2016). *Effective weight loss: An acceptance-based behavioral approach: Clinician guide*. Oxford University Press.

Fruzzetti, A. E. (2022). Dialectical thinking. *Cognitive and Behavioral Practice*, 29(3), 567–570. https://doi-org/10.1016/j.cbpra.2022.02.011

Gearhardt, A. N., Corbin, W. R., & Brownell, K. D. (2009). Preliminary validation of the Yale Food Addiction Scale. *Appetite*, 52(2), 430–436. https://doi.org/10.1016/j.appet.2008.12.003

Genin, M., Vinson, E., Lagrange, A., & Le Barbenchon, E. (2022). Self-compassion and resistance to persuasion. *Psychology & Health*, 37(10), 1241–1252. https://doi.org/10.1080/08870446.2021.1941959

Goodman, G. (2013). Is mentalization a common process factor in transference-focused psychotherapy and dialectical behavior therapy sessions? *Journal of Psychotherapy Integration*, 23(2), 179–192. https://doi-org.adelphi.idm.oclc.org/10.1037/a0032354

Hayes, S. C., Ciarrochi, J., Hofmann, S. G., Chin, F., & Sahdra, B. (2022). Evolving an idionomic approach to processes of change: Towards a unified personalized science of human improvement. *Behaviour Research and Therapy*, 156, 104155. https://doi.org/10.1016/j.brat.2022.104155

Hoover, L. V., Yu, H. P., Duval, E. R., & Gearhardt, A. N. (2022). Childhood trauma and food addiction: The role of emotion regulation difficulties and gender differences. *Appetite*, 177, 1–8. https://doi-org/10.1016/j.appet.2022.106137

Hutchinson E. (2011). Systems neuroscience: The stress of dieting. *Nature Reviews Neuroscience*, 12(2), 65. https://doi.org/10.1038/nrn2985

Kazmierski, K. F. M., Borelli, J. L., & Rao, U. (2022). Negative affect, childhood adversity, and adolescents' eating following stress. *Appetite*, 168, 105766. https://doi-org/10.1016/j.appet.2021.105766

Kearney, R. J. (1996). *Within the wall of denial: Conquering addictive behaviors*. W. W. Norton & Co.

King, B. M. (2013). The modern obesity epidemic, ancestral hunter-gatherers, and the sensory/reward control of food intake. *The American Psychologist*, 68(2), 88–96. https://doi.org/10.1037/a0030684

Latner, J. D., Puhl, R. M., Murakami, J. M., & O'Brien, K. S. (2014). Food addiction as a causal model of obesity. Effects on stigma, blame, and perceived psychopathology. *Appetite*, 77, 77–82. https://doi.org/10.1016/j.appet.2014.03.004

Linardon, J., Tylka, T. L., & Fuller-Tyszkiewicz, M. (2021). Intuitive eating and its psychological correlates: A meta-analysis. *The International Journal of Eating Disorders*, 54(7), 1073–1098. https://doi.org/10.1002/eat.23509

Marlatt, K. L., & Ravussin, E. (2018). Energy expenditure and obesity. In T. A. Wadden & G. A. Bray (Eds.), *Handbook of obesity treatment* (pp. 38–63). The Guilford Press.

Meneguzzo, P., Garolla, A., Bonello, E., & Todisco, P. (2022). Alexithymia, dissociation and emotional regulation in eating disorders: Evidence of improvement through specialized inpatient treatment. *Clinical Psychology & Psychotherapy*, 29(2), 718–724. https://doi.org/10.1002/cpp.2665

Miller, W. R., & Moyers, T. B. (2017). Motivational interviewing and the clinical science of Carl Rogers. *Journal of Consulting and Clinical Psychology*, 85(8), 757–766. https://doi.org/10.1037/ccp0000179

Moeseneder, L., Ribeiro, E., Muran, J. C., & Caspar, F. (2019). Impact of confrontations by therapists on impairment and utilization of the therapeutic alliance. *Psychotherapy Research: Journal of the Society for Psychotherapy Research*, 29(3), 293–305. https://doi.org/10.1080/10503307.2018.1502897

Norcross, J. C. & Lambert, M. J. (2019). *Psychotherapy relationships that work: Evidence-based therapist contributions.* Oxford University Press.

Puhl, R. M., & Brownell, K. D. (2006). Confronting and coping with weight stigma: An investigation of overweight and obese adults. *Obesity (Silver Spring, Md.)*, 14(10), 1802–1815. https://doi.org/10.1038/oby.2006.208

Rogers, C. R. (1951). *Client-centered therapy.* Houghton Mifflin.

Rogers, C. R. (1961). *On becoming a person.* Houghton Mifflin.

Romo, L. K. (2018). An examination of how people who have lost weight communicatively negotiate interpersonal challenges to weight management. *Health Communication*, 33(4), 469–477. https://doi.org/10.1080/10410236.2016.1278497

Ryan, R. M., & Deci, E. L. (2019). Supporting autonomy, competence, and relatedness: The coaching process from a self-determination theory perspective. In S. English, J. M. Sabatine, & P. Brownell (Eds.), *Professional coaching: Principles and practice* (pp. 231–245). Springer Publishing Company.

Tryon, G. S., Birch, S. E., & Verkuilen, J. (2018). Meta-analyses of the relation of goal consensus and collaboration to psychotherapy outcome. *Psychotherapy (Chicago, Ill.)*, 55(4), 372–383. https://doi.org/10.1037/pst0000170

Watkins, P. L., Clifford, D., & Souza, B. (2018). The Health At Every Size® paradigm: Promoting body positivity for all bodies. In E. A. Daniels, M. M. Gillen, & C. H. Markey (Eds.), *Body positive: Understanding and improving body image in science and practice* (pp. 160–187). Cambridge University Press. https://doi-org.adelphi.idm.oclc.org/10.1017/9781108297653.008

Yu, J., Song, P., Zhang, Y., & Wei, Z. (2020). Effects of mindfulness-based intervention on the treatment of problematic eating behaviors: A systematic review. *Journal of Alternative and Complementary Medicine*, 26(8), 666–679. https://doi.org/10.1089/acm.2019.0163

Zilcha-Mano, S., & Ben David-Sela, T. (2022). Is alliance therapeutic in itself? It depends. *Journal of Counseling Psychology*, 69(6), 786–793. https://doi.org/10.1037/cou0000627

Index

abstinence versus moderation 71–73
acceptance and commitment therapy 6, 54, 156
adaptationist perspective 83–86
advice 132–133
ambivalence 58–61, 157
anorexia nervosa 29
anti-obesity ideology 23
ascetic lifestyle 102
assertiveness towards stigmatizing behavior 170–173
attachment theory 53, 103
attitudes towards food 29
autonomy: child's 52; supporting patient's 27, 41–42, 56–61, 82–83, 132–135, 167

'bad' numbers: blaming self for 118–119; blood glucose 126–127; blood pressure 126–127; BMI and 123–124; calorie counting 125–126; cholesterol 126–127; confrontation about 119–122; overview 117–118
bariatric surgery 27
behavioral weight loss intervention: cognitive reappraisal 45–47; evidence which supports 5, 38; goal setting 41–42; learning theory 38–39; maladaptive cognitions 46–47; overview 37–38, 39–40; problem solving 44–47; resistance to 39–40; self-monitoring strategies 42–44
bias: confirmation 106; implicit 24–25; self-serving 106, 108, 159
blood glucose 126–127
blood pressure 126–127
Body Mass Index (BMI) 122–123, 152
body positivity 6, 25–28

calorie counting 41, 42–43, 99–100, 102–103, 106, 124–126
cheating 148–151
children/infants: attachment theory 53, 103; early food experiences 51–52
choice, freedom of 56–61
cholesterol 126–127
cognitive behavioral approaches 133
cognitive reappraisal 45–47

commercial weight-loss diets 12
communication, health 59–60
Compensatory Health Beliefs Scale 46
conditioning theory 38
confirmation bias 106
conflict discussions 121
confrontation ruptures 9, 10–11, 115–116, 119–122
confronting stigmatizing behavior 167–173
conscientiousness 91
consumer culture 47–48
counting calories 41, 42–43, 99–100, 102–103, 106, 124–126
cravings 42, 69–70, 101
cross-cultural differences 12
cultural humility 12

defiant self-destructiveness 139–140
demand characteristics 137
de-mentalization 166
denial 117
deVos, Kelly 29–30
Dialectical Behavior Therapy 10, 27, 40, 54, 156
dichotomous thinking 73, 100, 124, 150
dietary beliefs 12
dissociation 123–124, 138, 147–148
distress tolerance 156
divergent weight management stigma 2
dodo bird hypothesis 8–9
duration of treatment 13

eating disorders 7, 29, 33–34
emotional eating: as assertion of autonomy 56–61; and emotion regulation 53–56; overview 52–53
emotional support versus self-control 137–139
emotion regulation deficit 54–56
enablers 164
epistemic trust 98, 103–106
epistemic vigilance 107
evidence-based perspective to weight management 5, 8, 13

evolutionary perspective: adaptationist view 83–86; human eating habits/diet 86–89; pleasure in feeding others 89–90
excuses/rationalizations 45
exercise 13–14

fat phobia 2, 5
fat shaming 2, 5
feasting with others 89–90
food addiction: abstinence versus moderation 71–73; controversy around 67, 68; evidence for 67–71; overview 7–8, 66–67; and stigma 75–77; treatment 73–75; weight cycling and 154–155
food diary 105
'foodporn' 67
Freud, Sigmund 53

generalist psychotherapists 97–98, 131–135
glycemic index 101
goal consensus 10
goal setting 41–42, 156
guide versus traveling companion 131–135

health at any size model 6, 7, 28–30
health communication 59–60
high fat diet 101
hitting bottom 158–159
honesty 43
humility 12

ideal diet (concept of) 98–103
implicit bias 24–25
individual difference variables 5
informing the therapist of weight loss plans 144–148
insecure attachment 53, 103–104
internalized weight stigma 2, 5, 11, 24–25, 105
intuitive eating 6–7, 30–33, 163–164
Intuitive Eating Scale 31
Irby, Samantha 28
Irrational Food Belief Scale 46

lapses 155; *see also* relapse prevention; relapse recovery
learning theory: and overeating 38–39; *see also* behavioral weight loss intervention
low glycemic diet 101

maintenance of weight loss 41
maladaptive cognitions 46–47
mentalization 107
Merkin, Daphne 26
metabolic syndromes and weight 28–29, 30
mindful-based interventions (MBI) 7, 32
mindful eating 6–7, 30–33, 31–33, 54, 163–164

Mindful Eating Questionnaire 31
mindfulness 156
mindlessness 138–139
minority stress 75–77, 134
'model minority' 76
moderation versus abstinence 71–73
moralization 159–161
motivated reasoning 12, 43, 47, 106, 108
motivational interviewing 6, 58, 133, 157
motivation enhancement 156

neutrality 8
nondirective treatment approach 132–133
nutritional counseling 46

obesity epidemic 100–101
one-size-fits-all approach 8, 85
operant conditioning 39
oppositional defiant disorder 140
oral behavior and emotion regulation 53
orthorexia nervosa 7, 33–34
overconsumption, consumer culture and 47–48
Overeaters Anonymous 7, 73–75

Paleolithic diet 101
passing comments from patients 145
patient autonomy, respect for 27, 41–42, 56–61, 82–83, 132–135, 167
Pavlov's conditioning model 38
perfectionism 76, 90–92
permissive versus restrictive approach 135–137
person-centered therapy 132–133
pets 88
plateauing 151–152
preventative medicine 123
problem solving, in behavioral weight loss interventions 44–47
processed carbohydrates 100–101
psychotherapist as sounding board 97–98, 131–135

rate of weight loss 41
rationalizations/excuses 45
reactance theory 57, 59, 60–61
realistic goals 156
reasons for losing weight ('good') 23
relapse prevention 155–157
relapse rates 100
relapse recovery 158–159
re-moralization 159–161
restrictive versus permissive approach 135–137
risk tolerance 30
ruptures 9–11, 115–116

satiety set point 72
self-blame 118–119

self-control 138–139
self-control versus emotional support 137–139
self-destructiveness 139–140
self-determination 56–61
self-monitoring strategies 42–44, 143–152
self-serving bias 106, 108, 159
self-sufficient approach 144–148
Serenity Prayer 3, 150
shame 119
Sharpton, Al 42
shifts in thinking over lifespan 29–30
social eating 90, 165
social justice approaches 134
social status, body weight and 85
starvation diets 32–33, 41, 99–100, 146
stigma 2, 5, 11, 24–25, 26, 75–77, 105, 163–173
stigmatizing behavior 167–173
support, emotional 137–139
sustainability of weight loss 99

therapeutic alliance 2, 8, 9–11, 103–106, 119–122, 159–161
therapist biases 24–25

transference-focused psychotherapy 120–121
traveling companion versus guide 131–135
12-step precepts 7, 73–75, 154

'unconditional permission to eat' 31, 32

validation 10, 116
very low-calorie diets 32–33, 41, 99–100, 146
'virtue signaling' 164, 165

weight bias 24–25
weight cycling 7, 100, 126, 154, 160
weight moralization 159–161
weight stigma 2, 5, 11, 24–25, 26, 75–77, 105, 163–173
Weight Watchers 101–103
withdrawal 68, 69, 74, 100
withdrawal ruptures 9, 11
worldview defense 106–107

Yale Food Addiction Scale 67–69

zero-point diet 101–102, 104